AF815433

Physeo

TABLE OF CONTENTS

We would like to extend a special thanks to the following individuals who have spent countless hours and support to make Physeo possible.

Ajay Davidson, MD

Alexandra Galel, MD

Alexandra Harding

Anissa Laine Bayabos Amilhamja

Anne-Sophie van Wingerden
Medical Student
Columbia Vagelos College of Physicians and Surgeons

Antonio Acevedo

Ayan Agarwal
MBBS Student
Vardhman Mahavir Medical College and Safdarjung Hospital
New Delhi, India

Brianna Cocuzzo, MsC

Brooke Walsh, MS

Camelita Thrift

Christopher A. Price, MS

Emily Dinning, MD

Genevieve Saliuk
MD Candidate 2024
UTMB School of Medicine

George Myo Win, BS
University of Missouri-Columbia School of Medicine

Ghadeer Magdy Elshafey, MD

H. Robert Cannon, DO

Dr. Jabran Wasti, House Officer
Dr. Ruth K.M. Pfau Civil Hospital
Karachi, Pakistan

Jae Cheol Bae

Dr. James Nunn

Jennifer M. Locke, BA
MD Candidate

Justin Wong, DO

Kurestin Miller, BA
MD Candidate

Lauren S. Faber, MD

Lauren Schwartz

Lee Azolai

Leslie Jewett, MD

Logan B. Carlyle, OMS-II

Marisol Cárdenas Calderón, MD

Mark Parry, MD, Resident Physician
Department of Obstetrics and Gynecology
OhioHealth – Riverside Methodist
Columbus, Ohio

Mason T. Bennet

Mateo Betancourt Escobar
Universidad Autónoma de San Luis
Potosí, Mexico

Mohamed Elshennawy

Natalia Kerr, MD

Nijat Aliyev, MD

Nikoloz Karazanashvili

Nirupamaa Sivanushanthan
Medical Student

Ostapenko Karolina

Dr. Rahil Patel, Medical Officer
Sharda Hospital
New Delhi, India

Mr. Rishabh Goyal

Roaa Zayat, MD

Rojin Arefi, MD

Ryan Zia

Salikh Murtaliev, MD

Sarah Jaber, D.O.
Internal Medicine Physician

Sergio R. Ortiz, MD, MPH

Shawna-Kay Young
MD Student

Shelia Chandrahas

Soomal Zukhruf Memon

Sumit Raut

Syed Ali Haider

Syed Awais Ahmed, MD

Tori Walsh

Tamari Papidze

Telyn Peterson, OMS-III
Rocky Vista University
Southern Utah

Trey Edwards, DO

Warda Hameed, MD

Yasmeen Abdulrahman, MD

Yomna Dean, MS-4

Zurabi Zaalishvili, MD

DERMATOLOGY

Dermatology | Section 1: Malignant Skin Lesions

I. Basal Cell Carcinoma: Introduction
   A. Most common malignant skin cancer
   B. Arises from the basal layer of epidermis
   C. Locally invasive and aggressive
   D. Metastasis is rare
   E. Good prognosis

II. Basal Cell Carcinoma: Etiology
   A. Exposure to sunlight
   B. White racial population
   C. Albinism
   D. Xeroderma pigmentosum
   E. Arsenic exposure

III. Basal Cell Carcinoma: Types
   A. Nodular type (most common)
   B. Superficial type
   C. Morpheaform/sclerosing type

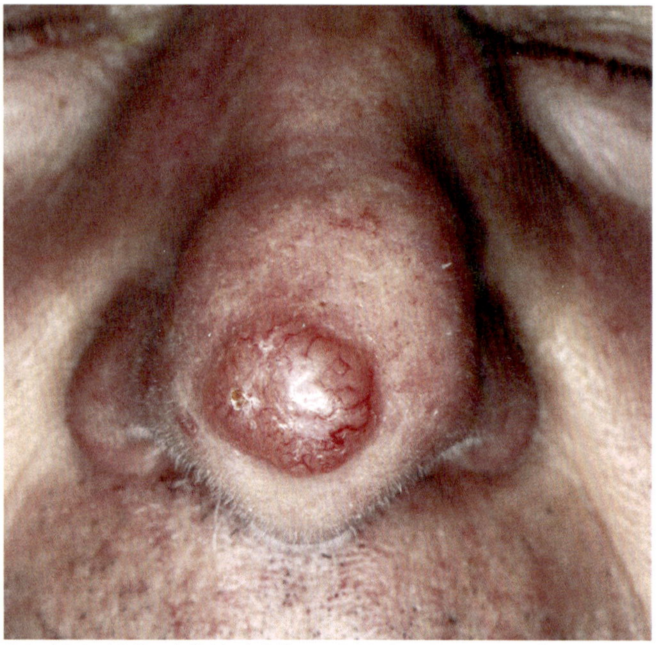

FIGURE 21.1.1 - Nodular Type of Basal Cell Carcinoma

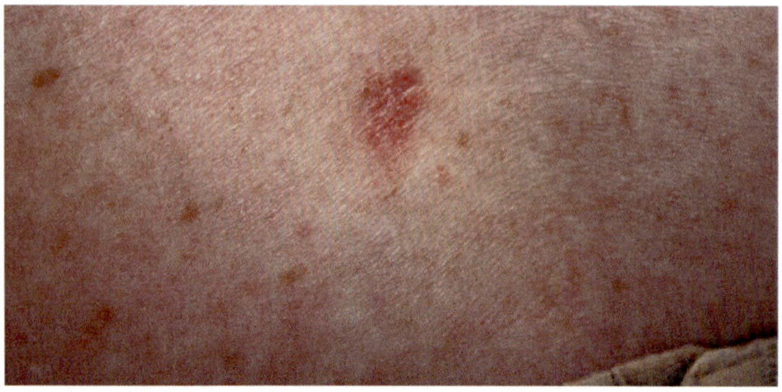

FIGURE 21.1.2 - Superficial Type of Basal Cell Carcinoma

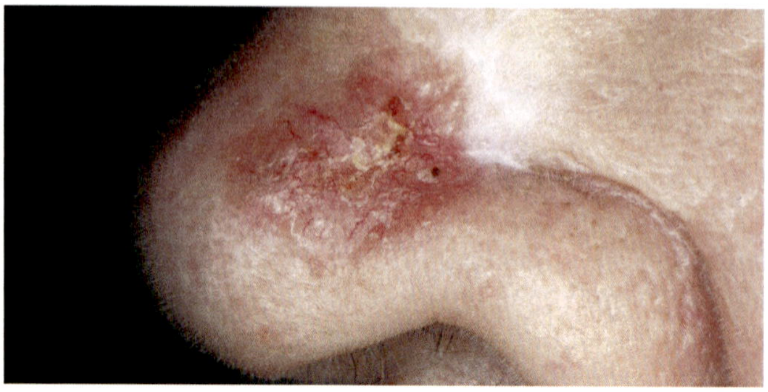

FIGURE 21.1.3 - Morpheaform Type of Basal Cell Carcinoma

IV. Basal Cell Carcinoma: Clinical Presentation
   A. Slow growing
   B. Pearly, pink, papule
   C. Telangiectasia
   D. Rodent ulcer and rolled out margins
   E. Sites: face (eyelids, nose, forehead, upper lip)

V. Basal Cell Carcinoma: Diagnosis
   A. Clinical examination
   B. Dermoscopy
   C. Skin biopsy
      1. Partial/full thickness biopsy
      2. Palisading pattern
      3. Nests of basophilic cells

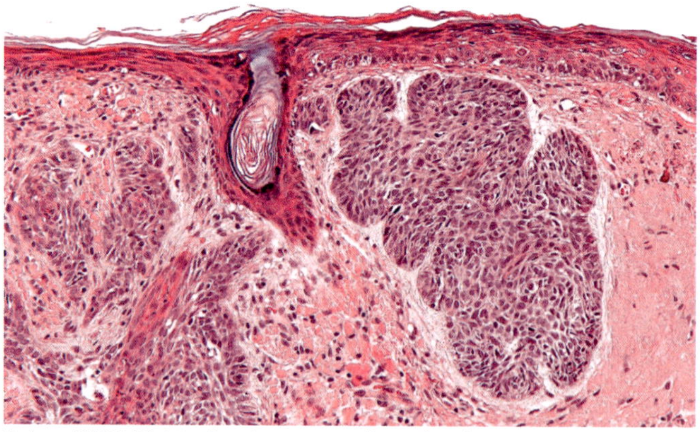

FIGURE 21.1.4 - Light Microscopy of Basal Cell Carcinoma

VI. Basal Cell Carcinoma: Management
   A. Surgical excision (standard)
      1. Remove lesion with 4 to 5 mm of surrounding healthy tissue
   B. Mohs micrographic surgery
   C. Topical therapy: imiquimod, fluorouracil
   D. Radiotherapy
   E. Cryotherapy

VII. Squamous Cell Carcinoma: Introduction
   A. Second most common skin cancer
   B. Arises from epidermal keratinocytes
   C. In the spinous layer of epidermis
   D. Incidence increases with age
   E. Metastasis to regional lymph nodes

VIII. Squamous Cell Carcinoma: Risk Factors
   A. Sun exposure
   B. Ionizing radiation
   C. Chemical carcinogens (e.g. arsenic, radon)
   D. Chronic inflammation (e.g. burn scars, ulcers)
   E. Immunosuppression
   F. Inherited disorders (e.g. albinism, xeroderma pigmentosum)
   G. Precancerous lesions (e.g. actinic keratosis, Bowen disease)

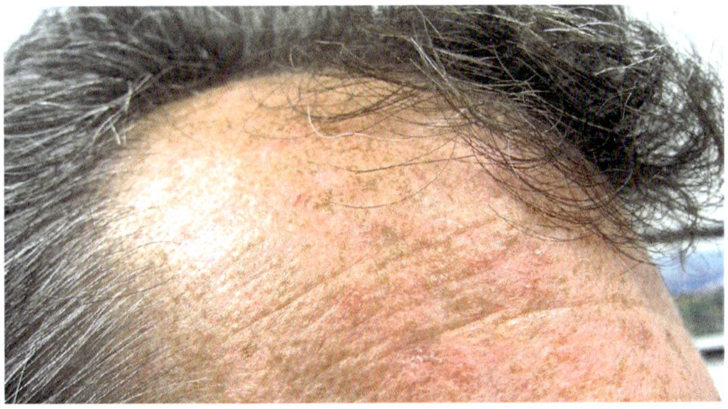

FIGURE 21.1.5 - Actinic Keratoses

IX. Squamous Cell Carcinoma: Clinical Presentation
   A. Erythematous, papule or nodule
   B. Non-healing ulcer with everted edges
   C. Cauliflower lesion
   D. Slow growing, locally invasive
   E. Sites: face (lower lip), neck, trunk

X. Squamous Cell Carcinoma: High Risk Features
   A. Size ≥ 10mm (face), ≥ 20mm (trunk)
   B. Ill-defined margins
   C. Rapidly growing
   D. Immunosuppression
   E. Previous radiation
   F. Neurological symptoms

XI. Squamous Cell Carcinoma: Clinical Variants
   A. Keratoacanthoma
   B. Verrucous carcinoma
   C. Marjolin's ulcer

XII. Squamous Cell Carcinoma: Diagnosis
   A. History and clinical examination
   B. Biopsy
      1. Method: shave/punch/excisional biopsy
      2. Atypical keratinocytes invading into dermis
      3. Keratin pearls
      4. Intercellular bridges

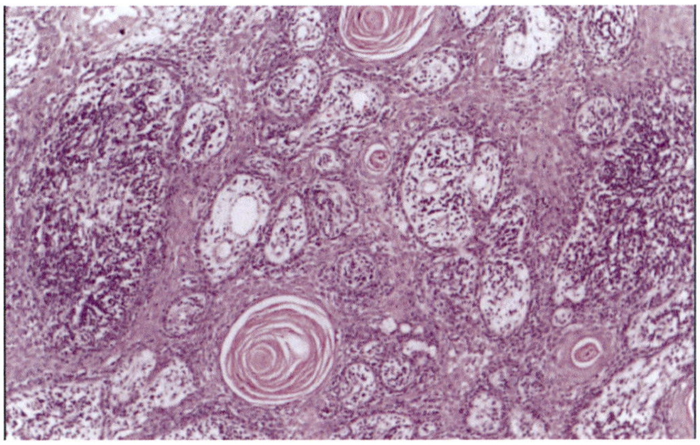

FIGURE 21.1.6 - Light Microscopy of Squamous Cell Carcinoma

XIII. Squamous Cell Carcinoma: Management
   A. Surgical methods
      1. Surgical excision
      2. Mohs micrographic surgery
   B. Cryotherapy
   C. Radiation
   D. Chemotherapy for metastasis

XIV. Melanoma: Introduction
   A. Highly malignant skin cancer
   B. Arises from melanocytes from epidermal layer
   C. Life-threatening
   D. Metastasis to lymph nodes, lungs, liver, brain

XV. Melanoma: Risk Factors
   A. Sun exposure
   B. Light skin complexion
   C. Albinism
   D. Congenital melanocytic nevi, dysplastic nevi
   E. Inherited skin conditions (FAMM syndrome)
   F. Immunosuppression

XVI. Melanoma: Types
   A. Superficial spreading melanoma
      1. Most common
      2. Predilection for back (men) and lower extremities (women)
      3. Pigmented macule with irregular borders
      4. Horizontal growth
   B. Nodular melanoma
      1. Pigmented, pedunculated nodule
      2. Vertical growth
      3. Worst prognosis
      4. Rapid metastasis
   C. Lentigo maligna melanoma
      1. Precancerous lesion: lentigo maligna
      2. Irregularly pigmented macule
   D. Acral lentiginous melanoma
      1. Common in dark-pigmented skin and Asians
      2. Palmar, plantar and subungual surfaces
      3. Rapidly progresses to vertical growth pattern: poor prognosis

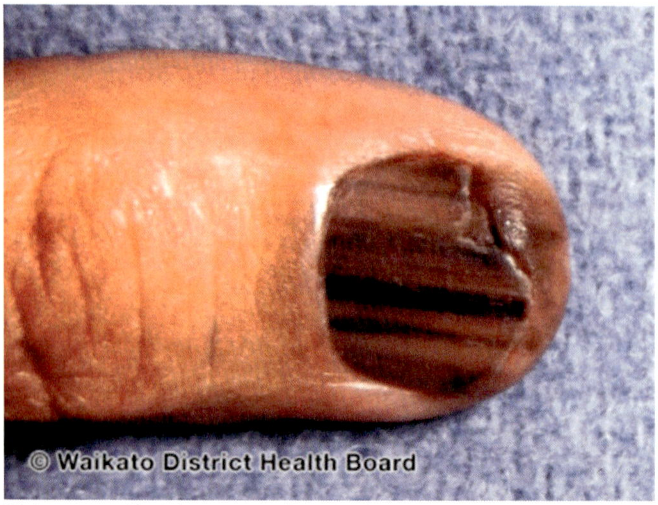

FIGURE 21.1.7 - Subungual Melanoma

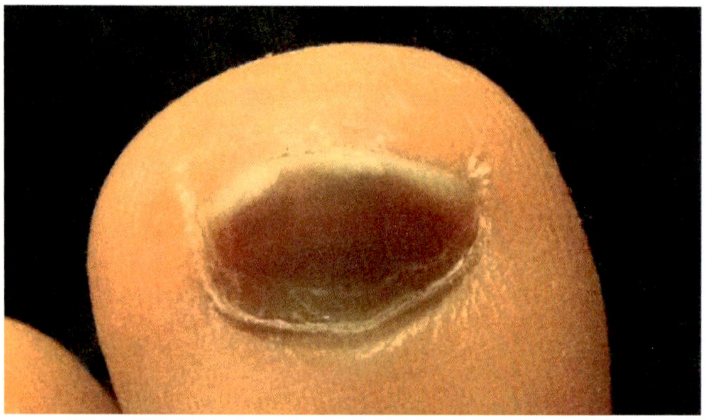

FIGURE 21.1.8 - Subungual Hematoma

XVII. Melanoma: Clinical Presentation
- A. ABCDE criteria
  1. A: Asymmetry
  2. B: Border irregularity
  3. C: Color changes (pink-blue-black)
  4. D: Diameter > 6mm
  5. E: Evolution (shape, size)
- B. "Ugly duckling" sign

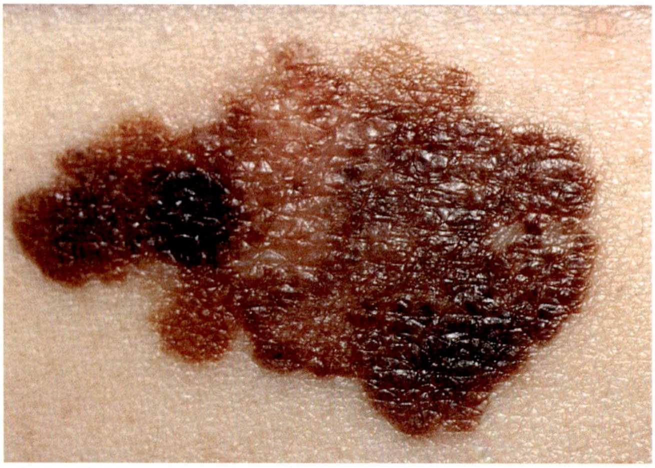

FIGURE 21.1.9 - Melanoma

XVIII. Melanoma: Diagnosis
- A. History and clinical examination
- B. Dermoscopy: ABCDE criteria
- C. Biopsy (diagnostic)
  1. Excisional biopsy of lesion with 1 to 3 mm of normal skin margin
  2. Presence of nests of atypical melanocytes
- D. Immunohistochemistry
  1. S-100 protein: positive

XIX. Melanoma: Management
- A. Surgery
  1. Full thickness excision of the lesion with narrow margin
  2. Allows to determine Breslow depth and invasion
  3. Breslow depth ≤ 1 mm: 1 cm safety margin
  4. Breslow depth > 1 mm: 2 cm safety margin and sentinel LN biopsy
- B. Immunotherapy (BRAF inhibitor)
- C. Radiation

XX. Mycosis Fungoides: Introduction
- A. Most common cutaneous CD^{4+} T cell lymphoma
- B. Progressive skin lesions
- C. Common in men
- D. Can progress to Sezary syndrome

XXI. Mycosis Fungoides: Clinical Presentation
- A. Initially scaly plaques and patches (variable size)
- B. Pruritic
- C. Alopecia
- D. Generalized erythroderma
- E. Sites: buttocks, trunk
- F. Systemic spread: lymph nodes, liver, spleen

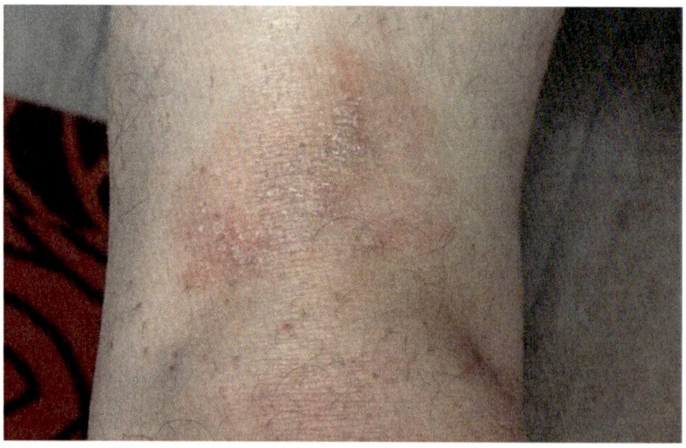

FIGURE 21.1.10 - Mycosis Fungoides

XXII. Mycosis Fungoides: Diagnosis
- A. Histopathology
- B. Pautrier microabscesses
  1. Pathognomonic
  2. Intraepidermal aggregates of atypical mononuclear cells (CD^{4+} T cells)
  3. Atypical cells also present in upper dermis
- C. Microscopy: Sezary cells (cerebriform nucleus)

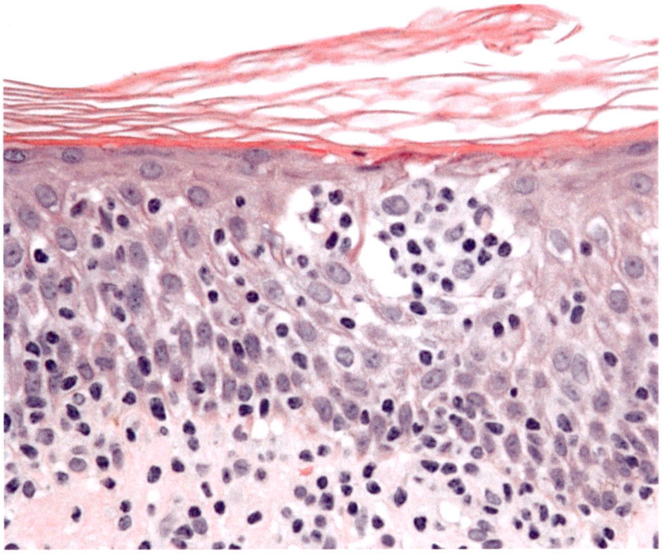

FIGURE 21.1.11 - Light Microscopy of Pautrier Microabscesses

XXIII. Mycosis Fungoides: Management
- A. Initial stage
  1. Topical treatments (corticosteroids)
- B. Advanced stage
  1. Combination therapy
  2. Total electron skin beam therapy
  3. Radiation therapy

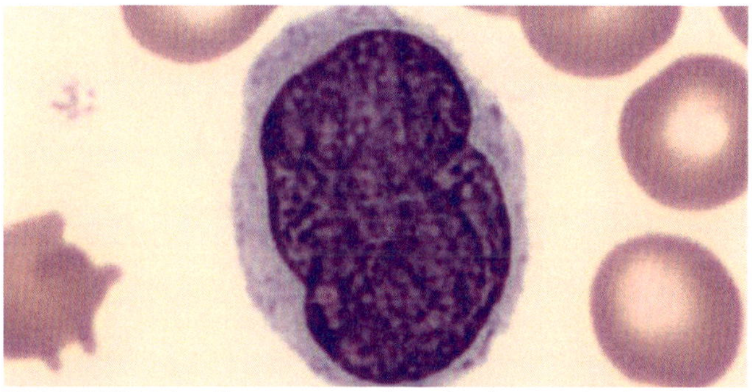

FIGURE 21.1.12 - Peripheral Blood Smear: Sezary Cell

REVIEW QUESTIONS

1. A 75-year-old man comes to the physician because of a skin lesion on his forehead. He first noticed the lesion 3 years ago and it has progressively enlarged. The man states he has been a farmer for over 50 years. Physical examination shows a whitish nodule with visible telangiectasias. A skin biopsy is performed. What findings would you expected to see on histology of the skin biopsy?
   - **Nests of basophilic cells with a palisading pattern are expected on skin biopsy.**
   - This patient presents with a 3 year history of a whitish nodule accompanied by telangiectasias.
   - This is a classic description of basal cell carcinoma.
   - BCC is characterized by intradermal nests of basophilic cells with a palisading pattern.

2. A 57-year-old woman comes to the physician because of a skin ulcer on her right thigh. She first noticed the ulcer 6 months ago. It disappeared at first after applying moisturizing cream, but then recently reappeared. She had a full thickness burn in the same area roughly 2 years ago. Biopsy of the ulcer shows keratin pearls and intercellular bridges. What is the most likely diagnosis of this patient's skin lesion?
   - **The most likely diagnosis is Marjolin ulcer.**
   - This patient presents with a relapsing skin ulcer.
   - Biopsy shows keratin pearls and intercellular bridges.
   - These findings indicate the presence of squamous cell carcinoma or SCC.
   - SCC commonly arises in the areas of chronic skin damage such as ulcers, previous burns, scars, and sinus tracts.

3. A 72-year-old woman comes to the physician because of a discolored nail on his right foot. He first noticed the color change 4 months ago and it has darkened progressively since. Physical examination shows the nail of the right second toe to be nontender, asymmetric, with brownish discoloration and color variation across the lesion. The patient has no previous history of trauma to his foot. What is the most likely diagnosis of this patient's nail lesion?
   - **The most likely diagnosis is subungual melanoma.**
   - This patient presents with a rapidly progressive lesion on his right toe nail.
   - It is nontender, asymmetric and there is a color variation across the lesion.
   - Additionally, there is no history of local trauma.
   - All of these findings are consistent with subungual melanoma, a subtype of acral lentiginous melanoma.
   - At first glance, subungual melanoma and subungual hematoma may look similar, however, subungual hematoma is symmetric, commonly tender, evenly brown in a patient with a history of nail trauma. These findings are not seen in this patient.

REVIEW QUESTIONS

4. A 36-year-old man comes to the physician because of a skin lesion on his right arm. He first noticed the lesion 5 months ago and it has enlarged and darkened since. He is a professional surfer for a living. Physical examination shows an 8 mm lesion with asymmetric borders and alternating brown and pink colors. He has many moles, but this mole does not look like the others. What is the next best step in the management of this patient?

- **The next best step is excisional biopsy.**
- This patient, a surfer with possibly prolonged sun exposure, has an 8 mm mole which is asymmetric, multi-colored, and it progressed rapidly.
- This lesion meets the ABCDE criteria for melanoma.
- This mole is different from his other moles.
- This is called the "ugly duckling" sign, which is also suggestive of melanoma.
- The next best step in the management of this patient with suspected melanoma is excisional skin biopsy with 1 to 3 mm of normal skin margins.

5. A 57-year-old man comes to the physician because of itchy skin lesions. He first noticed these lesions approximately 1 year ago and states they have enlarged since then. Physical examination shows diffuse pruritic plaques, generalized erythema, generalized lymphadenopathy, and hepatosplenomegaly. Complete blood count shows a leukocyte count of 50,000/mm^3 (N=4500-11000). What do expected to be seen on skin biopsy and blood smear?

- **Pautrier microabscesses and Sezary cells are expected to be found on skin biopsy and blood smear samples.**
- This patient presents with diffuse itchy skin plaques and erythema, lymphadenopathy and hepatosplenomegaly.
- Additionally, his leukocyte count is very high, specifically 50,000/mm^3.
- All of these findings are consistent with mycosis fungoides, with systemic dissemination which is also known as Sezary syndrome.
- Mycosis fungoides is a CD^{4+} T cell malignancy characterized by atypical CD4+ T cells aggregating in the epidermis.
- These aggregations are called Pautrier microabscesses.
- Since this patient also has signs of disseminated disease like generalized lymphadenopathy, hepatosplenomegaly and leukocytosis, his blood smear will also show these atypical CD^{4+} T cells with "cerebriform" or "cloverleaf" nuclei.

6. A 62-year-old woman comes to the physician because of a skin lesion on her upper lip. She first noticed the lesion approximately 8 months ago but did not pay attention until it enlarged. She has a past medical history of hypertension. She works landscape architect. Her vital signs include a temperature of 36.1° C (97° F), a blood pressure of 150/95 mmHg, a heart rate of 85 beats/min, and a respiratory rate of 16 breaths/min. The physical examination shows a pearly papule of 5 mm on the right upper lip accompanied by several telangiectasias. Biopsy of the lesion shows intradermal nests of basophilic cells with a palisading pattern. Which of the following is the best next step in the management of this patient?

   A. Mohs micrographic surgery
   B. Full-thickness surgical excision with wide margins
   C. Imiquimod
   D. Radiotherapy

- **The correct answer is option A.**
- This landscape architect with possibly prolonged sun exposure now presents with a 5 mm pearly papule accompanied by several telangiectasias.
- Biopsy of the lesion shows intradermal nests of basophilic cells with a palisading pattern.
- This presentation is most consistent with basal cell carcinoma or BCC.
- Since this patient's BCC is on the face which is an esthetically sensitive area, we need to choose a minimally invasive procedure to avoid tissue scarring.
- Mohs micrographic surgery is minimally invasive because it sequentially removes very thin layers of skin until there are no malignant cells in the tissue sample under the microscope.
- Option B is incorrect because this patient's basal cell carcinoma is on the face, an esthetically sensitive area, and we should try to be as minimally invasive as possible. Wide margin excision, on the other hand, will likely leave a large scar on the patient's lip.
- Option C is incorrect because it is only a second-line therapy for basal cell carcinoma.
- Option D is incorrect because it is mostly used for unresectable or large tumors. This patient's tumor is in a surgically accessible area and is only 5 mm in diameter.

CARDIOLOGY

Cardiology | Section 1: Acute Coronary Syndromes

I. Unstable Angina: Pathophysiology
   A. Oxygen demand is unchanged but supply is decreased secondary to reduced resting coronary blood flow
   B. Typically due to fixed atherosclerotic lesions
   C. Possible thrombosis, hemorrhage or plaque rupture

II. Unstable Angina: Clinical Features
   A. Chronic stable angina that is worsening
   B. New onset angina that is severe or worsening
   C. Chest pain at rest

III. Unstable Angina: Diagnosis
   A. CBC
   B. Cardiac biomarkers (e.g. troponin I)
   C. ECG
   D. Chest X-ray
   E. Cardiac stress test
   F. Cardiac catheterization (elective)

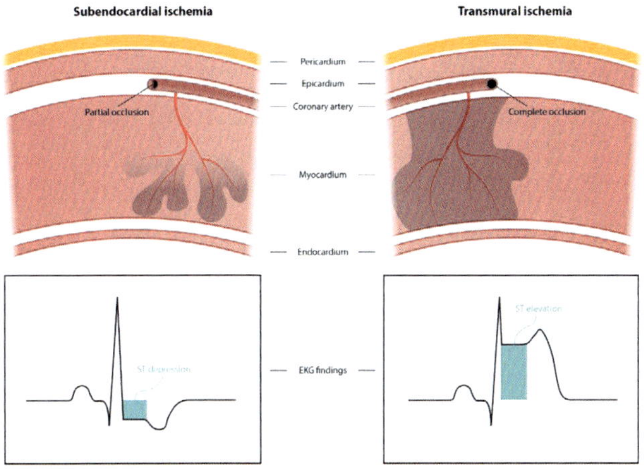

FIGURE 12.2.2 - Causes of Ischemia

IV. Unstable Angina: Treatment
   A. MONA-BASH: morphine, oxygen, nitrates, aspirin + clopidogrel, beta blockers, ACE inhibitor, statins, heparin
   B. Cardiac catheterization + PCI

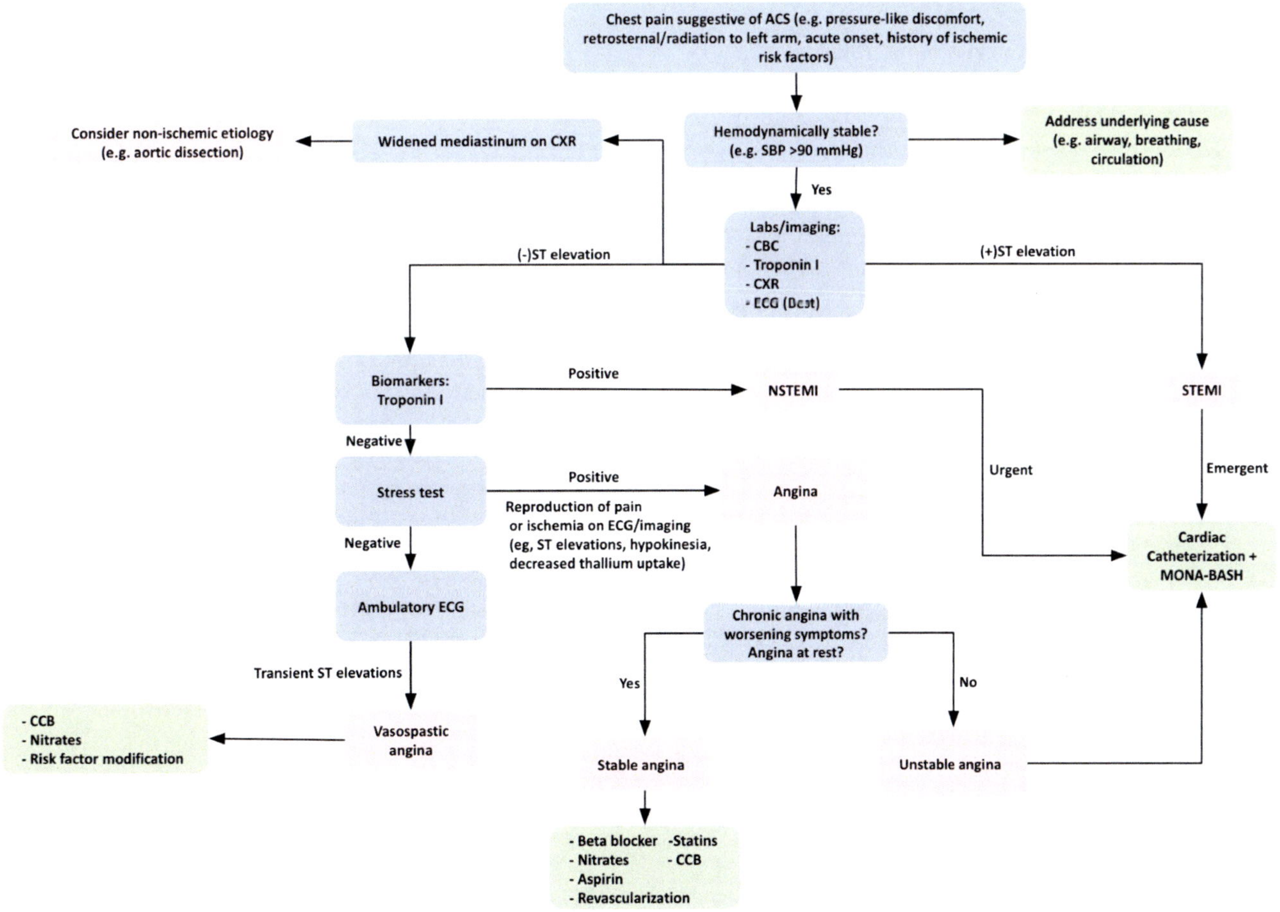

FIGURE 21.2.1 - Algorithm of Acute Coronary Syndrome: Diagnosis & Management

V. NSTEMI: Pathophysiology
   A. Imbalance of oxygen supply from coronary vessels and oxygen demand of myocardial tissues leading to cellular damage
   B. Usually due to rupture of atherosclerotic plaque and thrombosis formation occluding coronary arteries

VI. NSTEMI: Clinical Features
   A. Chest pain (> 20 minutes)
   B. Radiation to jaw, back or arms (mostly on left side)
   C. Epigastric discomfort
   D. Dyspnea, diaphoresis, weakness, nausea/vomiting, sense of impending doom, and syncope

VII. NSTEMI: Diagnosis
   A. CBC
   B. Cardiac biomarkers (e.g. troponin I)
   C. ECG
   D. Chest X-ray
   E. Cardiac catheterization (urgent)

VIII. NSTEMI: Treatment
   A. Medical
      1. MONA-BASH
      2. tPA not recommended
   B. Surgical
      1. Cardiac catheterization
      2. PCI or CABG
   C. Revascularization urgent if
      1. Hemodynamically unstable
      2. Severe LV dysfunction or heart failure
      3. Persistent angina at rest despite medical therapy
      4. Mitral regurgitation or ventricular septal defect
      5. Sustained ventricular arrhythmias

IX. STEMI: Pathophysiology
   A. Imbalance of oxygen supply from coronary vessels and oxygen demand of myocardial tissues leading to cellular damage
   B. Usually due to rupture of atherosclerotic plaque and thrombosis formation causing occlusion of coronary artery

X. STEMI: Clinical Features
   A. Chest pain (> 20 minutes)
   B. Radiation to jaw, back or arms (mostly on left side)
   C. Epigastric discomfort
   D. Dyspnea, diaphoresis, weakness, nausea/vomiting, sense of impending doom, and syncope

XI. STEMI: Diagnosis
   A. CBC
   B. Cardiac biomarkers (e.g. troponin I)
   C. ECG
   D. Chest X-ray
   E. Cardiac stress test
   F. Cardiac catheterization

XII. STEMI: Treatment
   A. Medical treatment
      1. MONA-BASH + fibrinolysis
      2. Give tPA if symptom onset within 12 hours and door to PCI time > 120 minutes
      3. Nitroglycerin contraindicated in signs of right sided STEMI
   B. Surgical treatment
      1. Emergent PCI or CABG

XIII. CABG vs PCI
   A. CABG: left main artery or ≥ 3 vessel involvement, PCI failure
   B. PCI: 1-2 vessel disease with door to balloon time < 90 minutes
   C. Drug eluting stent (DES): dual antiplatelet therapy 1 year
   D. Bare metal stent: dual antiplatelet therapy 1 month

XIV. Treatment Caveats for ACS
   A. Unfractionated heparin preferred in chronic kidney disease
      1. GFR < 30 mL/min or creatinine > 3.5 mmol/L
   B. No ACE inhibitors in
      1. Pregnancy
      2. Previous cough/angioedema
      3. AKI, bilateral RAS, CKD with creatinine > 3.5 mmol/L
      4. SBP < 90 mmHg or K+ > 5 mmol/L

REVIEW QUESTIONS ?

1. Why are cardiac enzymes typically not elevated in the case of unstable angina?
   - **Cardiac enzyme levels remain too low to be detected in unstable angina because the level of ischemia in this condition is not severe enough to cause cardiac muscle cells to release enough enzymes such as Troponin or CK-MB to be detected in the bloodstream.**
   - Unstable angina and NSTEMI may be indistinguishable within the first 12 hour of the presentation of a patient with clinical symptoms of ACS and no ST elevations on ECG.
   - This is because cardiac enzymes can take a while to build up to detectable levels within the blood.

2. Which patient populations are atypical presentations (e.g. epigastric pain, abnormal duration, isolated referred pain of neck or jaw) of NSTEMI most common in?
   - **Atypical presentations of NSTEMI are most common in women, elderly, and diabetic patients.**

REVIEW QUESTIONS

3. What could cause abdominal pain, blue discoloration of the distal end of the great toe on the left foot, an increased creatinine, and a mottled purple net-like rash after cardiac catheterization?

    - **The correct answer is a cholesterol embolism.**
    - No invasive procedure is free from potential complications.
    - In this case, a cardiac catheterization can disrupt cholesterol plaques which can then disseminate through the systemic circulation and cause partial or total arterial occlusion, leading to potential end organ damage from ischemia.

4. A 75-year-old man comes to the emergency department due to upper abdominal pain for the past 30 minutes. He has a past medical history of poorly controlled type II diabetes mellitus and hypertension. He has been smoking 2 packs of cigarettes per day for the past 50 years. His vital signs include temperature of 36° C (96.8° F), blood pressure of 155/95 mmHg, heart rate of 78 beats/min, and respiratory rate of 19 breaths/min. The physical exam shows intensive perspiration and epigastric pain without positional variation or precordial tenderness. ECG shows 3-mm ST-segment elevation in leads II, III, and aVF. Cardiac troponin I is negative. The best next step to definitively diagnose this patient's current condition is?

    A. Echocardiography
    B. Arterial blood gasses
    C. Cardiac catheterization
    D. Cardiac stress test

- **The correct answer is option C.**
- This elderly man presents with upper abdominal pain for the past 30 minutes.
- He has a past medical history of poorly controlled type II diabetes mellitus and hypertension.
- He has been smoking 2 packs of cigarettes per day for the past 50 years.
- His comorbidities and lifestyle habits predispose him to atherosclerotic vascular disease.
- The physical exam reveals intensive perspiration and the epigastric pain without positional variation or precordial tenderness.
- These findings suggest acute coronary syndrome.
- ECG shows 3-mm ST-segment elevation in leads II, III, and aVF.
- These findings indicate an acute inferior STEMI due to right coronary artery thrombosis.
- However, cardiac troponin I is negative.
- It's worth noting that initially negative troponins should not make one exclude NSTEMI or STEMI because troponins take time to increase.
- Since the pretest probability of myocardial infarction is high in this patient, the best next step to definitively diagnose him is cardiac catheterization.
- In patients with myocardial infarction, the cardiac catheterization typically shows an acute occlusion of the coronary artery along with regional wall motion abnormalities like myocardial stunning.
- Options A and B are incorrect because although echocardiography and arterial blood gasses are usually done in a patient with suspected myocardial infarction, they cannot definitively diagnose acute coronary syndrome.
- Option D is incorrect because cardiac stress test is used to screen the patients for stable angina. However, it is not used in patients with suspected acute coronary syndrome because a cardiac stress test can exacerbate the patient's symptoms.
- Additionally, even if this particular patient had a negative stress test, it would still not exclude the acute coronary syndrome. Therefore, he requires urgent cardiac catheterization.

Cardiology | Section 2: Pericardial Diseases: Pericardial Effusion & Cardiac Tamponade

I. Pericardial Effusion: Definition
   A. Acute or chronic fluid accumulation in the pericardial space
   B. Can progress to cardiac tamponade

II. Pericardial Effusion: Causes
   A. Transudative
      1. Cirrhosis
      2. Nephrotic syndrome
      3. Congestive heart failure (CHF)
   B. Exudative
      1. Malignancy
      2. Trauma
   C. Hemopericardium after MI

III. Pericardial Effusion: Clinical Presentation
   A. Chronic or small pericardial effusion
      1. Usually asymptomatic
   B. Acute or large pericardial effusion
      1. Chest pain
      2. Shortness of breath
      3. Jugular venous distention

IV. Pericardial Effusion: Diagnosis
   A. Transthoracic echocardiography (gold standard) in all patients with suspected pericardial effusion
      1. Normal pericardial fluid volume: 10 to 50 mL
      2. Small effusion: 50 to 100 mL
      3. Moderate effusion: 100 to 500 mL
      4. Large effusion: > 500 mL
   B. ECG: tachycardia, low voltage QRS
   C. Pericardial fluid analysis
      1. Cell count and differential, protein and glucose, cytology, microbiology (gram stain, acid fast stain, PCR)
   D. Laboratory studies to determine the underlying cause
      1. CBC (leukocytosis), inflammatory markers
      2. Troponins
      3. Basic metabolic panel: BUN, creatinine (uremic pericarditis)

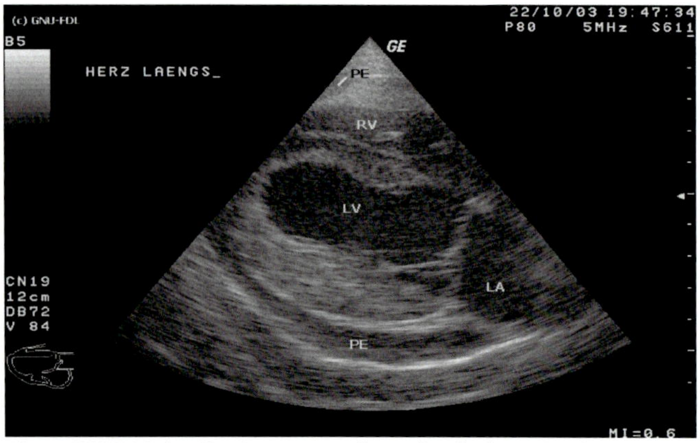

FIGURE 21.2.3 - Pericardial Effusion on Echocardiogram

V. Pericardial Effusion: Management
   A. Assess hemodynamic state
      1. Unstable (tamponade): urgent pericardiocentesis
      2. Stable: elective pericardial fluid drainage
   B. Asymptomatic: monitor with serial echocardiography

VI. Cardiac Tamponade: Definition
   A. Rapid accumulation of pericardial fluid causing obstructive shock
   B. Hemorrhagic or nonhemorrhagic

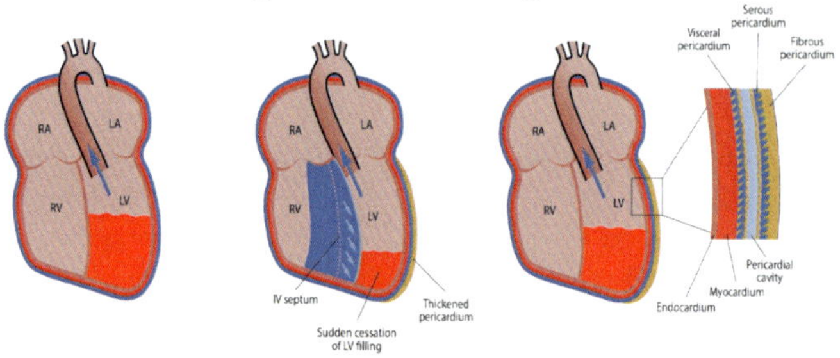

FIGURE 21.2.4 - Layers of Pericardium

VII. Cardiac Tamponade: Causes
   A. Hemorrhagic
      1. Chest trauma (e.g. gunshot, stab wound)
      2. Post-MI free wall rupture
      3. Stanford type A aortic dissection
      4. Iatrogenic (e.g. central line placement)
   B. Non-hemorrhagic
      1. Pericarditis and pericardial effusion

VIII. Cardiac Tamponade: Clinical Presentation
   A. Beck's triad
      1. Hypotension, muffled heart sounds, and elevated JVP
   B. Pulsus paradoxus (↓ in SBP > 10 mmHg during inspiration)
   C. Signs of obstructive shock
      1. Pallor
      2. Cold and clammy skin
   D. Normal lung auscultation

IX. Cardiac Tamponade: Diagnosis
   A. Echocardiography
      1. Large pericardial effusion
      2. Collapse of right atrium and ventricle
   B. ECG
      1. Low-voltage QRS complexes; electrical alternans
   C. Right heart catheterization
      1. Equalization of diastolic pressures within all chambers

X. Cardiac Tamponade: Management
   A. Acute and unstable: urgent pericardiocentesis even before echocardiography
   B. Subacute and stable
      1. Close monitoring
      2. Serial echocardiography
   C. Surgery: traumatic tamponade (hemorrhagic) unlikely to resolve only by pericardiocentesis

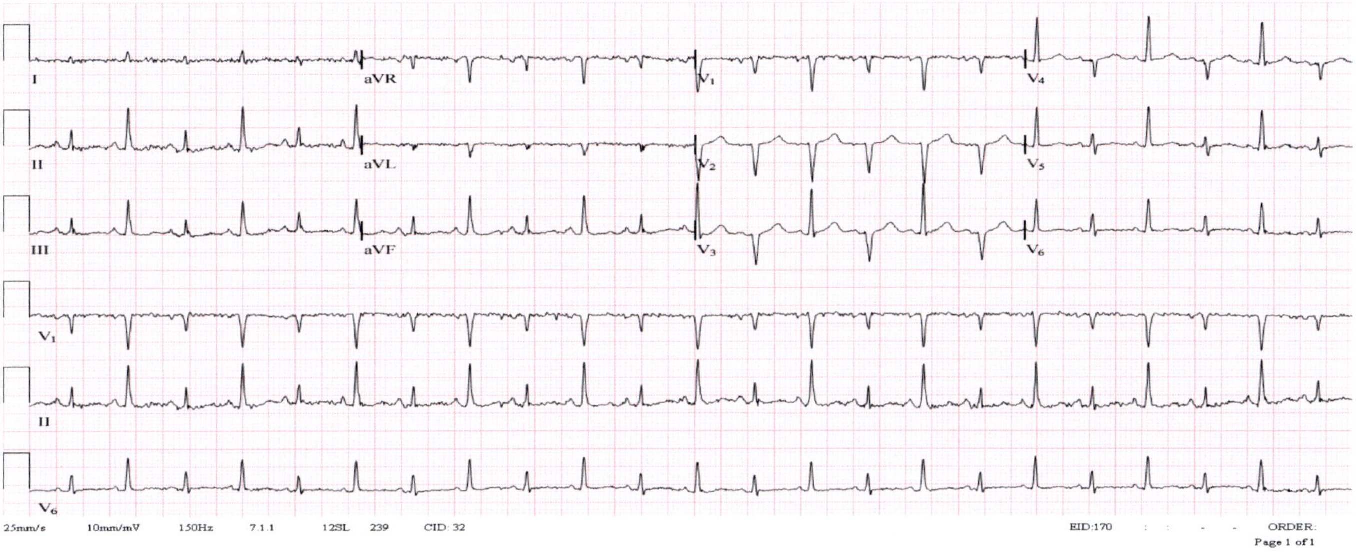

FIGURE 21.2.5 - ECG Showing Electrical Alternans

Condition	Key Features	Management
Acute pericarditis	- Idiopathic (most common) - Viral infections - Pleuritic chest pain relieved by sitting up and leaning forward - Diffuse ST elevation and PR depression on ECG	- Treat underlying cause (e.g. dialysis for uremia) - NSAIDs (first line) - Colchicine - Corticosteroids typically avoided due to risk of recurrence
Constrictive pericarditis	- Idiopathic (most common) - Cardiac surgery - Chest radiation - Miliary TB - Kussmaul sign - Thick and calcified pericardium on imaging	- NSAIDs - Colchicine - Pericardiectomy
Pericardial effusion	- Transudative: cirrhosis, nephrotic syndrome, CHF - Exudative: malignancy, trauma - Post-MI hemopericardium - Chronic and/or small effusion: asymptomatic - Acute and/or large effusion: chest pain, SOB, JVD	- Hemodynamically unstable: urgent pericardiocentesis - Hemodynamically stable: elective pericardiocentesis - Asymptomatic: serial echocardiography
Cardiac tamponade	- Hemorrhagic and nonhemorrhagic - Beck's triad (hypotension, muffled heart sounds, JVD) - Pulsus paradoxus - Electrical alternans on ECG - Equalization of diastolic pressures	- Hemodynamically unstable: urgent pericardiocentesis - Hemodynamically stable: serial echocardiography - Traumatic hemorrhagic tamponade: surgery

TABLE 21.2.1 - Pericardial Diseases

REVIEW QUESTIONS

1. A 79-year-old man comes to the physician because of shortness of breath and chest pain for the past 2 weeks. He has chronic kidney disease, and has missed the last three hemodialysis sessions. His BUN is 80 mg/dL (7-18 mg/dL). Echocardiography shows hypoechoic space between visceral and parietal pericardium, and the ECG shows QRS complexes with low amplitude. What is the most likely mechanism of the ECG finding in this patient?

   - **The most likely mechanism of the ECG finding is pericardial effusion → pericardial fluid interferes with myocardial electrical impulses reaching electrodes → low-voltage QRS complexes.**
   - This patient reports shortness of breath and chest pain for the past 2 weeks.
   - He has chronic kidney disease, and he has missed the last three hemodialysis sessions.
   - BUN is 80 mg/dL.
   - Echocardiography shows hypoechoic space between visceral and parietal pericardium.
   - All these findings suggest uremic pericarditis with pericardial effusion.
   - ECG shows QRS complexes with low amplitude.
   - Low-voltage QRS complexes in case of pericardial effusion is present because pericardial fluid interferes with myocardial impulses reaching the electrodes.

2. A 65-year-old man comes to the emergency department due to chest pain, altered mental status, and shortness of breath for the past hour. He had anterior wall myocardial infarction 10 days ago. His vital signs include temperature of 36° C (96.8° F), blood pressure of 70/50 mmHg, heart rate of 150 beats/min, and respiratory rate of 29 breaths/min. Systolic blood pressure drops by 15 mmHg on inspiration. ECG shows low-voltage QRS complexes with the amplitude alternating from beat to beat. Which of the following is the best next step in the management of this patient?

   A. Pericardiocentesis
   B. Thoracentesis
   C. Echocardiography
   D. Chest X-ray

   - **The correct answer is A.**
   - This patient presents with chest pain, shortness of breath, and hemodynamic instability evidenced by severe hypotension and tachycardia.
   - He has a history of anterior wall myocardial infarction 10 days ago.
   - His systolic blood pressure drops by 15 mmHg on inspiration.
   - A drop in systolic blood pressure by more than 10 mmHg on inspiration is called pulsus paradoxus.
   - ECG shows low-voltage QRS complexes with the amplitude alternating from beat to beat. This sign is known as electrical alternans.
   - All these findings suggest cardiac tamponade presumably due to free myocardial wall rupture.
   - The best next step in the management of the patient with high suspicion of tamponade is emergent pericardiocentesis.
   - Option B, thoracentesis, is incorrect because thoracentesis drains fluid from the pleural, rather than the pericardial cavity. Patients with tamponade do not have fluid in the pleural cavity.
   - Option C, echocardiography, is incorrect because although echocardiography is used to diagnose tamponade, time should not be wasted confirming the cardiac tamponade because this patient is severely unstable and needs emergent intervention.
   - Option D, chest X-ray, is incorrect because it is time-consuming and not sensitive enough to diagnose cardiac tamponade.

Cardiology | Section 3: Valvular Heart Disease: Aortic Regurgitation & Stenosis

Condition	Etiology	Key Features
Aortic regurgitation	- Regurgitant backflow of blood across incompetent aortic valve	- Dyspnea, palpitations, angina, bifid pulse, corrigan pulse, S3 - Diastolic decrescendo murmur
Aortic stenosis	- Thickening of aortic valve leaflets resulting in partial obstruction	- Dyspnea, palpitations, angina, syncope, delayed peripheral pulses, delayed carotid upstroke - Crescendo-decrescendo systolic murmur

TABLE 21.2.2 - Aortic Regurgitation and Aortic Stenosis

I. Aortic Regurgitation: Definition
   A. Inadequate closure of the aortic valve leading to regurgitant blood flow

II. Aortic Regurgitation: Pathophysiology
   A. Regurgitant flow leads to increase in:
      1. LV end diastolic volume
      2. LV dilation
      3. LV wall thickness
   B. Compensatory mechanisms fail over time

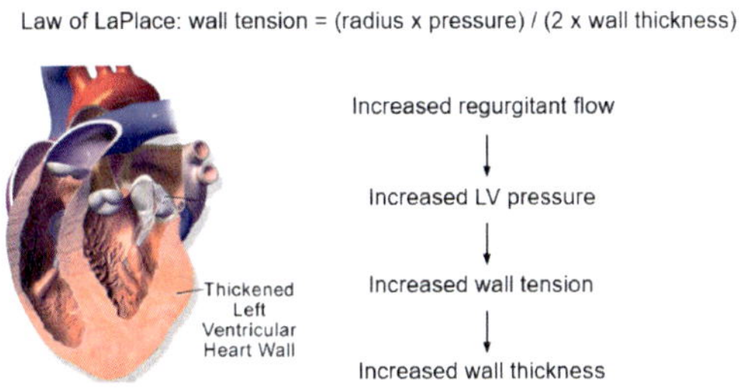

FIGURE 21.2.6 - Pathophysiology of Aortic Regurgitation

III. Aortic Regurgitation: Risk Factors
   A. Valvular disease
      1. Rheumatic heart disease
      2. Congenital bicuspid valve
      3. Calcified valve
   B. Aortic root dilation
      1. Marfan syndrome
      2. Hypertension

IV. Aortic Regurgitation: Presentation
   A. Asymptomatic for years
   B. Symptoms
      1. Palpitations, dyspnea, angina, orthopnea
   C. Findings
      1. Widened pulse pressure, Corrigan pulse, bifid pulse, head bobbing
      2. Decrescendo diastolic murmur at lower left sternal border

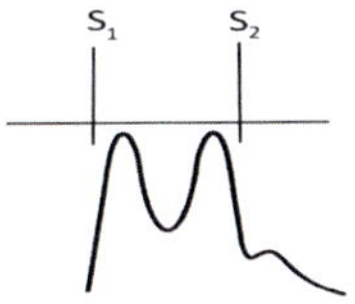

FIGURE 21.2.7 - Bifid Pulse

V. Aortic Regurgitation: Diagnosis
   A. Imaging
      1. Echocardiogram: aortic valve leaflet thickening, vegetations, sclerosis, bicuspid valve, aortic sinus dilation, regurgitant jet on doppler
      2. ECG: left ventricular hypertrophy such as increased QRS amplitude or Cornell criteria (add R wave in aVL and S wave in V3, positive if > 28 mm in males and > 20 mm in females)

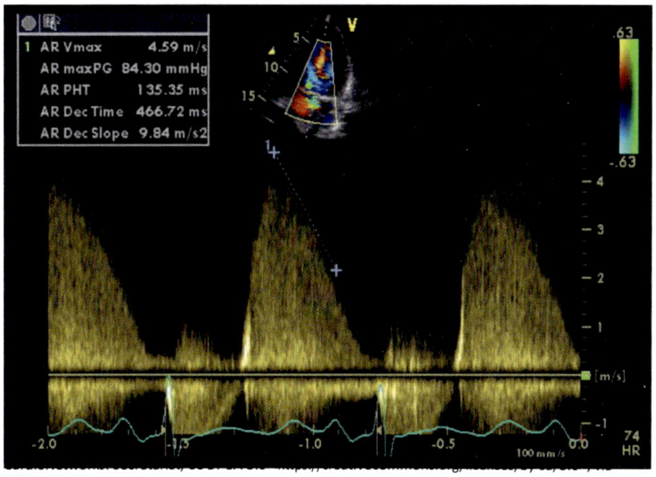

FIGURE 21.2.8 - Aortic Regurgitation on Echocardiogram

VI. Aortic Regurgitation: Management
   A. Asymptomatic with no LV dysfunction
      1. No therapy
   B. Asymptomatic with severe regurgitation and LV dysfunction
      1. ACE inhibitor or ARB for afterload reduction
   C. Symptomatic
      1. Salt restriction, diuretics, ACEi/ARB, beta blocker, surgical valve replacement for definitive treatment
   D. Acute aortic regurgitation is a medical emergency
      1. Requires immediate surgical intervention

VII. Aortic Stenosis: Definition
   A. Narrowing of aortic valve leading to obstruction of outflow of blood from the left ventricle

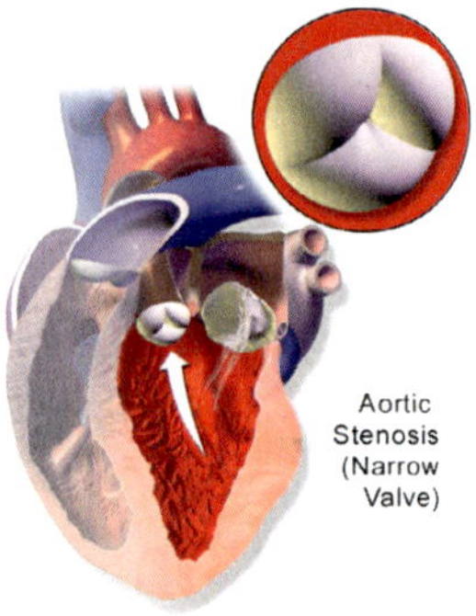

FIGURE 21.2.9 - Aortic Stenosis

VIII. Aortic Stenosis: Pathophysiology
- A. Aortic valve sclerosis (seen in elderly due to stress on valve over time)
- B. Rheumatic disease
- C. Narrowed aortic outflow tract causes concentric hypertrophy
    1. Increased oxygen demand and impaired filling
    2. Can lead to left heart failure

IX. Aortic Stenosis: Risk Factors
- A. Bicuspid aortic valve
- B. Rheumatic heart disease
- C. Atherosclerosis
    1. Age > 75, smoking, diabetes, hypertension, hyperlipidemia

X. Aortic Stenosis: Presentation
- A. Asymptomatic for years
- B. Symptoms
    1. Dyspnea, palpitations, angina, syncope
- C. Findings
    1. Delayed peripheral pulses, delayed carotid upstroke, S4 heart sound
    2. Crescendo-decrescendo murmur at upper right sternal border

XI. Aortic Stenosis: Diagnosis
- A. Imaging
    1. Chest X-ray (look for signs of CHF)
    2. Echocardiogram demonstrates thickened and/or calcified aortic leaflets with reduced systolic motion and small orifice
    3. Echocardiogram may also show bicuspid aortic valve or LV hypertrophy

XII. Aortic Stenosis: Management
- A. Asymptomatic
    1. Medical treatment of risk factors, echocardiogram every 3-5 years
- B. Severe stenosis defined as: maximum aortic jet velocity ≥ 4 m/s or transvalvular gradient ≥ 40 mmHg or valve area < 1.0 cm^2
- C. Replace valve if: LVEF < 50%, onset of symptoms, concurrent cardiac procedure
- D. Use diuretics, beta blockers, vasodilators with caution

REVIEW QUESTIONS ?

1. What type of cardiac hypertrophy would be present in chronic aortic regurgitation?
    - **Eccentric hypertrophy would be present in chronic aortic regurgitation.**
    - Eccentric hypertrophy is a type of cardiac remodeling associated with dilated cardiomyopathy where sarcomeres are added in series causing muscle fibers to increase in length and width.
    - This dilation occurs in response to the increased left ventricular end diastolic volumes and increased pressures.

2. Why is left ventricular oxygen demand increased in chronic aortic stenosis?
    - **Left ventricular oxygen demand is increased in chronic aortic stenosis because of increased heart rate, additional muscular tissues, and reduced coronary flow reserve.**
    - The heart will respond to the decreased cardiac output caused by the stenotic valve obstructing the outflow tract by increasing the heart rate. Cardiac output equals stroke volume multiplied by heart rate. This increased rate will cause the myocardium to need more cellular energy and therefore more oxygen demand.
    - As the heart remodels and hypertrophies, the added cardiac muscular tissues will require more oxygen as well.
    - The hypertrophied heart paired with a faster heart rate will lead to impaired diastolic fillings. This will further reduce the coronary flow reserve and contribute to increased oxygen demand.

3. How is pulse pressure affected by aortic stenosis?
    - **Pulse pressure is narrowed in the setting of aortic stenosis.**
    - There may be a lesser difference in the systolic and diastolic pressures, this is typically due to decreases in stroke volume caused by the valve obstructing blood flow.

Cardiology | Section 4: Valvular Heart Disease: Mitral Valve Diseases

Condition	Etiology	Key Features
Mitral valve prolapse	- Myxomatous degeneration of valve tissue, connective tissue disorder (Marfan syndrome)	- Usually asymptomatic, possible palpitations or atypical chest pain - Mid-systolic click with mid to late systolic murmur
Mitral stenosis	- Thickening of mitral valve leaflets usually due to rheumatic disease	- Dyspnea, orthopnea, palpitations, angina, hemoptysis - Diastolic opening snap with diastolic murmur
Mitral regurgitation	- Regurgitant backflow of blood across incompetent mitral valve	- Dyspnea, orthopnea, PND, palpitations, pulmonary edema - Holosystolic murmur with radiation to axilla

TABLE 21.2.3 - Valvular Heart Conditions

I. Mitral Valve Prolapse: Definition
   A. Structural defect in mitral valve leading to the bulging of mitral leaflets into left atrium during systole (> 2mm above annular plane)
   B. Mostly idiopathic
   C. Most common cause of mitral regurgitation

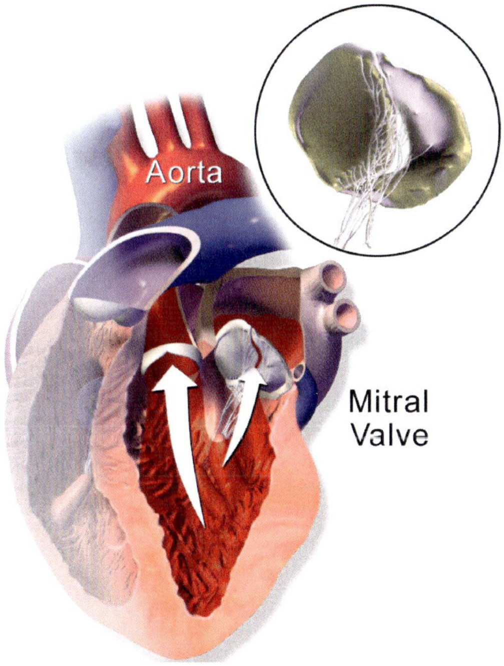

FIGURE 21.2.10 - Mitral Valve Prolapse

II. Mitral Valve Prolapse: Pathophysiology
   A. Myxomatous degeneration
   B. Long, unstable valve leaflets with excess valvular tissue
   C. Mitral annulus dilation lead to possible chordae tendinae rupture
   D. Valve leaflets flail into left atrium and cause mitral regurgitation

III. Mitral Valve Prolapse: Risk Factors
   A. Other valvular abnormalities (e.g. tricuspid, aortic)
   B. Thoracic skeletal abnormalities
   C. Von Willebrand disease
   D. Family history
   E. Connective tissue disorders (e.g. Marfan, Ehlers-Danlos syndromes)
   F. Infective endocarditis or Rheumatic disease
   G. Myocardial infarction

IV. Mitral Valve Prolapse: Presentation
   A. Typically asymptomatic
   B. Symptoms
      1. Atypical chest pains, palpitations
   C. Findings
      1. Midsystolic click followed by mid to late systolic murmur at mitral area

V. Mitral Valve Prolapse: Diagnosis
   A. Imaging
      1. Echocardiogram shows flailing of faulty mitral valve leaflets
      2. Defined by leaflets > 2 mm above mitral annulus

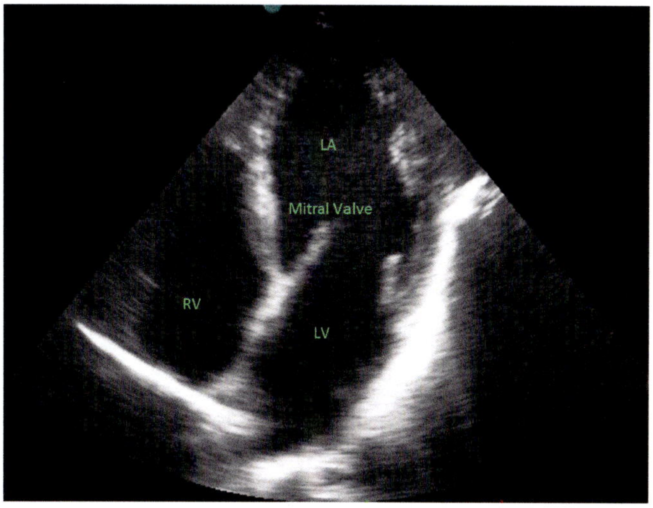

FIGURE 21.2.11 - Mitral Valve Prolapse on Echocardiogram

VI. Mitral Valve Prolapse: Management
   A. Asymptomatic: reassurance
   B. Symptomatic
      1. Give beta blockers for chest pain and palpitations

VII. Mitral Stenosis: Definition
   A. Thickening of mitral leaflets leading to obstruction of blood flow from left atrium to left ventricle
   B. Almost always caused by rheumatic heart disease
      1. Age-related calcification or radiation induced fibrosis

VIII. Mitral Stenosis: Pathophysiology
   A. Stenotic valve leads to obstruction of blood flow into the left ventricle
   B. Decrease in left ventricular end diastolic volume (decrease SV)
   C. Increase in left atrial pressure
   D. Increase in pulmonary capillary pressure → cardiogenic pulmonary edema

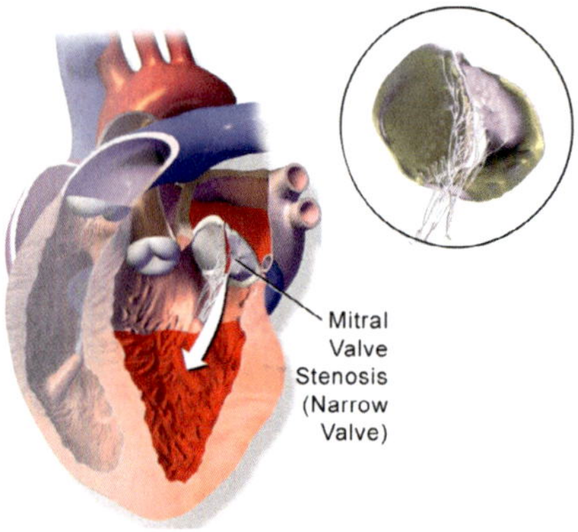

FIGURE 21.2.12 - Mitral Valve Stenosis

IX. Mitral Stenosis: Risk Factors
   A. History of rheumatic disease
   B. Congenital defects (rare)

X. Mitral Stenosis: Presentation
   A. Asymptomatic for years
   B. Symptoms
      1. Exertional dyspnea, orthopnea, palpitations, angina
   C. Findings
      1. Diastolic opening snap followed by low pitched murmur best heard over cardiac apex

XI. Mitral Stenosis: Diagnosis
   A. Imaging
      1. Chest X ray shows left atrial enlargement
      2. Echocardiogram shows narrowing of mitral orifice
      3. Echocardiogram in setting of rheumatic heart disease shows commissural fusion with diastolic doming

   B. Mitral Stenosis: Management
      1. Asymptomatic: no therapy
      2. Symptomatic
   C. Medical: diuretics for pulmonary congestion, beta blockers for rate control
   D. Anticoagulation: if history of embolic event or AF present
   E. Surgical: valve replacement indicated for severe disease

XII. Mitral Regurgitation: Definition
   A. Inadequate closure of the mitral valve leading to regurgitant blood flow across valve during systole

XIII. Mitral Regurgitation: Pathophysiology
   A. Defect in any part of mitral apparatus
   B. Burdens left ventricle with excess volume load (increased EDV)
   C. Heart will compensate to maintain adequate output (e.g. increase HR)
   D. Left ventricle will dilate and hypertrophy to balance wall stress
   E. Decompensation may occur leading to symptoms

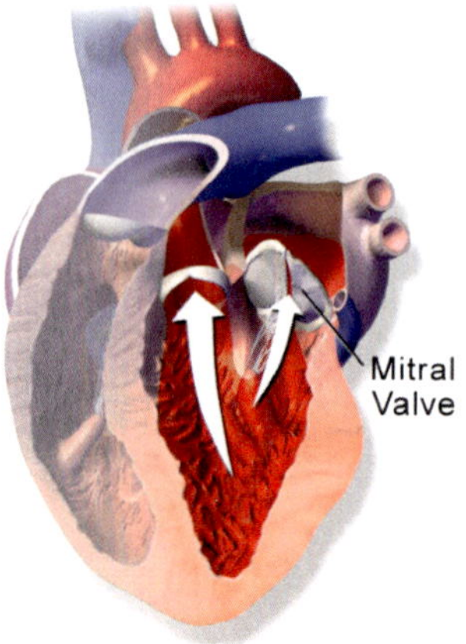

FIGURE 21.2.13 - Mitral Valve Regurgitation

XIV. Mitral Regurgitation: Risk Factors
   A. Mitral valve prolapse is the most common cause
   B. Acute
      1. Endocarditis, papillary muscle or chordae tendinae rupture
   C. Chronic
      1. MVP, rheumatic disease, connective tissue disorders, cardiomyopathy, coronary artery disease, valvular calcification

XV. Mitral Regurgitation: Presentation
   A. Symptoms
      1. Exertional dyspnea, orthopnea, paroxysmal nocturnal dyspnea, palpitations
   B. Findings
      1. Decreased or absent S1, S3, holosystolic murmur at cardiac apex with radiation to axilla

XVI. Mitral Regurgitation: Diagnosis

A. Imaging

1. Echocardiogram shows backflow of blood across valve during systole on doppler and/or flail leaflets of the valve

XVII. Mitral Regurgitation: Management

A. Asymptomatic: surgery if LVEF 30-60% and/or LVESD > 40 mm

B. Symptomatic

1. Medical: reduced afterload with vasodilators, anticoagulation if atrial fibrillation present
2. Surgical: repair or replacement of valve is definitive, indicated in chronic regurgitation if LVEF > 30% or LVEF < 30% with high likelihood of successful repair

REVIEW QUESTIONS

1. What effect would standing maneuver have on murmur heard in mitral valve prolapse?

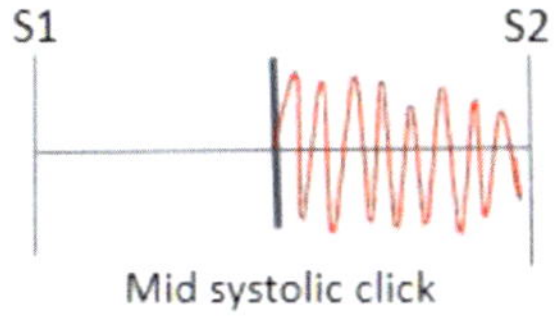

- **On standing, the classic mid-systolic click would occur slightly earlier in systole and the murmur would also lengthen.**
- Standing reduces venous return and therefore slightly less blood will fill the ventricle.
- When this happens the mitral valves take slightly less time to flail into the left atrium due to the fact that the smaller ventricular volume leads to less stretch on the mitral annulus and a more easily compliant mitral valve leaflet.
- This can be simplified by imagining the valve as a rubber band stretched as far as possible between two points. If those two points are brought closer together, the rubber band flops around more easily.

2. Which extra heart sound may be present in worsening mitral valve prolapse?

- **The extra heart sound that may be present in worsening mitral valve prolapse is S3 heart sound.**
- It can develop as a result of left ventricular volume overload if mitral valve prolapse progresses to mitral regurgitation.
- S3 is typically heard immediately after S2 during early diastole and may be described as a low-frequency sound.
- It typically reflects an increase in atrial pressures leading to increased flow rates of blood filling the left ventricle.
- It can be imagined as a large amount of blood entering the left ventricle rapidly striking against a very compliant left ventricle.

3. Why may a patient with longstanding mitral valve stenosis have trouble swallowing?

- **Chronic long standing mitral valve stenosis can lead to left atrial dilation and can cause cardiovascular dysphagia.**
- This occurs when the enlarged left atrium is displaced posteriorly causing external compression of the esophagus.
- On rare occasions, this can also cause compression of the left recurrent laryngeal nerve and lead to chronic cough or voice hoarseness.

4. Why is atrial fibrillation associated with mitral stenosis? What is this often a warning sign of?

- **Mitral stenosis leads to left atrial dilatation which results in atrial fibrillation due to disruption of electrical conduction through the atria. Atrial fibrillation in the setting of mitral stenosis often precipitates acute decompensation.**
- This is because not enough pressure can be generated to overcome the elevated left atrial pressures and provide adequate blood flow across the stenotic valve.

5. Which neurocutaneous disorder has been associated with mitral regurgitation?

- **Tuberous sclerosis is associated with mitral regurgitation.**
- The individuals with this condition can often have cardiac rhabdomyomas around the mitral annulus and lead to regurgitation.

6. Why do arterial vasodilators improve symptoms of mitral regurgitation?

- **Arterial vasodilators improve systems of mitral regurgitation because they decrease afterload, increase forward blood flow, and decrease regurgitant flow.**

REVIEW QUESTIONS

7. A 43-year-old man comes to the emergency room after an episode of palpitations on his walk this morning which resolved after about 10 minutes. He has had recurrent shortness of breath upon exertion over the last 3 months, but never experienced palpitations. He has mild trouble breathing while going to bed at night. He denies any cough or chest pain. The patient states he has never smoked and has a remote history of rheumatic fever as a child. He is otherwise healthy. On physical examination, his temperature is 37.3° C (99.1° F), respiratory rate is 15 breaths/min, heart rate is 80 beats/min, and blood pressure is 129/79 mmHg. His lungs are clear to auscultation bilaterally and a systolic cardiac murmur is heard at the apex of the heart, which decreases with the valsalva maneuver. He has mild lower extremity swelling. CBC, troponin, ECG and chest X-ray are all unremarkable. What is the most likely diagnosis?

   A. Aortic regurgitation
   B. Chronic mitral regurgitation
   C. Pulmonary embolism
   D. Congestive heart failure
   E. Ventricular septal defect

- **The correct answer is B.**
- This patient has exertional dyspnea, palpitations, mild edema and orthopnea.
- On physical examination, a systolic murmur is heard at the cardiac apex that decreases with valsalva.
- He has a normal cardiac workup otherwise.
- All of these findings make mitral regurgitation the most likely diagnosis.
- This diagnosis would need to be confirmed with an echocardiogram.
- Aortic regurgitation may present with similar clinical symptoms. However, a history of rheumatic disease would more likely affect the mitral valve.
- Option A is incorrect because a systolic murmur at the apex of the heart which decreases with valsalva maneuver is not expected in the case of aortic regurgitation.
- Also, the physical exam is more in alignment with mitral valve regurgitation.
- A description of classic aortic regurgitation murmur may mention a decrescendo diastolic murmur heard loudest at the right sternal border.
- Option C is incorrect because a pulmonary embolism would likely present in a more acute manner than this patient's chronic presentation.
- Option D is incorrect because congestive heart failure could also present with orthopnea, shortness of breath and palpitations but a murmur would not necessarily be anticipated.
- A patient with symptomatic congestive heart failure may also have jugular venous distention or edema of lower extremities which this patient does not have.
- Option E is incorrect because a ventricular septal defect is less likely to fit the history of rheumatic disease and the murmur would likely be described as a holosystolic blowing murmur located at the left sternal border.

Cardiology | Section 5: Valvular Heart Diseases: Tricuspid Regurgitation

I. Tricuspid Regurgitation: Definition
   A. Inadequate closure of the tricuspid valve leading to regurgitant blood flow across valve during systole
   B. Usually secondary to annular dilation
      1. Leaflet tethering in setting of increased right ventricular pressure/volume overload

II. Tricuspid Regurgitation: Pathophysiology
   A. Backflow of blood into compliant right atrium
   B. Right atrial pressures can rise in severe cases
   C. Right sided heart failure is possible
   D. Renal failure from elevated central venous pressure

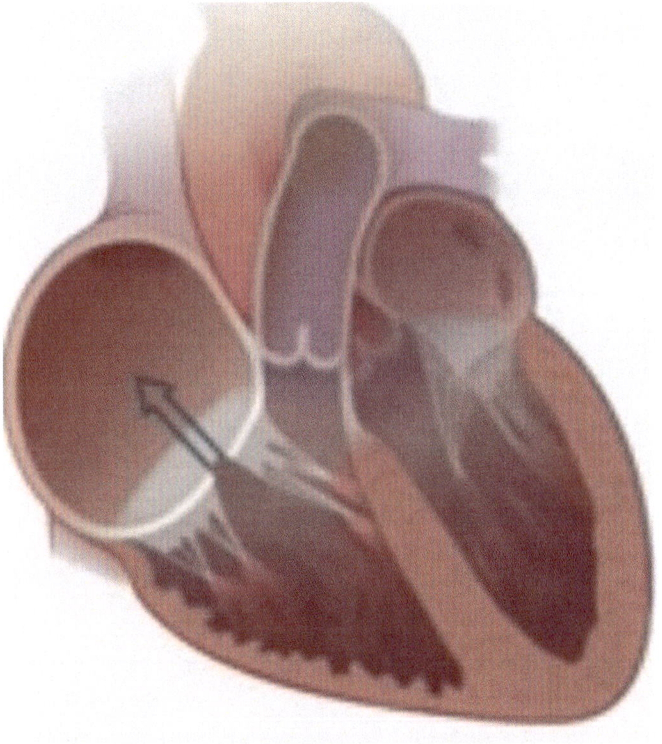

FIGURE 21.2.14 - Tricuspid Regurgitation

III. Tricuspid Regurgitation: Risk Factors
   A. Most cases secondary (i.e. in setting of increased RV pressure and/or volume)
      1. Heart failure, mitral stenosis/regurgitation, carcinoid syndrome, primary pulmonary disease
   B. Primary disease risk factors
      1. Pacemaker/ICD, IV drug use, rheumatic disease, history of chest wall trauma, Ebstein's anomaly

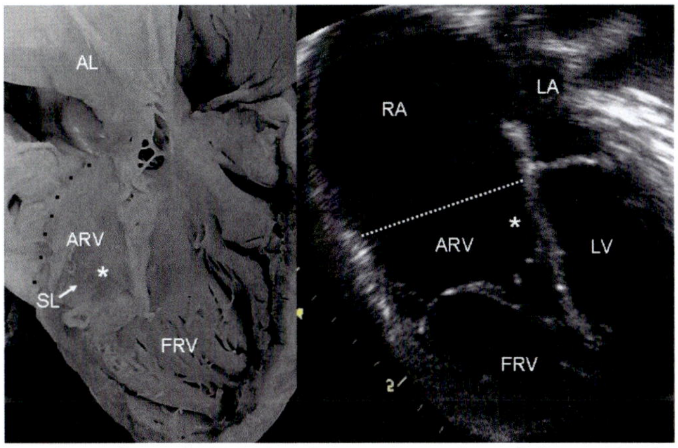

FIGURE 21.2.15 - Ebstein's Anomaly

IV. Tricuspid Regurgitation: Presentation
   A. Typically asymptomatic
   B. Findings
      1. Ascites, hepatomegaly, JVD, edema
      2. Inspiratory S3
      3. Prominent V wave with rapid Y descent
      4. Blowing holosystolic murmur at left lower sternal border

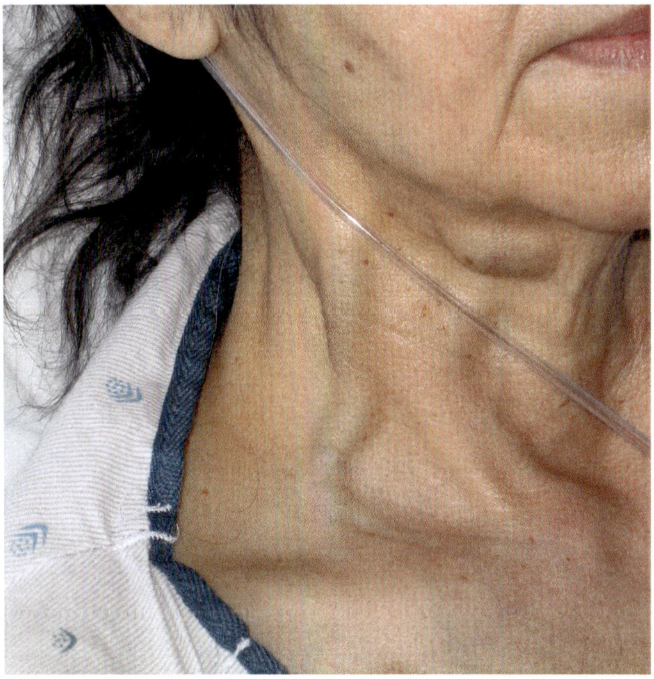

FIGURE 21.2.16 - Jugular Venous Distension

V. Tricuspid Regurgitation: Diagnosis
   A. Imaging
      1. Echocardiogram shows dilation of right atrium/ventricle and backflow of blood on doppler

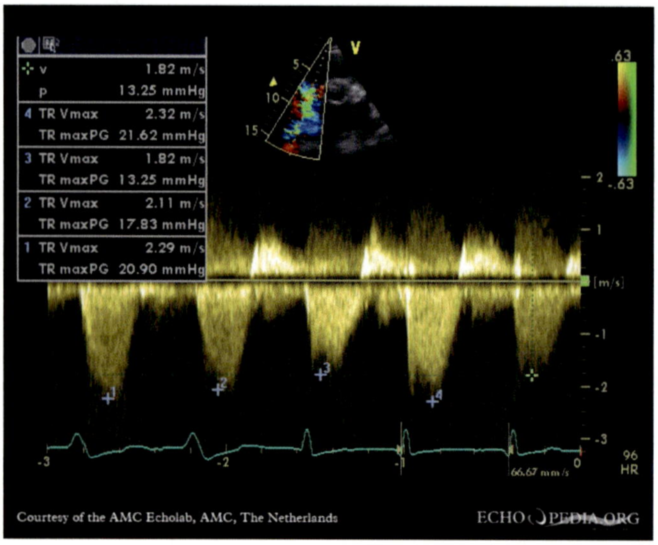

FIGURE 21.2.17 - Tricuspid Regurgitation on Echocardiogram

VI. Tricuspid Regurgitation: Management
   1. Treat underlying etiology
   2. Medical: diuretics for volume overload
   3. Surgical: replacement in symptomatic severe primary disease despite medical therapy without severe right ventricular dysfunction

Condition	Etiology	Key Features
Tricuspid regurgitation	- Regurgitant backflow of blood across incompetent tricuspid valve	- Usually asymptomatic, signs of right ventricular failure (ascites, hepatomegaly, JVD, edema) - Blowing holosystolic murmur
Infective endocarditis	- Infection of endocardial surface	- Fever, constitutional symptoms, predisposing factors, heart failure
Non-infective endocarditis	- Systemic illness creates vegetations on leaflets	- Sterile vegetations on valve leaflets, murmurs, symptoms of underlying illnesses

TABLE 21.2.4 - Tricuspid Regurgitation vs. Infective and Non-Infective Endocarditis

REVIEW QUESTIONS

1. Why might liver function tests be elevated in a patient with tricuspid regurgitation?
   - **In severe tricuspid regurgitation, elevated liver function tests such as AST, ALT, and hyperbilirubinemia may be present due to the progression of right-sided cardiac congestion.**
   - In tricuspid regurgitation, the decrease in forward movement of blood flow from the right side of the heart to the pulmonary vasculature would lead to backflow of blood into the superior vena cava and congestion of blood flow within the liver.

2. Why may an ablation for atrial flutter lead to tricuspid regurgitation?
   - **Tricuspid regurgitation may be caused by iatrogenic injury during a radiofrequency ablation procedure due to the proximity of the tricuspid valve to the cavotricuspid isthmus.**
   - Ablations for atrial flutter often target the cavotricuspid isthmus between the IVC and the tricuspid annulus because the isthmus may give rise to flutter waves.
   - All invasive procedures come with a small risk of causing valvular damage.

3. A 36-year-old man comes to the physician due to shortness of breath and bilateral leg swelling for the last week. He has had high fevers for two weeks. He has been using heroin since the age of 20 years. His vital signs include temperature of 38° C (100.4° F), blood pressure of 110/80 mmHg, heart rate of 110 beats/min, and respiratory rate of 15 breaths/min. The physical examination shows track marks on both antecubital fossa along with bilateral pitting edema up to the knees. Cardiac auscultation shows S3 heart sound and a blowing, holosystolic murmur at the left lateral sternal border. Which of the following is the best next step in the management of this patient?

   A. Echocardiography
   B. Right heart catheterization
   C. Chest X-ray
   D. Chest CT scan

   - **The correct answer is option A.**
   - **This patient has had high fevers for two weeks and now he presents with shortness of breath and bilateral leg swelling for the last week.**
   - **S3 heart sound and the bilateral pitting edema are likely due to right heart failure and volume overload.**
   - **The blowing, holosystolic murmur at the left lateral sternal border is suggestive of tricuspid regurgitation.**
   - **Considering that he is a chronic heroin user, he likely introduced bacteria into his venous blood.**
   - **The first heart valve that the venous blood comes into contact with is the tricuspid valve.**
   - **Therefore, bacteria in the blood caused infective endocarditis of the tricuspid valve.**
   - **Infective endocarditis of the tricuspid valve resulted in tricuspid regurgitation and right heart failure.**
   - **The best next test to diagnose any valvular abnormality, including tricuspid regurgitation, is echocardiography.**
   - **Option B, right heart catheterization, is incorrect because although it can definitively diagnose tricuspid regurgitation, it is an invasive procedure and should be avoided as the initial test.**
   - **Options C and D are incorrect because although chest X-ray and chest CT scan can identify the dilated right atrium and ventricle, these imaging modalities are not sensitive enough to definitively diagnose the tricuspid regurgitation.**

Cardiology | Section 6: Infective Endocarditis

I. Definition
   A. Infection of the endocardial surface of the heart
   B. Usually one or more heart valves are affected
   C. Infective endocarditis can be classified by
      1. Type of affected valve (native vs. prosthetic)
      2. Acuity of the infection (acute vs. subacute)
      3. Location of the infection (right-sided vs. left-sided)

II. Pathophysiology
   A. Endocardial injury (damaged valve) → adherence of platelet and fibrin → secondary infection → immune activation and further clot formation → valve destruction and loss of function
   B. Infection with highly virulent organism → binds to endothelial cell → bacterial proliferation → tissue destruction
   C. Bacterial vegetation and platelet thrombi on the valve can embolize
   D. Valvular destruction by bacteria and immune cells → loss of normal valve function → regurgitation

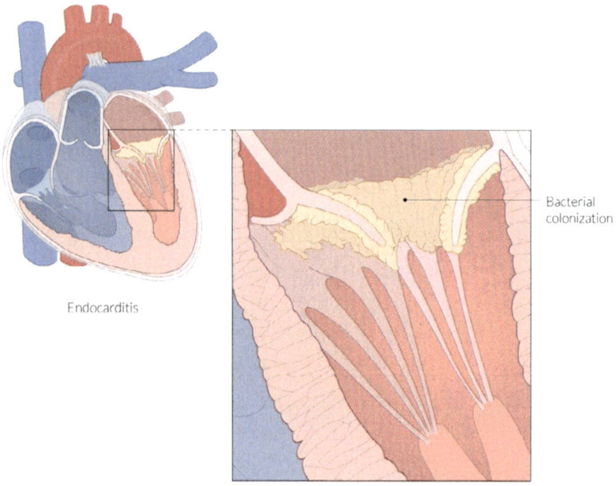

(c) AMBOSS Used under special agreement. Accessed December 21, 2021

FIGURE 21.2.18 - Bacterial Colonization on Mitral Valve in Infective Endocarditis

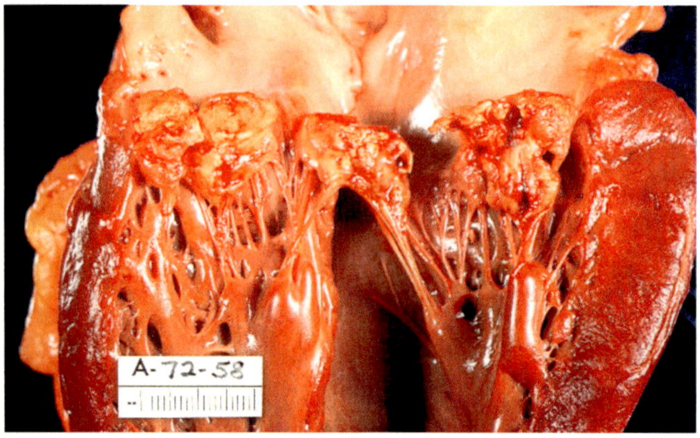

CDC/Public Domain

FIGURE 21.2.19 - Valvular Vegetations in Bacterial Endocarditis

III. Risk Factors
   A. Male sex
   B. Age > 60 yrs
   C. Valvular disease
   D. Prosthetic heart valves
   E. Congenital heart defects
   F. Previous endocarditis
   G. Poor dental status
   H. Dental procedures
   I. IV drug use
   J. IV catheter use
   K. Hemodialysis
   L. Immunocompromised status

IV. Clinical Features
   A. May present acutely or subacutely
   B. Constitutional symptoms: fever, chills, weight loss, malaise, arthralgias
   C. Cardiac symptoms
      1. New-onset heart murmur or change in an existing murmur
      2. Symptoms of heart failure: dyspnea, orthopnea, LE edema
      3. Arrhythmias
   D. Systemic symptoms arise due to embolization
   E. Splinter hemorrhages
   F. Janeway lesions: nontender macules
   G. Osler nodes: painful nodules
   H. Roth spots
   I. Acute kidney injury, splenomegaly, pulmonary embolism (right-sided)
   J. Neurological manifestations: seizures, paresis, altered mental status

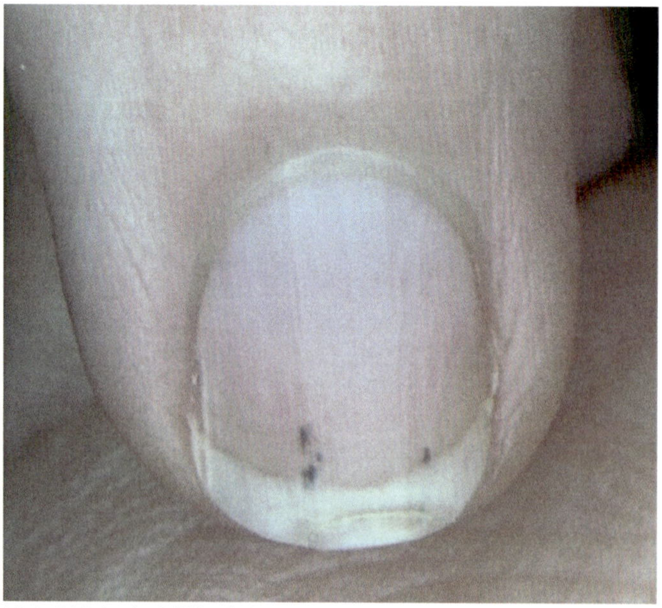

Splarka, Public domain, via Wikimedia Commons

FIGURE 21.2.20 - Splinter Hemorrhages due to Systemic Embolization

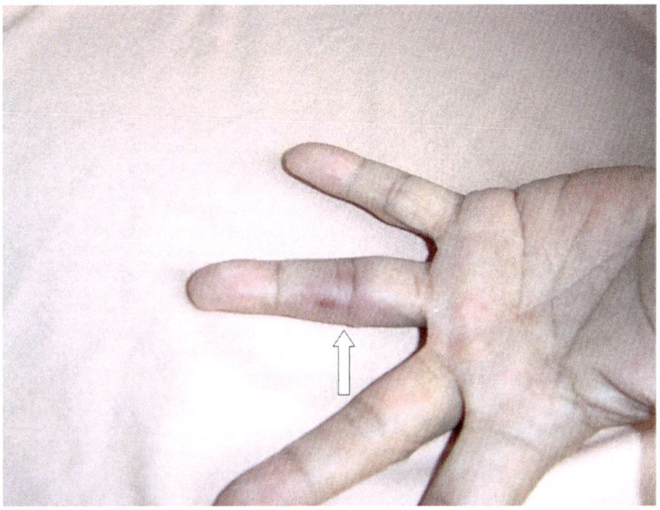

FIGURE 21.2.21 - Osler Node due to Deposition of Circulating Immune Complexes

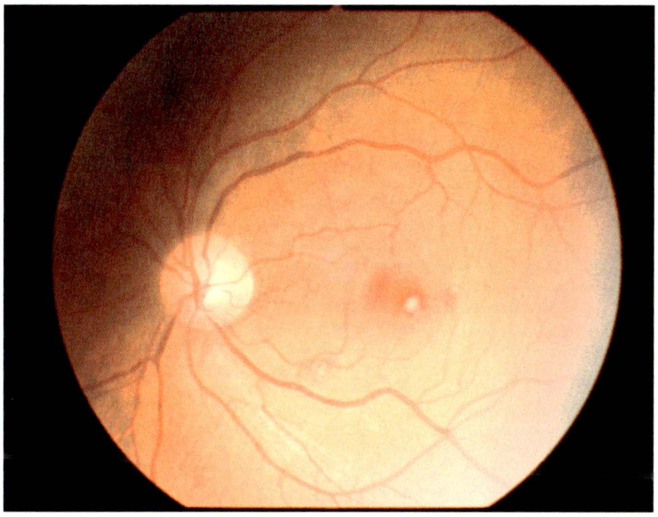

FIGURE 21.2.23 - Roth Spot due to Septic Embolus

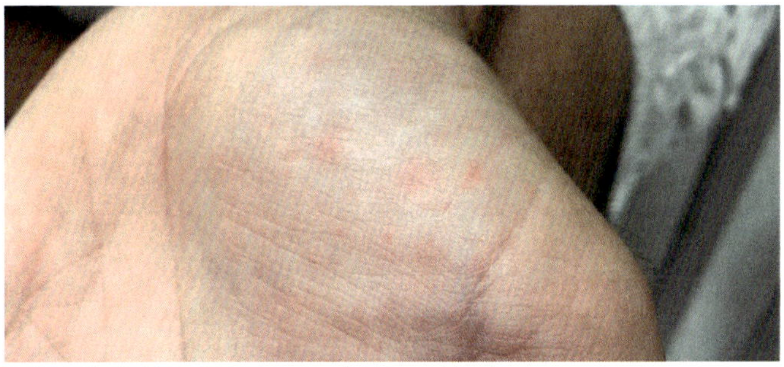

FIGURE 21.2.22 - Janeway Lesions in Infective Endocarditis

	Acute Bacterial Endocarditis	Subacute Bacterial Endocarditis
Clinical features	- Onset disease within days to weeks - Severe symptoms (high-grade fever, anorexia, malaise, and arthralgia)	- Onset within weeks to months - Mild symptoms (low-grade fever, back pain, weight loss)
Etiology	- Highly virulent organisms - Most commonly *S. aureus* - Can also be caused by group A streptococcus and *S. pneumoniae*	- Viridans Streptococci - Enterococci - HACEK organisms
Type of valve	- Undamaged native valves	- Damaged native valves or congenital valvular defects

TABLE 21.2.5 - Acute vs Subacute Bacterial Endocarditis

	Right-Sided Endocarditis	Left-Sided Endocarditis
Type of valve	- Tricuspid - Pulmonic	- Mitral - Aortic
Clinical features	- Symptoms due to pulmonary thromboemboli: dyspnea and hemoptysis - Symptoms of right heart failure: pitting edema, abdominal pain from hepatic congestion	- Symptoms due to systemic embolization - Symptoms of left heart failure: dyspnea and orthopnea due to pulmonary congestion
Etiology	- Associated with IV catheters and drug use - Mainly caused by *S. aureus* and coagulase-negative staphylococci	- *S. aureus* - Viridans Streptococci

TABLE 21.2.6 - Right-sided vs Left-sided Bacterial Endocarditis

V. Diagnosis
   A. Should be suspected in patients with fever and appropriate risk factors
   B. Modified Duke criteria are used to stratify patients based on the likelihood of disease
      1. Used in conjunction with clinical, pathological, microbiological, and imaging findings
   C. All patients receive multiple sets of blood cultures and echocardiography
   D. 3 sets of blood cultures and transthoracic echocardiography before initiation of treatment
   E. Additional evaluation: electrocardiogram, chest radiography, and routine lab tests such as a CBC and inflammatory markers
   F. Transthoracic echocardiography is the initial test of choice
   G. Transesophageal echocardiography only in selected cases
   H. Echocardiographic findings suggestive of endocarditis
      1. Valvular vegetation
      2. Abscess
      3. New valvular regurgitation
      4. Dehiscence of prosthetic valve

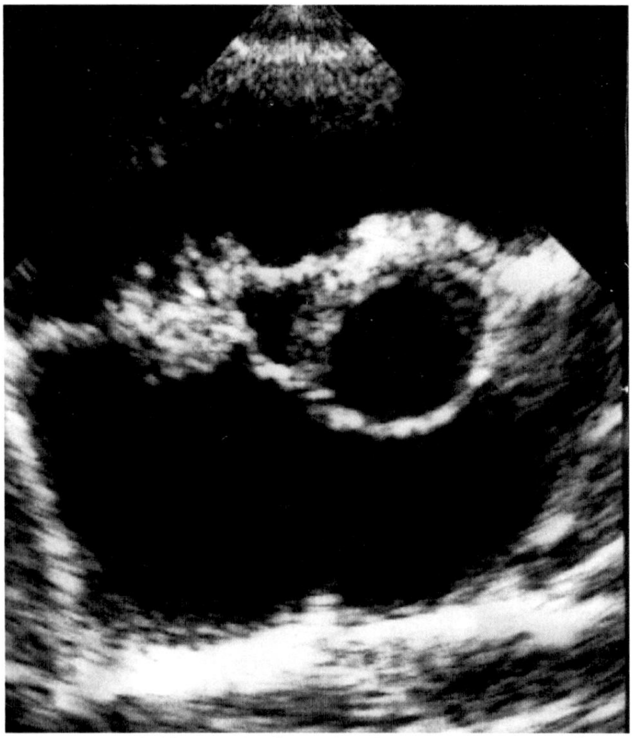

FIGURE 21.2.24 - Echocardiography Showing Valvular Vegetation in Infective Endocarditis

Modified Duke Criteria	
Major Criteria	- Typical microorganisms for infective endocarditis (Viridans streptococci, *S. aureus*, *S. gallolyticus,* HACEK group, community-acquired enterococci) - Persistently positive blood-cultures consistent with infective endocarditis[1] - One positive blood culture for Coxiella burnetii OR an anti-phase 1 IgG titer > 1:800 - Characteristic echocardiographic findings
Minor Criteria	- Predisposing condition; - Fever > 38°C - Vascular abnormalities[2] - Immunologic phenomena[3] - Positive blood cultures not fulfilling major criteria or serological evidence of infection with a common organism
Pathological Criteria	- Tissue culture or histology showing microorganism - Characteristic histologic feature of active endocarditis
1 - ≥ 2 positive blood cultures drawn at least 12 hours apart; All 3 or majority of ≥ 4 separate blood cultures; 2 - Major arterial emboli, septic pulmonary infarction, mycotic aneurysm, intracranial hemorrhage, conjunctival hemorrhages and janeway lesions; 3 - Glomerulonephritis, Roth spots, Osler nodes and rheumatoid factor	

TABLE 21.2.7 - Modified Duke Criteria

VI. Treatment
   A. Targeted antibiotic therapy is the mainstay of treatment
      1. Use blood culture results to guide selection
      2. Continue therapy for 4-6 weeks
   B. Empiric antibiotic therapy should not be started unless the patient is acutely ill with symptoms strongly suggestive of endocarditis
      1. Obtain blood cultures before starting
   C. Empiric antibiotic therapy for native valves
      1. Acute bacterial endocarditis: vancomycin + cefepime
      2. Subacute endocarditis: vancomycin + ampicillin-sulbactam
   D. Empiric antibiotic therapy for prosthetic valves
      1. Vancomycin + gentamicin + rifampin + cefepime
      2. > 1 year after placement: vancomycin + ceftriaxone
   E. Surgery indicated for
      1. Prosthetic valve endocarditis
      2. Valvular dysfunction or peri-valvular disease
      3. Heart failure
      4. Annular or aortic abscess
      5. New heart block
      6. Fungal endocarditis

VII. Management
   A. Antibiotic prophylaxis for the prevention of endocarditis is indicated for patients undergoing certain dental procedures
      1. Prosthetic valves
      2. History of endocarditis
      3. Unrepaired congenital heart disease
      4. Repaired congenital heart disease with residual effects
      5. Cardiac transplant with valvular regurgitation

VIII. Complications
   A. Heart failure: secondary to valvular insufficiency
   B. Perivalvular abscess: suspect if conduction abnormalities develop
   C. Pericarditis: can lead to tamponade
   D. Intracardiac fistula: secondary of extension of infection to myocardium
   E. Septic embolization: prevent by administering IV antibiotics ASAP
      1. Brain: stroke, paralysis, blindness, encephalopathy, mycotic aneurysm
      2. Lungs: pulmonary embolism
      3. Spleen: splenic or renal abscesses and/or infarctions
      4. Musculoskeletal: osteomyelitis, septic arthritis

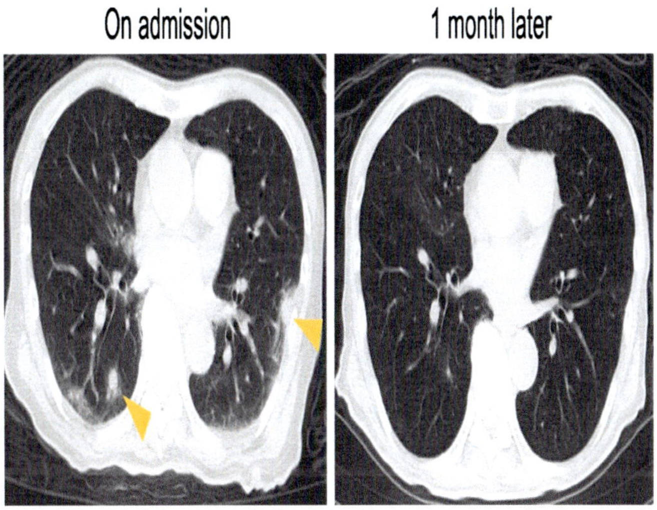

FIGURE 21.2.25 - Septic Pulmonary Emboli (Yellow Arrows) Due to Infective Endocarditis

REVIEW QUESTIONS

1. A 37-year-old man comes to the physician due to fever and palpitations for the past 3 days. He is an intravenous heroin user. Vital signs include temperature of 40° C (104° F) and heart rate of 120 beats/min. The physical examination shows violaceous tender nodes on the finger pads. The echocardiography shows vegetations on the tricuspid valve. Does this patient meet enough criteria for a definitive diagnosis of infective endocarditis?

    - **This patient meets enough criteria for a definitive diagnosis of infective endocarditis.**
    - In order to definitively diagnose endocarditis, the patient should meet at least 2 major criteria, 1 major and 3 minor criteria, or 5 minor criteria.
    - This patient is an intravenous heroin user which is a predisposing condition and minor criteria for endocarditis.
    - Additionally, he has a fever of more than 38° C which is another minor criteria.
    - The physical examination reveals violaceous tender nodes on the finger pads, finding consistent with Osler nodes. Osler nodes represent immunologic phenomena and are considered minor criteria.
    - The echocardiographic evidence of the vegetation is a major criteria.
    - So this patient meets 1 major and 3 minor criteria that are enough for a definitive diagnosis of infective endocarditis.

2. A 37-year-old woman comes to the emergency department after having an episode of left-sided weakness. She states that this morning she woke up to numbness in her entire left arm and slurred speech. This episode lasted approximately 5 minutes and then spontaneously resolved. She denies prior similar episodes. She has a history of a recent heart attack 3 months ago. Her vitals include temperature of 38.2° C (100.7° F), respiratory rate of 15 breaths/min, heart rate of 99 beats/min, and blood pressure of 129/79 mmHg. On physical examination, her lungs are clear to auscultation bilaterally and a new cardiac murmur is heard at the apex of the heart. She has tender red raised lesions on her toe pads.Her fundoscopy shows white spots on her retina surrounded by hemorrhage. What is the most likely cause of her morning weakness?

    A. Subarachnoid hemorrhage
    B. Epidural hematoma
    C. Septic embolization
    D. Atherosclerosis of middle cerebral artery

- **The correct answer is option C.**
- This patient had a new onset left arm weakness and numbness associated with slurred speech that spontaneously resolved after five minutes.
- She likely suffered a transient ischemic attack, also known as a TIA.
- Her fever, roth spots represented by her fundoscopy findings, new cardiac murmur, history of recent cardiac damage, Osler nodes on her toe pads, and stroke-like symptoms would fulfill the 5 minor findings of Duke's modified diagnostic criteria.
- In some instances, the vegetations developed in infective endocarditis can embolize and lead to ischemic strokes or transient ischemic attacks.
- Answer choice A, subarachnoid hemorrhage, commonly presents in a patient as the "worst headache of their life", or "thunderclap headache" and will not resolve after only five minutes. Additionally, it would not lead to any of the other systemic symptoms the patient has.
- Answer choice B is incorrect because an epidural hematoma often occurs secondary to trauma leading to damage to the middle meningeal artery, which this patient does not have. Additionally, symptoms related to an epidural hematoma would not be expected to resolve within 5 minutes or be associated with her other systemic symptoms.
- Answer choice D is incorrect because atherosclerosis of the middle cerebral artery could lead to a TIA with symptoms like the patient is describing, but would not be expected to have the other systemic symptoms such as new cardiac murmur or fever.

Cardiology | Section 7: Atrial Septal Defect & Ventricular Septal Defect

I. Atrial Septal Defect: Introduction
   A. Defect in the interatrial septum
      1. Ostium primum ASD
      2. Ostium secundum ASD (more common)
   B. Left-to-right shunt
   C. Associated with Down syndrome, fetal alcohol syndrome, and Holt-oram syndrome

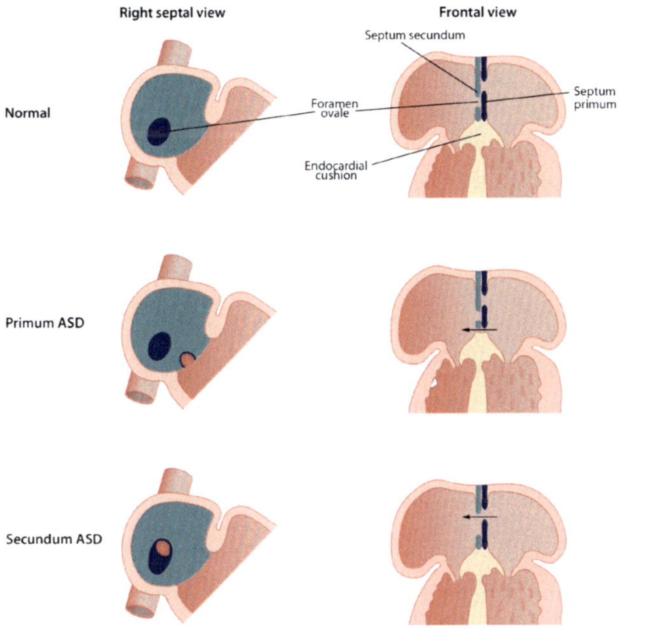

FIGURE 21.2.26 - Primum ASD vs. Secundum ASD

II. Atrial Septal Defect: Clinical Presentation
   A. Asymptomatic if small defect
   B. Poor weight gain, exercise intolerance, bronchopulmonary infections, hepatomegaly
   C. Cyanosis (right-to-left shunt: Eisenmenger syndrome)
   D. Clinical clues
      1. Systolic ejection murmur at left second intercostal space
      2. Wide fixed splitting of S2
      3. Parasternal heave

III. Atrial Septal Defect: Diagnosis
   A. Chest X-ray
      1. Enlargement of right atrium, right ventricle, and pulmonary arch
      2. Increased pulmonary vascular markings
   B. ECG: P pulmonale, right axis deviation, right bundle branch block
   C. Echocardiography: interatrial communication; most accurate test

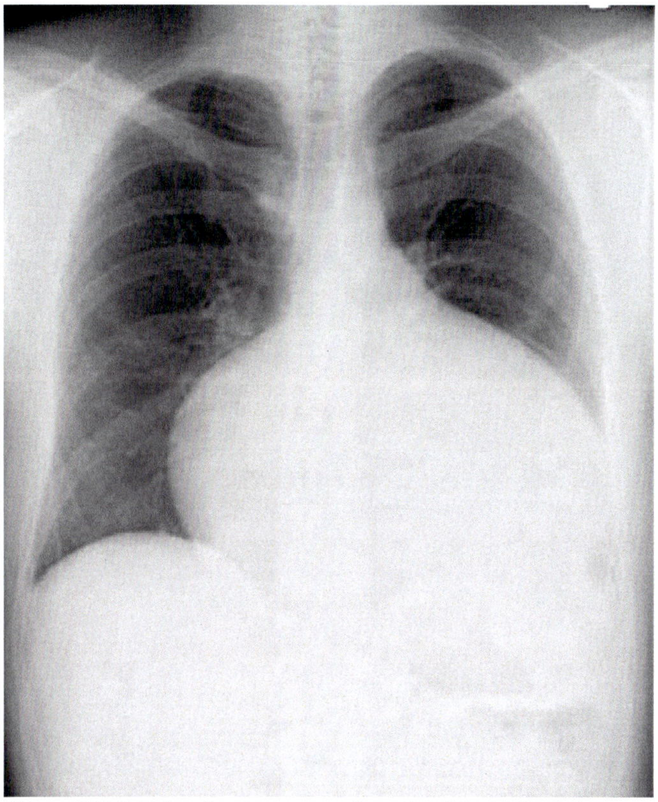

FIGURE 21.2.27 - Chest X-Ray: Enlarged RA and RV with Prominent Pulmonary Vascular Markings

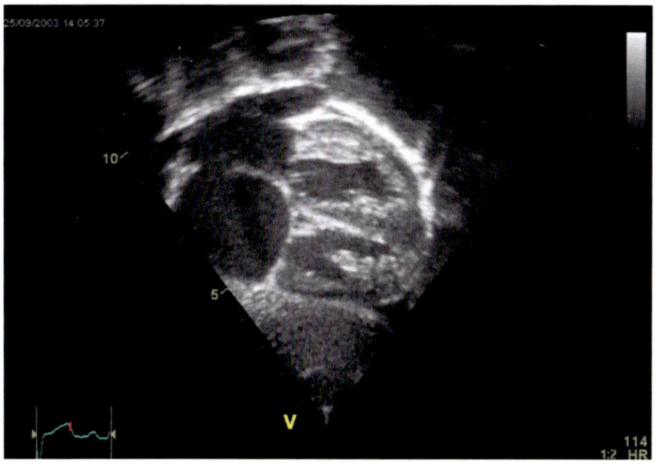

FIGURE 21.2.28 - Echocardiogram: Atrial Septal Defect

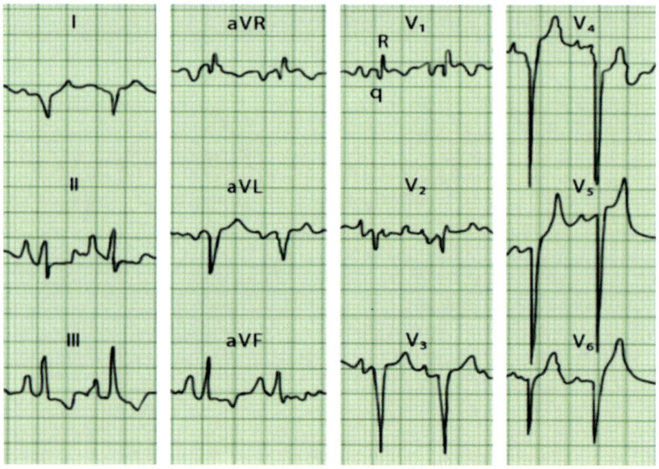

FIGURE 21.2.29 - ECG: P Pulmonale; Right Axis Deviation

IV. Atrial Septal Defect: Treatment
   A. Most cases undergo spontaneous closure
   B. Surgery or percutaneous transcatheter closure
      1. Symptomatic patients
      2. Significant left-to-right shunt

V. Atrial Septal Defect: Complications
   A. Paradoxical embolization: stroke
   B. Atrial arrhythmias
   C. Pulmonary hypertension
   D. Heart failure

VI. Ventricular Septal Defect: Introduction
   A. Most common congenital heart defect
   B. Defect in the interventricular septum
      1. Most commonly in the membranous part of the septum
   C. Associated with Down syndrome, Patau syndrome, and Edward syndrome

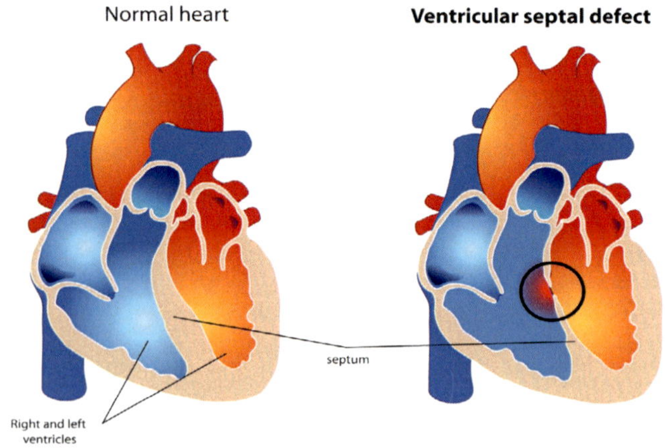

FIGURE 21.2.30 - VSD

VII. Ventricular Septal Defect: Clinical Presentation
   A. Small defect: mostly asymptomatic
   B. Medium to large defect: failure to thrive, fatigue, dyspnea with respiratory distress
   C. Clinical clues
      1. High-pitched holosystolic murmur over lower left sternal border
      2. Mid-diastolic flow murmur at the apex
      3. Loud pulmonic component of S2

VIII. Ventricular Septal Defect: Diagnosis
   A. Chest X-ray: enlarged LA and LV with increased pulmonary vascular markings; enlarged RV in advanced cases
   B. ECG
      1. Left axis deviation: LV hypertrophy due to volume overload
      2. Right axis deviation: RV hypertrophy in Eisenmenger syndrome
   C. Echocardiography: interventricular communication; most accurate test

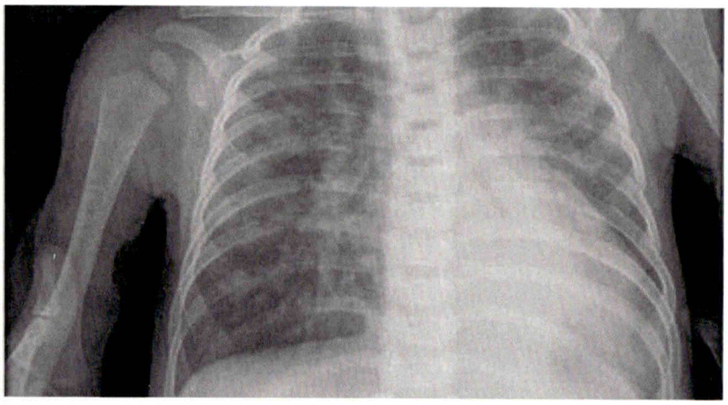

FIGURE 21.2.31 - Chest X-Ray: Enlarged RV with Prominent Pulmonary Vascular Markings

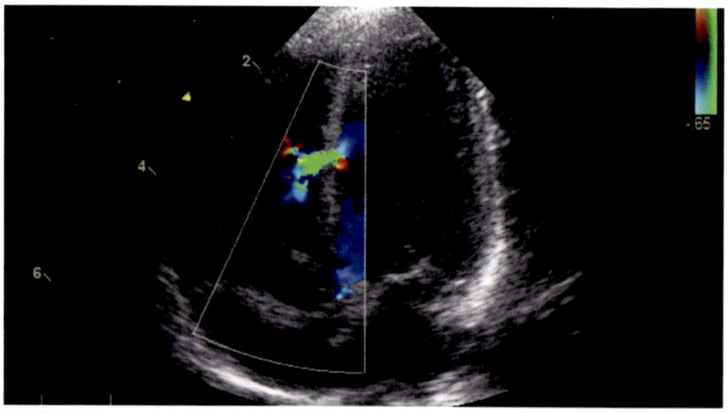

FIGURE 21.2.32 - Echocardiogram: VSD

IX. Ventricular Septal Defect: Treatment
   A. Small defect close spontaneously; consider follow-up echocardiography
   B. Indications for surgical intervention (patch repair)
      1. Large VSD and uncontrolled symptoms
      2. Signs of mild/moderate pulmonary hypertension
      3. Significant left-to-right shunting with LV dilation

X. Ventricular Septal Defect: Complications
   A. Heart failure
   B. Pulmonary hypertension
   C. Arrhythmias
   D. Infective endocarditis

REVIEW QUESTIONS

1. A 45-year-old woman is evaluated in the hospital for right facial droop and right arm weakness for 1 hour. Four days ago, she was admitted with a swollen and erythematous left leg. Initial Doppler ultrasound showed impaired blood flow in the deep femoral vein. She was started on intravenous unfractionated heparin. The physical examination today shows right facial and arm weakness along with sensory loss. Cardiac auscultation is significant for fixed split of S2. Which congenital cardiac anomaly most likely accounts for this patient's current condition?

- **The most likely congenital cardiac anomaly is atrial septal defect.**
- This woman was initially admitted with a swollen and erythematous left leg.
- Initial ultrasound revealed impaired blood flow in the deep femoral vein, suggesting DVT.
- She was started on IV unfractionated heparin.
- The physical exam shows right facial and arm weakness along with sensory loss, which are signs of left middle cerebral artery stroke.
- Cardiac auscultation is significant for a fixed split of S2, which is a sign of an atrial septal defect.
- This patient's stroke was caused by her venous thrombus.
- When the venous thrombus enters systemic circulation and causes end-organ ischemia, this is known as paradoxical embolism.
- The atrial septal defect is the most likely underlying cardiac anomaly that accounts for the paradoxical embolism in this patient.

2. A 6-year-old girl is brought to the physician by her parents for a routine check-up. She has no specific complaints. The cardiac auscultation shows a holosystolic murmur at the left sternal border along with loud P2. ECG shows right axis deviation. Chest X-ray is significant for enhanced pulmonary vascular markings. What is the most likely diagnosis?

- **The diagnosis is ventricular septal defect.**
- This patient has a holosystolic murmur at the left sternal border along with loud P2.
- ECG shows right axis deviation.
- X-ray shows enhanced pulmonary vascular markings.
- These findings suggest the diagnosis of ventricular septal defect.
- Ventricular septal defect allows blood flow from the left ventricle to the right ventricle leading to right ventricular hypertrophy with axis deviation.
- Increased right ventricular preload leads to pulmonary hypertension that accounts for loud P2 and enhanced pulmonary vascular markings.

3. A newborn girl is brought to the office because her parents noticed persistent gasping for air for one day. On physical examination, there is a high pitched holosystolic murmur present when auscultating the lower left sternal border. The patient is sent for a chest X-ray which shows a dilated left atrium and left ventricle as well as increased vascular markings in the lung fields bilaterally. Which of the following conditions is most often associated with this patient's current presentation?

   A. Down syndrome
   B. Turner syndrome
   C. Klinefelter syndrome
   D. Triple X syndrome

- **The correct answer is option A.**
- A newborn presents to the office due to a persistent gasping for air which shows that the infant is dyspneic and possibly in respiratory distress.
- The patient has a high pitched holosystolic murmur heard best over the lower left sternal border, a dilated left atrium and ventricle, and increased vascular lung markings.
- All of the above are signs of a ventricular septal defect, or VSD.
- VSDs are most commonly associated with Trisomy 13, 18, and 21, also known as Patau syndrome, Edward syndrome, and Down syndrome respectively.
- Option B is incorrect because Turner syndrome is associated with bicuspid aortic valve and aortic root dilatation, not VSD.
- Option C is incorrect because Klinefelter syndrome is associated with symptoms of decreased testosterone, not VSD.
- Option D is incorrect because triple X syndrome is associated with few or no symptoms, not VSD.

I. Complete AV Septal Defect: Introduction
   A. Also known as endocardial cushion defect
   B. Defects in atrioventricular valves, atrial septum, and ventricular septum due to failure of endocardial cushion development
   C. Mostly associated with Down syndrome

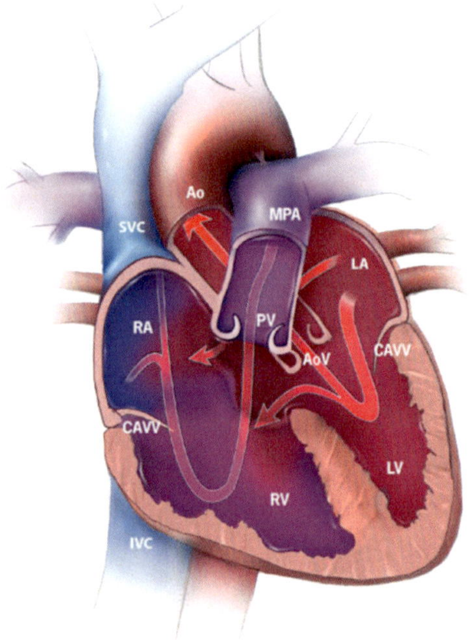

FIGURE 21.2.33 - AV Septal Defect

1. Complete AV Septal Defect: Clinical Presentation
   a. Nonspecific findings: failure to thrive, exercise intolerance, dyspnea, and diaphoresis
   b. Clinical clues
      i. Loud pulmonic S2 (pulmonary HTN)
      ii. Systolic ejection murmur (↑ flow across pulmonary valve)
      iii. Holosystolic murmur of VSD

II. Complete AV Septal Defect: Diagnosis
   A. Chest X-ray: cardiomegaly and increased pulmonary vascular markings
   B. ECG: left axis deviation
   C. Echocardiography: detects size of the defect and volume of the shunt; most accurate test
      1. Prenatal echo is helpful for early diagnosis; screening for Down syndrome should follow

III. Complete AV Septal Defect: Treatment
   A. Supportive therapy
      1. Diuretics and inotropes
   B. Surgical correction
      1. Perform before pulmonary HTN develops in infancy

IV. Complete AV Septal Defect: Complications
   A. In absence of surgery
      1. Pulmonary HTN
      2. Heart failure
   B. In presence of surgery
      1. Arrhythmias
      2. Congenital heart block

V. Coarctation of the Aorta: Introduction
   A. Luminal narrowing of aortic arch near the aortic isthmus
   B. Can be preductal or postductal
   C. Commonly associated with Turner syndrome

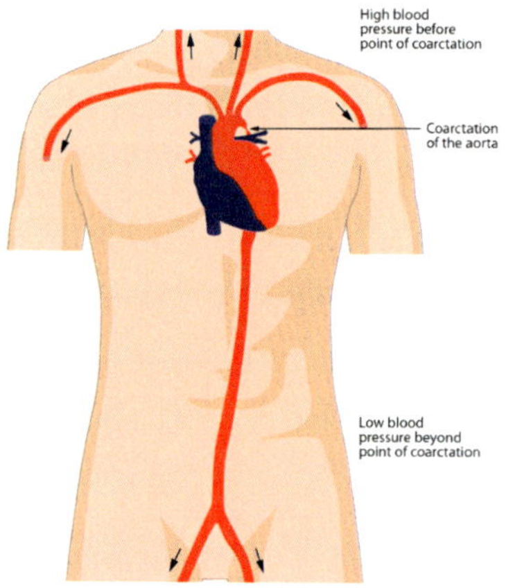

FIGURE 21.2.34 - Coarctation of the Aorta

VI. Coarctation of the Aorta: Clinical Presentation
   A. Irritability, poor feeding, exercise intolerance
   B. Clinical clues
      1. Upper extremity hypertension (e.g. headache, epistaxis)
      2. Brachial-femoral delay (decreased femoral pulse), ↓ blood pressure of lower extremities, lower extremity claudication
      3. Systolic ejection murmur at the left interscapular area

VII. Coarctation of the Aorta: Diagnosis
   A. Chest X-ray: cardiomegaly, rib notching, figure of 3 sign
   B. ECG: left axis deviation
   C. Echocardiography: stenosis of the aortic arch and its extent; most accurate test

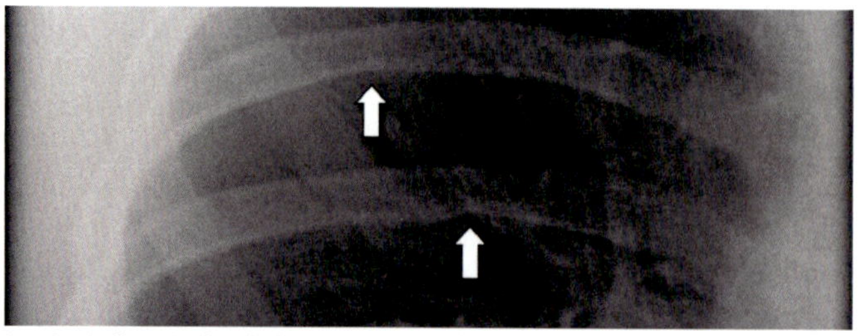

FIGURE 21.2.35 - Chest X-Ray: Rib Notching

VIII. Coarctation of the Aorta: Treatment
   A. Prostaglandin E1: to maintain ductus arteriosus patency until surgery
   B. Choice of treatment
      1. Surgical repair
      2. Balloon angioplasty with or without stent placement

IX. Coarctation of the Aorta: Complications
   A. Shock
   B. Secondary hypertension
   C. Aortic dissection and rupture
   D. Cerebral hemorrhage (rupture of berry aneurysms)

REVIEW QUESTIONS

1. A 2-year-old boy with Down syndrome is brought to the physician by his mom due to easy fatigability since birth. He cannot keep up with his elder siblings while playing and running with them. The cardiac auscultation shows a fixed split of S2 and a holosystolic murmur at the left sternal border with loud P2. Which embryological structure is most likely affected in this patient's condition?

   - **The embryological structure most likely affected is endocardial cushion defect.**
   - This boy with presents with easy fatigability.
   - The cardiac auscultation reveals a fixed split of S2 which suggests an atrial septal defect and a holosystolic murmur at the left sternal border with loud P2 which indicates ventricular septal defect. Therefore, this patient most likely has a complete atrioventricular septal defect.
   - Since the interatrial septum and the membranous part of interventricular septum are derived from endocardial cushion, complete AV septal defect signifies an endocardial cushion defect.

2. A 12-year-old girl is brought to the physician by her parents due to intermittent leg pain since the age of 6 years. She cannot keep up with her peers while running due to leg cramps. The physical examination shows brachiofemoral delay along with systolic ejection murmur at the left interscapular area. Which findings are likely expected on this patient's chest X-ray?

   - **Chest X-ray findings are expected to show rib notching, sign of "3", and cardiomegaly.**
   - This patient presents with intermittent leg pain. She cannot keep up due to leg cramps.
   - The physical exam shows brachiofemoral delay along with systolic ejection murmur at the left interscapular area.
   - These findings point to aortic coarctation.
   - Aortic coarctation is a narrowing near the aortic isthmus that restricts the blood flow to the lower extremities. Reduced blood flow to the legs accounts for the leg cramps and the brachiofemoral delay.
   - The chest X-ray findings include rib notching due to collateral circulation, sign of "3" due to aortic narrowing, and cardiomegaly.

3. A 3-hour-old girl is assessed in the neonatal intensive care unit due to lethargy and poor feeding. She was born at 38 weeks of gestation via spontaneous vaginal delivery. Her vital signs are within normal limits. The physical examination shows pink skin over the upper trunk, head, and upper extremities. The skin is pale on the lower trunk and lower extremities. The brachial pulses are strong while femoral pulses are weak. Cardiac auscultation shows a systolic ejection murmur at the left interscapular area. Which of the following is the best immediate next step in the management of this patient?

   A. Intravenous normal saline
   B. Intravenous PGE_1
   C. Balloon angioplasty with stent placement
   D. Balloon angioplasty without stent placement

   - **The correct answer is option B.**
   - This girl admitted for lethargy and poor feeding.
   - The physical examination shows pink skin over the upper trunk, head, and upper extremities. The lower extremities are pale. This pattern of skin discoloration is known as differential cyanosis which indicates insufficient blood flow.
   - The brachial pulses are strong, while femoral pulses are weak.
   - Cardiac auscultation shows a systolic ejection murmur at the left interscapular area.
   - These are classic findings of coarctation of the aorta.
   - The best immediate next step in the management of a neonate with aortic coarctation is intravenous PGE_1 administration. This is because prostaglandins E_1 and E_2 keep the ductus arteriosus open.
   - Patent ductus arteriosus can provide blood flow to the lower extremities before definitive surgery is performed
   - Option A is incorrect because giving intravenous normal saline to a stable patient with aortic coarctation may further increase the cardiac afterload and the proximal aortic diameter leading to heart failure, aortic dissection, or aortic rupture.
   - Options C and D are incorrect because the neonate with aortic coarctation needs to receive intravenous PGE_1 before balloon angioplasty with or without stent placement is performed.

Cardiology | Section 9: Patent Ductus Arteriosus & Pulmonic Valve Stenosis

I. Patent Ductus Arteriosus: Introduction
   A. Failure of spontaneous closure of ductus arteriosus postnatally
      1. Normally, functional closure occurs within 18-24 hours
   B. Associated with prematurity and congenital rubella syndrome

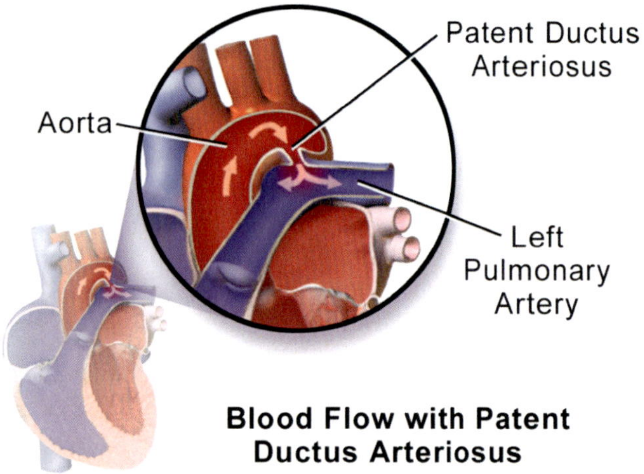

FIGURE 21.2.36 - Patent Ductus Arteriosus

II. Patent Ductus Arteriosus: Clinical Presentation
   A. Irritability, failure to grow, exercise intolerance
   B. Differential cyanosis when Eisenmenger syndrome develops
   C. Clinical clues
      1. Bounding pulses
      2. Wide pulse pressure
      3. Loud machine-like continuous murmur; best heard in the left infraclavicular area

III. Patent Ductus Arteriosus: Diagnosis
   A. Chest X-ray: cardiomegaly, prominent pulmonary artery
   B. ECG: left axis deviation (left ventricular hypertrophy)
   C. Echocardiography: evaluate pulmonary artery pressure and volume of shunted blood; most accurate test

IV. Patent Ductus Arteriosus: Treatment
   A. Conservative management: small PDA and absence of left heart volume overload
      1. Indomethacin for the closure of PDA unless patency is required for survival (e.g. TOF)
   B. Surgical closure or percutaneous catheter occlusion
      1. Failure of pharmacological therapy
      2. Child on maximal ventilator support

V. Patent Ductus Arteriosus: Complications
   A. Infective endocarditis
   B. Pulmonary hypertension
   C. Heart failure

VI. Pulmonary Valve Stenosis: Introduction
   A. Stenosis of the pulmonary valve leading to right ventricular outflow obstruction
   B. Isolated congenital defect

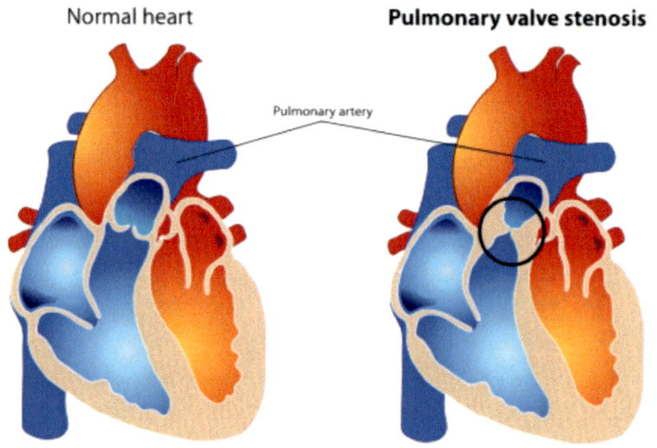

FIGURE 21.2.37 - Pulmonary Valve Stenosis Leading to Right Ventricular Outflow Obstruction

VII. Pulmonary Valve Stenosis: Clinical Presentation
   A. Can be asymptomatic
   B. Angina and dyspnea when symptomatic
   C. Clinical clues
      1. Crescendo-decrescendo systolic murmur at second left ICS (increases on inspiration)
      2. S2 wide splitting

VIII. Pulmonary Valve Stenosis: Diagnosis
   A. Chest X-ray: poststenotic dilation of pulmonary artery
   B. ECG: right axis deviation
   C. Echocardiography: evaluate the grade of stenosis; most accurate test

IX. Pulmonary Valve Stenosis: Treatment
      1. No treatment required for mild cases
      2. Percutaneous balloon pulmonary valvuloplasty
      3. Surgery in some critical cases and child with multiple heart defects

X. Pulmonary Valve Stenosis: Complications
   A. Infective endocarditis
   B. Heart failure

REVIEW QUESTIONS

1. A 7-year-old boy is brought to the physician by his parents due to bilateral leg swelling for the past 2 weeks. He was born with a congenital cardiac defect. The physical examination shows 1+ pitting edema in the lower extremities. The cardiac auscultation shows crescendo-decrescendo systolic murmur at the left second intercostal space along with wide splitting of S2. What is the most likely diagnosis?

- **The most likely diagnosis is congenital pulmonary valve stenosis.**
- This young boy presents with 1+ pitting edema in the lower extremities.
- He was born with a congenital cardiac defect which most likely accounts for his edema.
- The cardiac auscultation shows crescendo-decrescendo systolic murmur at the left second intercostal space along with wide splitting of S2.
- Left second intercostal space is the pulmonary area.
- Therefore, this patient likely has a defect of the pulmonary valve.
- Given the systolic crescendo-decrescendo murmur and wide splitting of S2, the patient most likely has congenital pulmonary valve stenosis

2. A 10-year-old girl is brought to the physician due to easy fatigability since she has started playing sports. She joined the school runners' team but she cannot keep up with her peers due to severe leg cramps while running. Her vital signs include temperature of 36° C (96.8° F), blood pressure of 110/40 mmHg, heart rate of 75 beats/min, and respiratory rate of 16 breaths/min. The physical examination shows bounding radial pulse and a harsh murmur throughout the cardiac cycle best heard at the left infraclavicular area. Which of the following is the most likely diagnosis in this patient?

   A. Coarctation of aorta
   B. Patent ductus arteriosus
   C. Ventricular septal defect
   D. Atrial septal defect

- **The correct answer is B.**
- This young girl presents with easy fatigability.
- She joined the school runners' team but she cannot keep up with her peers due to severe leg cramps while running.
- Her vital signs are significant for a wide pulse pressure of 70 mmHg.
- The pulse pressure is the difference between systolic and diastolic blood pressures. This patient's systolic blood pressure is 110 mmHg while diastolic blood pressure is 40 mmHg. So, the pulse pressure would be 70 mmHg.
- The physical examination shows bounding radial pulses and the harsh murmur throughout the cardiac cycle, best heard at the left infraclavicular area.
- Wide pulse pressure, bounding pulse, and a continuous murmur best heard at the left infraclavicular area are consistent with patent ductus arteriosus.
- Option A is incorrect because coarctation of aorta is associated with the systolic ejection murmur at the left interscapular, rather than infraclavicular, area.
- Option C is incorrect because ventricular septal defect is usually not associated with leg claudication
- Additionally, ventricular septal defect causes a holosystolic murmur at the left sternal border.
- Option D is incorrect because atrial septal defect is typically not associated with leg claudication. Also, it causes fixed splitting of S2 which is absent in this patient.

Cardiology | Section 10: Tetralogy of Fallot & Transposition of the Great Vessels

I. Tetralogy of Fallot: Introduction
   A. Most common cyanotic congenital heart defect
   B. Combination of
      1. Overriding of aorta
      2. Pulmonary stenosis (most important prognostic factor)
      3. Right ventricular hypertrophy
      4. Ventricular septal defect
   C. Mostly sporadic; associated with Down and DiGeorge syndromes

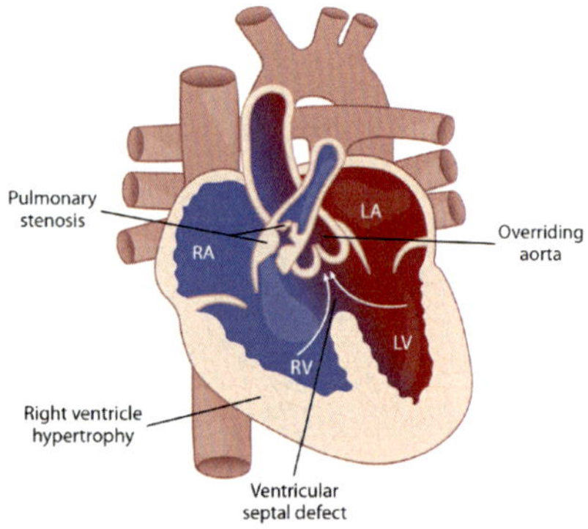

FIGURE 21.2.38 - Tetralogy of Fallot

II. Tetralogy of Fallot: Clinical Presentation
   A. Cyanosis and hypercyanotic tet spells
   B. Irritability, poor feeding, lethargy
   C. Clinical clues
      1. Harsh crescendo-decrescendo systolic murmur at left lower sternal border
      2. Single S2

III. Tetralogy of Fallot: Diagnosis
   A. Hyperoxia test: helps to rule out pulmonary causes of cyanosis
   B. Chest X-ray: boot-shaped heart, decreased pulmonary vascular marking
   C. ECG: right axis deviation due to right ventricular hypertrophy
   D. Echocardiography: confirmatory test
      1. Detects pressure gradient of right ventricular outflow tract

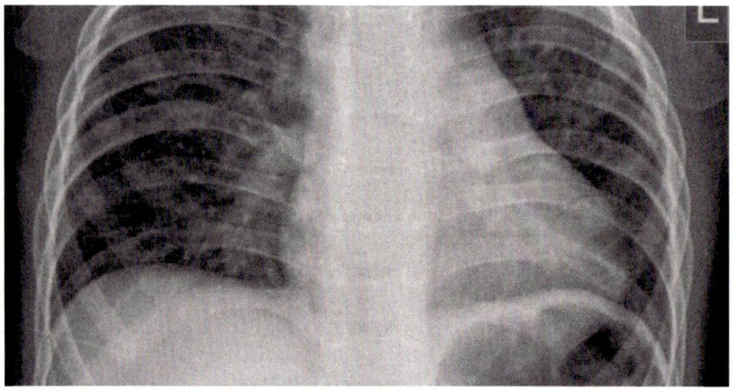

FIGURE 21.2.39 - Chest X-Ray: Boot-Shaped Heart

IV. Tetralogy of Fallot: Treatment
   A. Knee-chest position or squatting: ↑ systemic vascular resistance
   B. Supportive measures: morphine, oxygen, IV fluids, beta blockers
   C. Surgical intervention: by age of 1 year
      1. VSD repair, resection of infundibular muscle bundles to relief RVOT obstruction
      2. If early surgery is not possible: Blalock-Taussig shunt (connection between subclavian artery and pulmonary artery)

V. Tetralogy of Fallot: Complications
   A. Heart failure
   B. Infective endocarditis
   C. Arrhythmias (post surgical repair)

VI. Transposition of the Great Vessels: Introduction
   A. Arterial switch: deoxygenated blood from right ventricle enters the aorta; oxygenated blood from left ventricle enters the pulmonary artery
      1. The aortopulmonary septum fails to spiral
   B. A shunt is needed for survival (e.g. ASD, VSD, PDA)
   C. Mostly seen in infants of diabetic mothers; more common in males

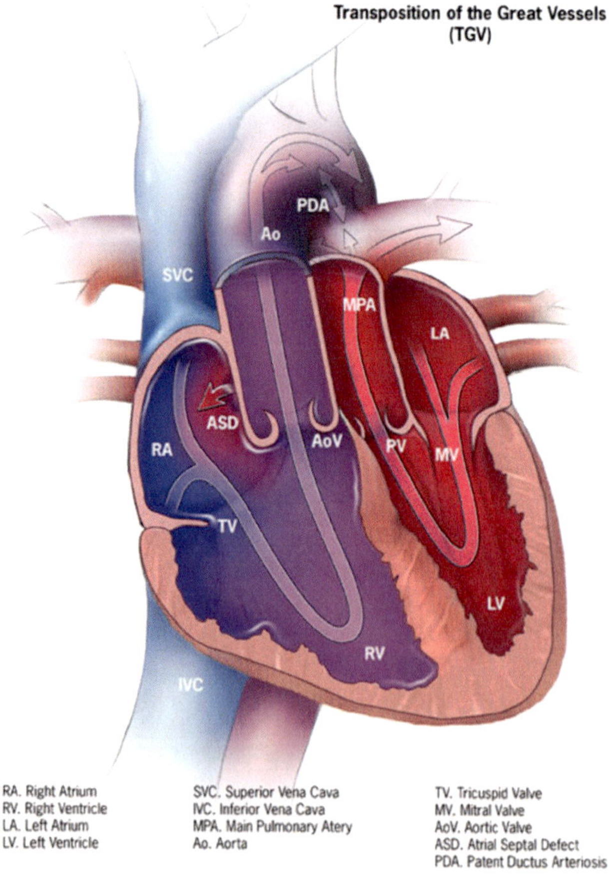

FIGURE 21.2.40 - Transposition of the Great Vessels

VII. Transposition of the Great Vessels: Clinical Presentation
   A. Cyanosis
   B. Clinical clues
      1. Loud, single S2
      2. No murmur, unless there is other defect such as VSD

VIII. Transposition of the Great Vessels: Diagnosis
   A. CXR: "egg on a string" appearance of heart, increased pulmonary vascular markings
   B. ECG: mostly normal findings
   C. Echocardiography: confirmatory test
      1. Detection of abnormal location of aorta and pulmonary artery

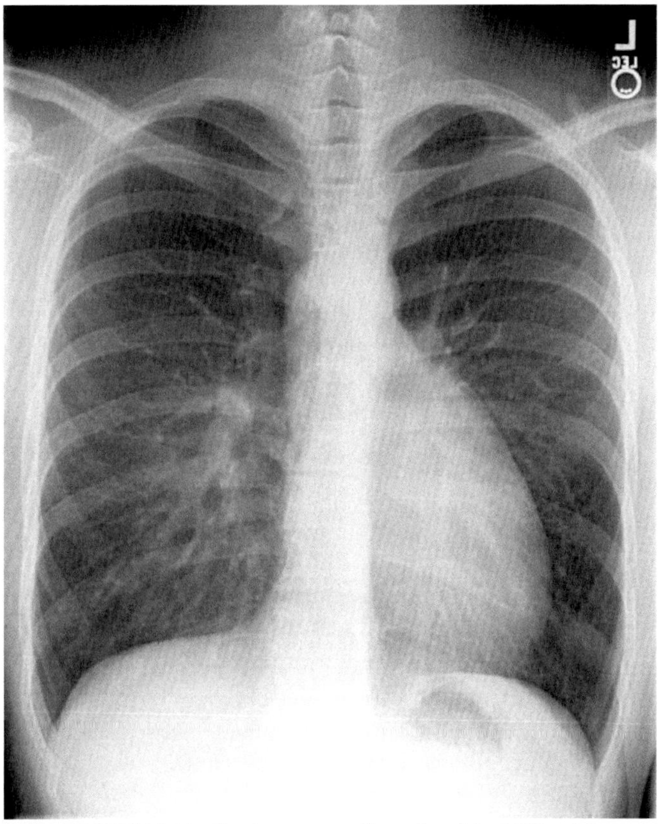

FIGURE 21.2.41 - Chest X-Ray: "Egg on a String" Appearance of Heart

IX. Transposition of the Great Vessels: Treatment
   A. PGE1 infusion to maintain patency of PDA
   B. Avoid NSAIDs
   C. Surgical intervention within first two weeks

REVIEW QUESTIONS

1. Surgical procedure is determined by the presence of other cardiac defects such as VSD and left ventricular outflow tract obstructionA 1-year-old boy is brought to the physician by his parents due to poor feeding and lethargy since birth. He was born at home at 39 weeks of gestation. Mother reports that her baby becomes blue whenever he cries, and she has to push his legs close to his chest to relieve bluish discoloration. An echocardiography shows ventricular septal defect, overriding aorta, pulmonary infundibular stenosis, and right ventricular hypertrophy. What is the most likely diagnosis?

   - **The most likely diagnosis is tetralogy of Fallot.**
   - This infant is brought to the physician due to poor feeding and lethargy.
   - Mother reports that her baby becomes blue whenever he cries, a phenomenon known as "tet spell" and caused by right ventricular outflow obstruction in patients with tetralogy of Fallot.
   - The mother has to push the infant's legs close to his chest to relieve bluish discoloration. This is because squatting increases systemic vascular resistance, decreases right-to-left shunt, and improves oxygenation by encouraging blood in the right ventricle to flow through pulmonary arteries.
   - An echocardiography shows ventricular septal defect, overriding aorta, pulmonary infundibular stenosis, and the right ventricular hypertrophy, which are the classic components of tetralogy of Fallot.

REVIEW QUESTIONS

2. A 2-hour-old newborn boy is evaluated in the newborn intensive care unit due to diffuse cyanosis and lethargy. He was born at term without any complications. Echocardiography shows the aorta arising from the right ventricle and the pulmonary trunk arising from the left ventricle, and patent ductus arteriosus. Which medication should be immediately administered to enhance this patient's survival until surgery?

- **The medication that should be immediately administered to enhance this patient's survival until surgery is a PGE_1 analog like misoprostol or alprostadil.**
- This 2-hour-old infant is evaluated in the newborn intensive care unit due to diffuse cyanosis and lethargy.
- Echocardiography shows the aorta arising from the right ventricle and the pulmonary trunk arising from the left ventricle, and patent ductus arteriosus.
- These findings are classic for transposition of great vessels.
- This condition involves complete separation of systemic and pulmonary circuits so it is incompatible with life unless a shunt like PDA is present.
- Therefore, the patent ductus arteriosus needs to be maintained until surgery is performed.
- Ductus arteriosus is kept open by prostaglandins E_1 and E_2, so, a PGE_1 analog like misoprostol or alprostadil needs to be administered.

3. A 2-hour-old newborn girl is evaluated in the nursery for diffuse cyanosis. She was born at 38 weeks of gestation via spontaneous vaginal delivery. The pregnancy was uncomplicated. The patient's vital signs include temperature of 37° C (98.6° F), blood pressure of 65/50 mmHg, heart rate of 145 beats/min, and respiratory rate of 50 breaths/min. The physical exam shows exacerbation of cyanosis during strong cry. Cardiac auscultation shows holosystolic murmur at the left lower sternal border as well as crescendo-decrescendo systolic murmur at the right upper sternal border. The echocardiography shows right ventricular hypertrophy as well as overriding aorta. Which of the following is the most important prognostic factor in this patient?

   A. Ventricular septal defect
   B. Right ventricular hypertrophy
   C. Pulmonary infundibular stenosis
   D. Overriding aorta

- **The correct answer is option C.**
- This 2-hour-old newborn is evaluated in the nursery for diffuse cyanosis.
- Her vital signs are normal for the newborn.
- The physical exam shows exacerbation of cyanosis during strong cry, a phenomenon known as a "tet spell."
- Cardiac auscultation shows holosystolic murmur at the left lower sternal border which suggests ventricular septal defect.
- There is also a crescendo-decrescendo systolic murmur at the right upper sternal border which is consistent with pulmonary stenosis.
- The echocardiography shows right ventricular hypertrophy as well as overriding aorta.
- Ventricular septal defect, pulmonary infundibular stenosis, right ventricular hypertrophy, and overriding aorta are consistent with tetralogy of Fallot.
- The most important prognostic factor for tetralogy of Fallot is the degree of pulmonary infundibular stenosis.
- In other words, the more stenotic the right ventricular outflow tract is, the less oxygenation occurs in the lungs which leads to increased risk of death.
- Options A, B, and D are incorrect because although ventricular septal defect, right ventricular hypertrophy, and overriding aorta are all present in tetralogy of Fallot, none of them is the most important prognostic factor for the patient's survival.

Cardiology | Section 11: Total Anomalous Pulmonary Venous Return, Persistent Truncus Arteriosus & Tricuspid Atresia

I. Total Anomalous Pulmonary Venous Return (TAPVR): Introduction
   A. Congenital anomaly of pulmonary veins where oxygenated blood is drained into systemic venous circulation (e.g. coronary sinus, SVC)
   B. Two forms
      1. Obstruction of pulmonary venous return is present
      2. Obstruction of pulmonary venous return is absent
   C. ASD, PFO, or PDA is needed for survival

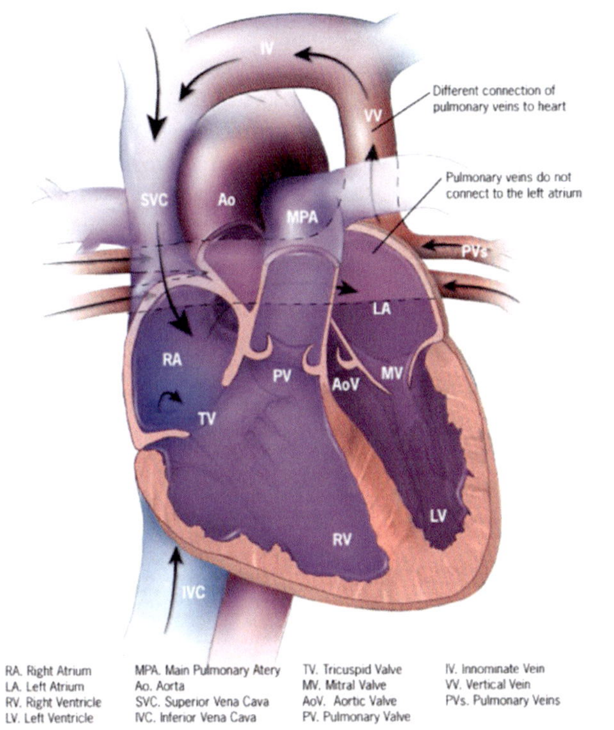

FIGURE 21.2.42 - Total Anomalous Pulmonary Venous Return

II. Total Anomalous Pulmonary Venous Return: Clinical Presentation
   A. TAPVR with obstruction
      1. Presents early in life with cyanosis and respiratory distress
   B. TAPVR without obstruction
      1. Presents in first or second year of life with poor feeding, irritability, and growth failure

III. Total Anomalous Pulmonary Venous Return: Diagnosis
   A. TAPVR with obstruction
      1. CXR reveals pulmonary edema
      2. Echocardiography is confirmatory
   B. TAPVR without obstruction
      1. CXR reveals "snowman" or "figure 8" sign
      2. Echocardiography is confirmatory

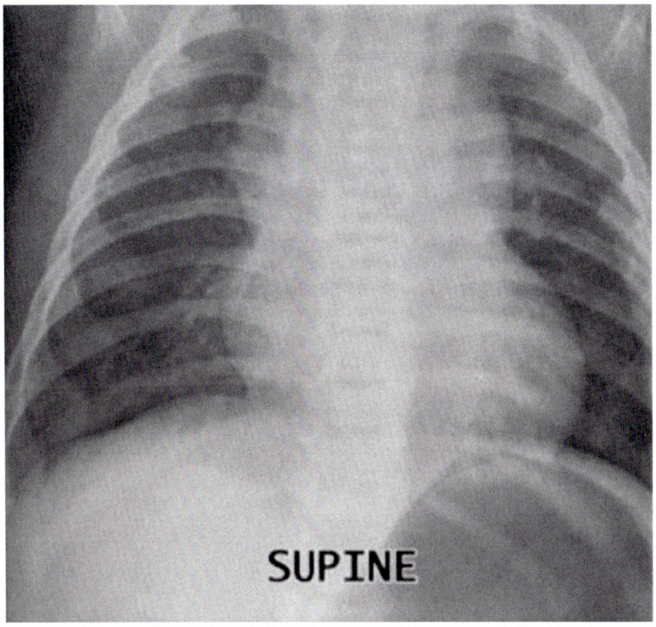

FIGURE 21.2.43 - Chest X-Ray: Snowman Sign

IV. Total Anomalous Pulmonary Venous Return: Treatment
   A. Supportive measures for cardio-respiratory stabilization (e.g. oxygen, ventilation)
   B. Surgical repair: definitive treatment

V. Persistent Truncus Arteriosus: Introduction
   A. Single trunk arises from both right and left ventricles
   B. Poor development of aorticopulmonary septum due to failure of migration of neural crest cells
   C. Most commonly associated with DiGeorge syndrome

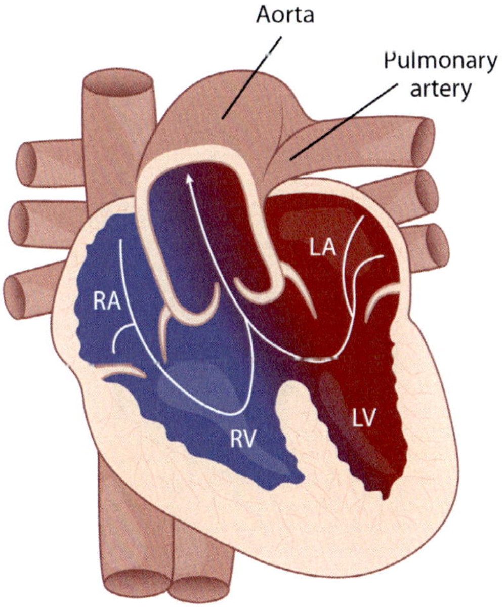

FIGURE 21.2.44 - Persistent Truncus Arteriosus

VI. Persistent Truncus Arteriosus: Clinical Presentation
   A. Cyanosis
   B. Irritability, poor feeding and growth, diaphoresis
   C. Clinical clues
      1. Loud, single S2
      2. Bounding peripheral pulses
      3. Systolic ejection murmur with loud ejection click at the left sternal border

VII. Persistent Truncus Arteriosus: Diagnosis
   A. Can be detected prenatally by fetal echocardiography
   B. CXR: cardiomegaly with increased pulmonary vascular markings
   C. ECG: normal findings; right or left axis deviation
   D. Echocardiography: confirmatory test
      1. Detection of single trunk

VIII. Persistent Truncus Arteriosus: Treatment
   A. Supportive measures for cardio-respiratory stabilization (e.g. ventilation, diuretics)
   B. Surgical correction: performed in the neonatal period in order to prevent pulmonary hypertension

IX. Tricuspid Atresia: Introduction
   A. Absent or poorly developed tricuspid valve
   B. Restricted blood flow from right atrium to right ventricle
   C. Associated with Down syndrome, congenital rubella syndrome, and maternal diabetes mellitus
   D. ASD, VSD or PDA is required for survival

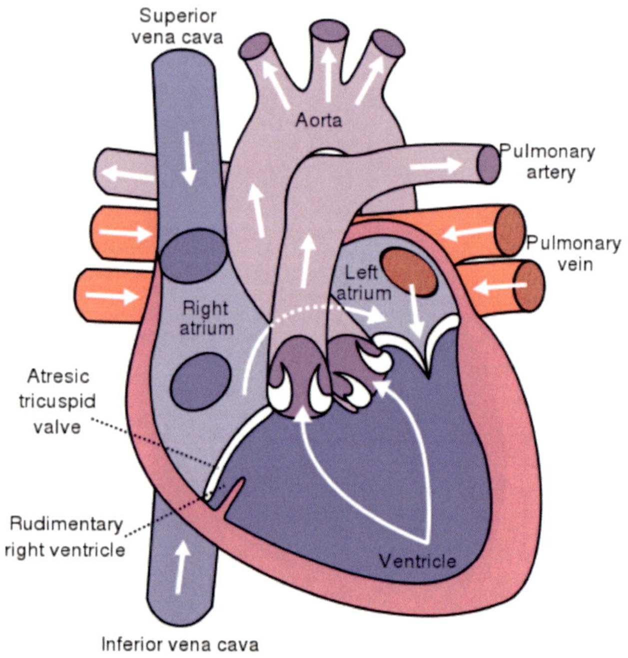

FIGURE 21.2.45 - Tricuspid Atresia

X. Tricuspid Atresia: Clinical Presentation
   A. Cyanosis
   B. Clinical clues
      1. Single S2
      2. Holosystolic murmur at lower left sternal border if VSD is present
      3. Prominent "a" wave in JVP

XI. Tricuspid Atresia: Diagnosis
   A. Can be detected prenatally through fetal echocardiography
   B. CXR: decreased pulmonary vascular markings and normal heart size
   C. ECG: left axis deviation
   D. Echocardiography: gold standard

XII. Tricuspid Atresia: Treatment
   A. PGE1 administration (e.g. alprostadil): to ensure patency of ductus arteriosus
   B. Supportive measures for cardio-respiratory stabilization (e.g. oxygen, ventilation, inotropes)
   C. Surgical correction: palliative procedures of three stages

REVIEW QUESTIONS

1. A 4-hour-old infant is evaluated in the nursery for cyanosis and poor feeding. She was born at 40 weeks of gestation via spontaneous vaginal delivery without any complications. Cardiac auscultation shows a fixed splitting of S2. The echocardiography reveals pulmonary veins entering the coronary sinus. What is the most likely diagnosis?

- **The most likely diagnosis is total anomalous pulmonary venous return.**
- This 4-hour-old infant is evaluated for cyanosis and poor feeding.
- Cardiac auscultation shows a fixed splitting of S2, which suggests the presence of atrial septal defect.
- The echocardiography reveals pulmonary veins entering the coronary sinus, which is classic for total anomalous pulmonary venous return.
- This is when pulmonary veins drain into the right heart, either through the superior vena cava or coronary sinus.
- The patient should have an atrial septal defect to allow for right-to-left shunting and maintenance of cardiac output.

2. A 3-hour-old infant is evaluated in the nursery due to diffuse cyanosis. He was born at 36 weeks of gestation via spontaneous vaginal delivery. The delivery was uneventful. On physical examination, a holosystolic murmur is heard over the left lower sternal border. The echocardiography shows one vessel arising from both left and right ventricles, along with a ventricular septal defect. What is the most likely pathophysiology of this patient's underlying condition?

- **The most likely pathophysiology of this patient's underlying condition is failure of aorticopulmonary septum formation → persistent truncus arteriosus.**
- This 3-hour-old infant is evaluated due to diffuse cyanosis.
- The echocardiography reveals one vessel arising from both left and right ventricles, along with ventricular septal defect, which are classic findings of persistent truncus arteriosus.
- Normally, the formation of an aorticopulmonary septum divides the truncus arteriosus into ascending aorta and the pulmonary trunk.
- Therefore, failure of aorticopulmonary septum formation leads to persistent truncus arteriosus.

3. A 2-hour-old boy is assessed in the neonatal intensive care unit for diffuse cyanosis. He was born at 39 weeks of gestation via spontaneous vaginal delivery. The delivery was uneventful. Mother did not have regular prenatal care. Apgar scores were 5 and 7 at 1 and 5 minutes, respectively. The physical examination shows diffuse cyanosis and lethargy. Cardiac auscultation shows a single S2 and holosystolic murmur at the left lower sternal border. Chest X-ray is remarkable for decreased pulmonary vascular markings while ECG shows left axis deviation. Echocardiography reveals absent blood flow from the right atrium to the right ventricle along with atrial and ventricular septal defects. Which of the following is the most likely diagnosis?

   A. Total anomalous pulmonary venous return
   B. Persistent truncus arteriosus
   C. Tricuspid atresia
   D. Tricuspid regurgitation

- **The correct answer is option C.**
- This 2-hour-old boy is evaluated for diffuse cyanosis.
- Apgar scores were 5 and 7 at 1 and 5 minutes, respectively.
- Cardiac auscultation shows a single S2 and holosystolic murmur at the left lower sternal border.
- Chest X-ray is remarkable for decreased pulmonary vascular markings while ECG shows the left axis deviation.
- Echocardiography reveals absent blood flow from the right atrium to the right ventricle along with atrial and ventricular septal defects.
- Absent blood flow from the right atrium to the right ventricle along with all the other findings are classic for tricuspid atresia.
- Option A is incorrect because although total anomalous pulmonary venous return can cause early postnatal cyanosis, it is characterized by pulmonary veins entering the right heart.
- Option B is incorrect because although persistent truncus arteriosus may account for diffuse cyanosis, it is not characterized by absent blood flow from the right atrium to the right ventricle.
- Option D is incorrect because although tricuspid regurgitation can cause the holosystolic murmur at the left lower sternal border, it does not account for cyanosis or the other findings mentioned in this question.

Cardiology | Section 12: Aortic Dissection

I. Definition
  A. Tear in the tunica intima of the aorta that extends down the vessel
  B. Does not involve the outer layers, media, or adventitia

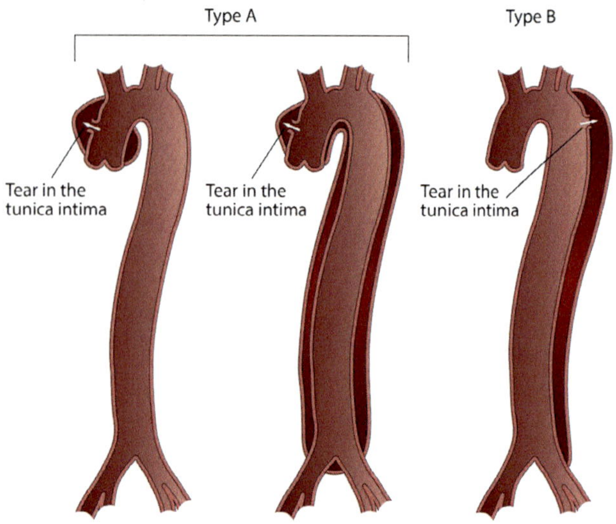

FIGURE 21.2.46 - Classification Systems for Aortic Dissections

II. Pathophysiology
  A. Aortic wall inflammation → apoptosis of smooth muscle cells → tunica media weakening and elastin disruption → tearing of the intima → creation of a flap → disruption of blood flow to various organs

III. Risk Factors
  A. Pre-existing conditions with degeneration of the tunica media
    1. Connective tissue disorders (e.g. Marfan syndrome)
    2. Atherosclerosis
    3. Tertiary syphilis
  B. Hypertension
  C. Deceleration injuries

IV. Clinical Features
  A. Ripping or tearing chest pain radiating to the back or shoulder
  B. Syncope
  C. Hypotension, tachycardia
  D. Complications of disrupted blood flow
    1. Acute kidney injury
    2. Cardiac tamponade, pleural effusion, aortic regurgitation
    3. Pulse deficits > 20 mmHg between left and right arms

V. Diagnosis
  A. Widening of the mediastinum on chest X-ray
    1. Present in 60-90% of patients
  B. Transesophageal echocardiogram
  C. CT with IV contrast
  D. MRI with gadolinium

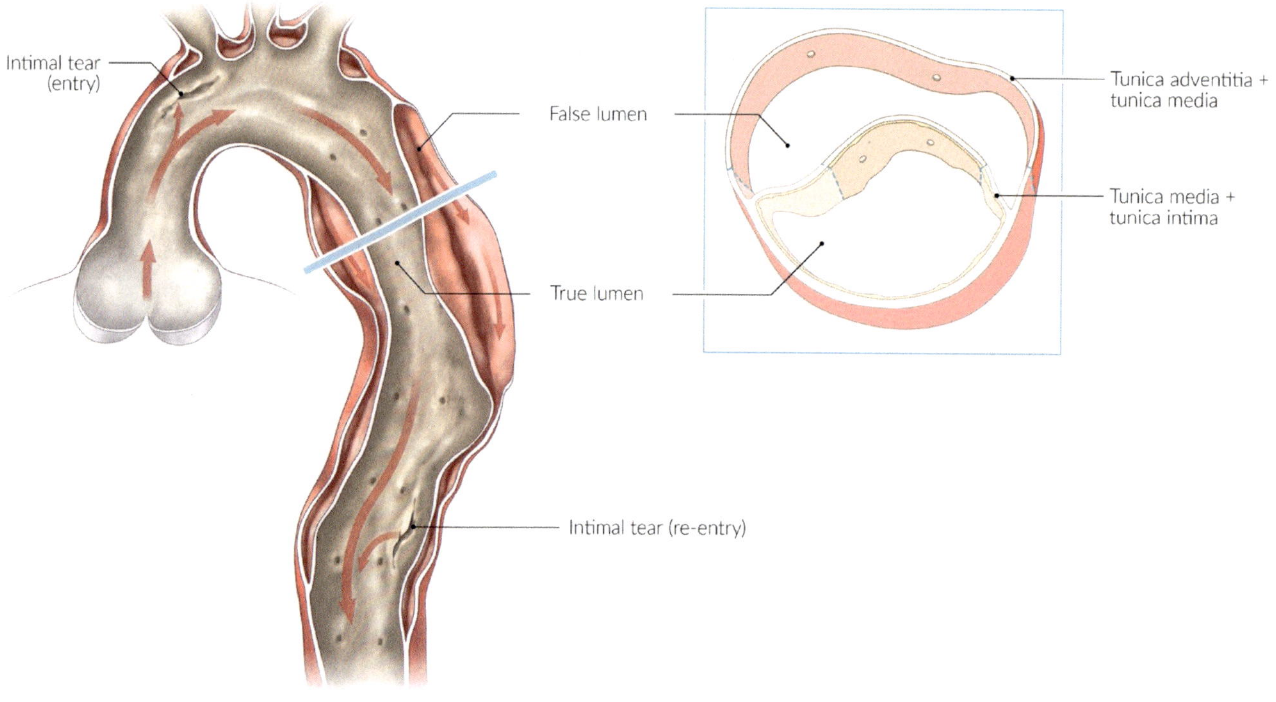

FIGURE 21.2.47 - Tearing of the Intima

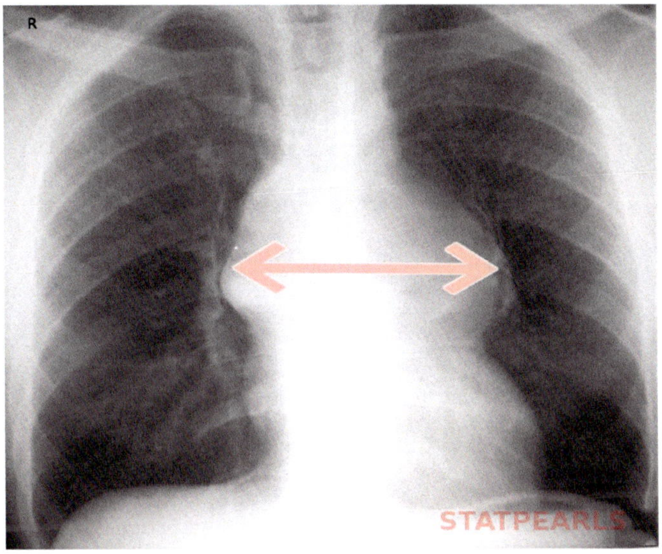

FIGURE 21.2.48 - Chest X-Ray Showing a Widening of the Mediastinum

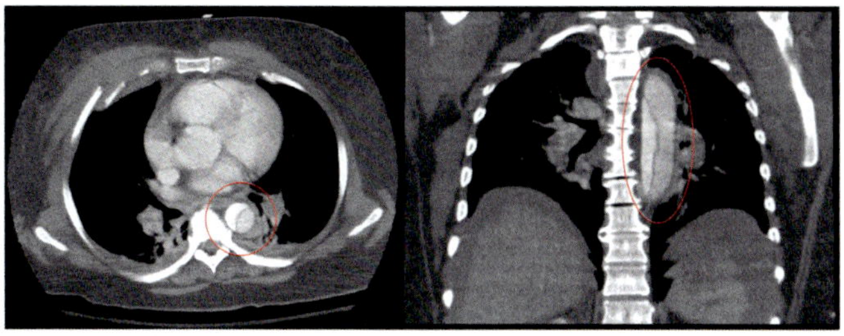

FIGURE 21.2.50 - CT scan Showing Thoracic Aortic Dissection

VI. Management
   A. Surgical repair
      1. Type A dissection
      2. Type B dissection if medical management fails
      3. Open or endovascular
   B. Medical management
      1. Type B dissection
      2. Blood pressure lowering agents such as esmolol or labetalol

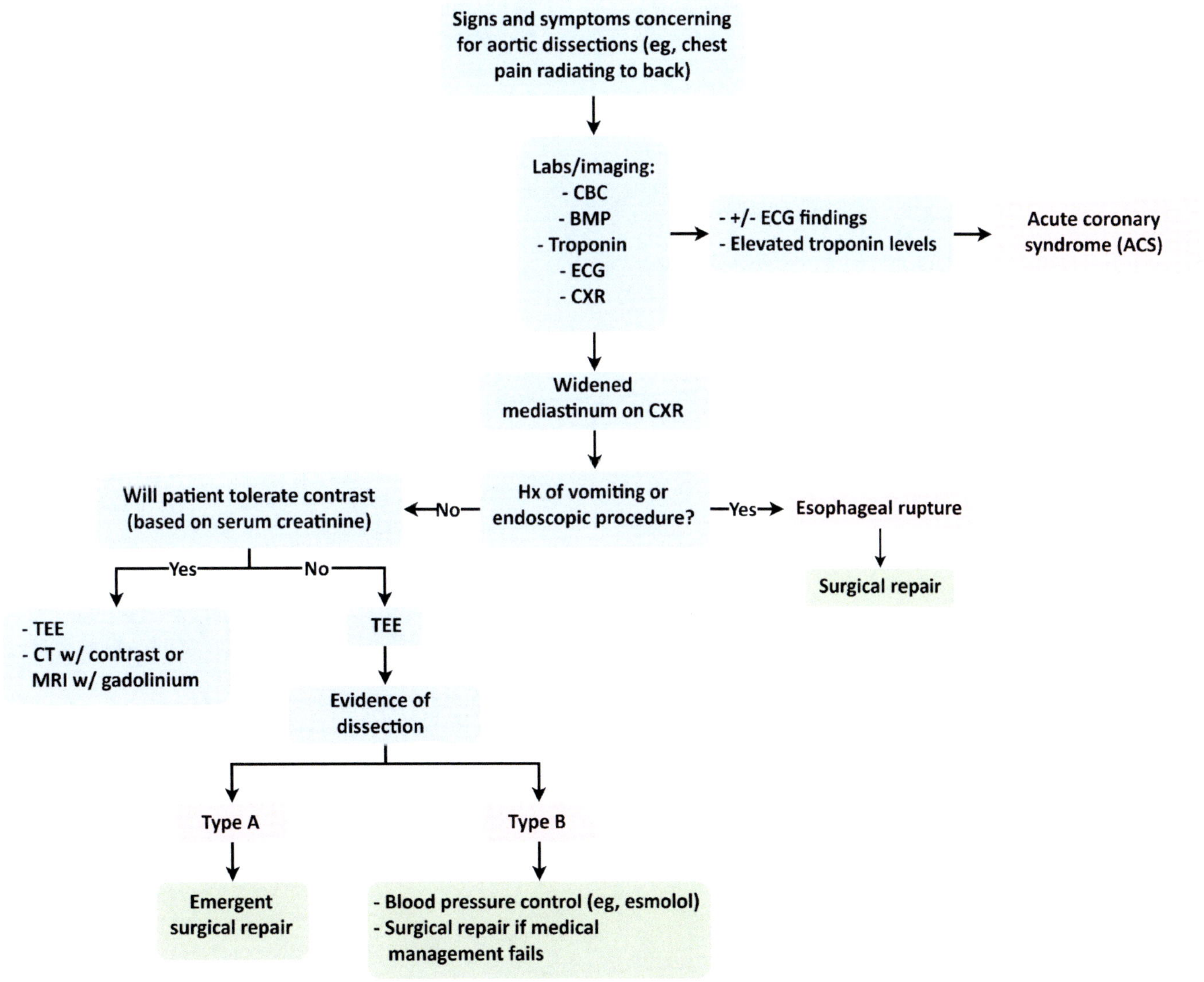

FIGURE 21.2.49 - Algorithm Showing Evaluation and Management of Aortic Dissections

REVIEW QUESTIONS

1. A CT scan demonstrates an aortic dissection consistent with this diagram. Using the Stanford classification system, what kind of dissection is shown?

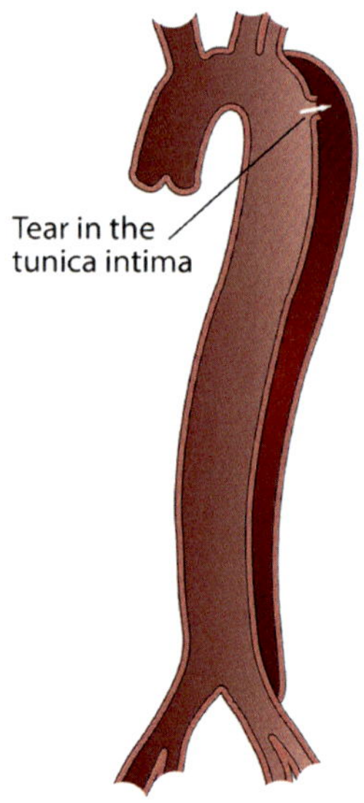

- **This diagram shows a Type B dissection according to the Stanford classification system.**
- The torn intima involves only the descending aorta.

2. How can an aortic dissection lead to acute kidney injury?

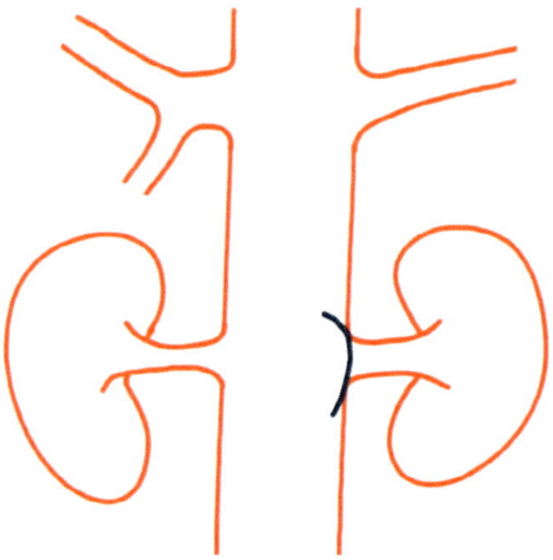

- **An aortic dissection can lead to an acute kidney injury by disrupting the blood flow to that kidney, leading to ischemia.**
- In the image above is the aorta and its branches. This shows the kidneys with their blood supply from the renal arteries. There is a dissection as drawn by the dark blue line.

3. Why would a patient with an aortic dissection have ST-segment changes and an elevated serum troponin?

- **In a patient with an aortic dissection, ST-segment changes and elevations in serum troponin are suggestive of cardiac ischemia, or myocardial infarction.**
- While myocardial infarctions are frequently caused by clots in the coronary vessels, they can also be caused by aortic dissection if the dissection extends through one of the coronary vessels.

4. A 57-year-old man comes to the emergency department due to severe chest pain for 20 minutes. The patient reports the pain started while driving to work, and describes the pain as "tearing". He has a past medical history of hypertension, and stage IV chronic kidney disease. Vital signs show blood pressure of 98/45 mmHg, pulses are asymmetric between the right and left arms, respiratory rate of 18 breaths/min, and oxygen saturation of 94%. He is diagnosed with aortic dissection via TTE. The patient fails first-line treatments and is then taken to the operating room for definitive repair. Involvement of which of the following vessels would likely also be seen on imaging?

   A. Involvement of the celiac trunk on transesophageal echo
   B. Involvement of the brachiocephalic artery on transesophageal echo
   C. Involvement of the superior mesenteric artery on MRI
   D. Involvement of the left subclavian artery on MRI
   E. Involvement of the celiac trunk on CTA

- **The correct answer is option A.**
- This patient has a dissection where first-line treatment failed and was then taken to the operating room.
- This means the patient had a type B dissection, which is first medically managed. If it's a type B dissection then the ascending aorta cannot be involved which eliminates answer options B and D.
- The patient has stage IV kidney disease, and therefore would be unable to tolerate CTA/MRI which uses contrast, making a transesophageal echocardiogram (TEE) the best option.

Cardiology | Section 13: Abdominal Aortic Aneurysm

I. Definition
  A. Full thickness dilatation of a blood vessel that is greater than 50% increase past the baseline
  B. Average diameter of abdominal aorta in adults is 2 cm
  C. > 3 cm aneurysmal

II. Pathophysiology
  A. Failure of structural proteins such as elastin resulting in weakness of the aortic wall
  B. Contributing factors to aortic wall weakening
    1. Genetics
    2. Marked inflammation
    3. Proteolytic degradation of the aortic wall connective tissue

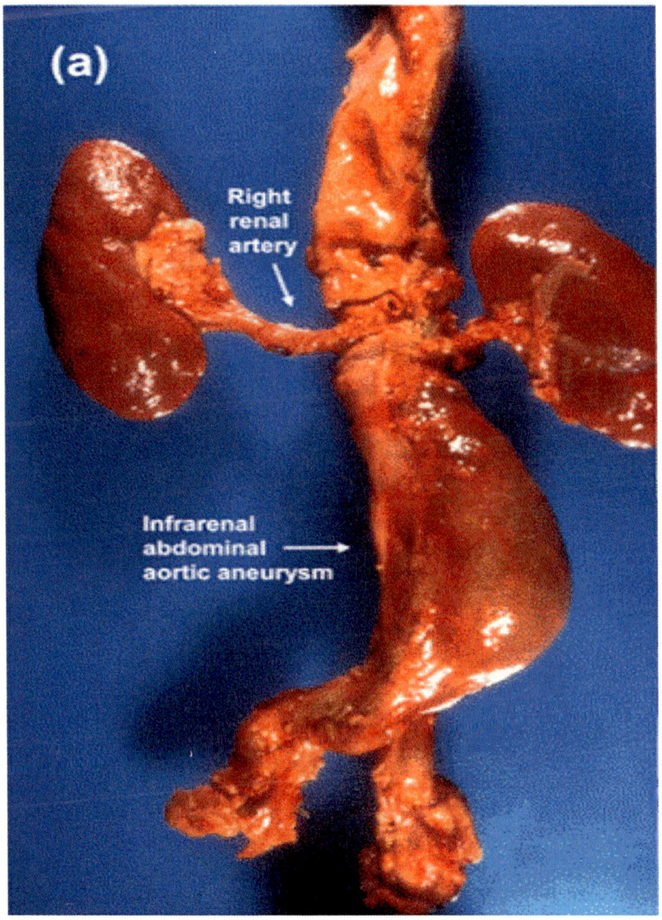

FIGURE 21.2.51 - Gross Image of an Infrarenal Aneurysm

III. Risk Factors
  A. Tobacco use
  B. Male gender
  C. Age > 60
  D. Caucasian
  E. Family history

IV. Clinical Features
  A. Usually asymptomatic
    1. Found on routine screening
    2. Incidental finding
  B. Ruptured abdominal aortic aneurysms
    1. Pulsatile abdominal mass
    2. Sudden and severe abdominal pain
    3. Hypotension

V. Diagnosis
  A. Abdominal aorta diameter on CT or ultrasound
    1. > 3 cm aneurysmal
    2. 4.0-5.5 cm medium aneurysm
    3. > 5.5 cm large aneurysms
    4. > 6.0 cm very large
  B. Ruptured abdominal aortic aneurysms
    1. Triad of hypotension, pulsatile abdominal mass, and sudden and severe abdominal pain
    2. Hypotension with sudden and severe abdominal pain and imaging showing an abdominal aneurysm

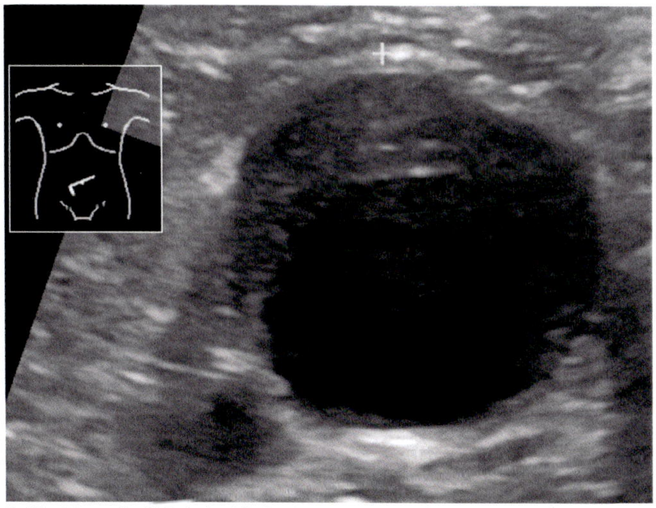

FIGURE 21.2.52 - Abdominal Ultrasound of the Aorta

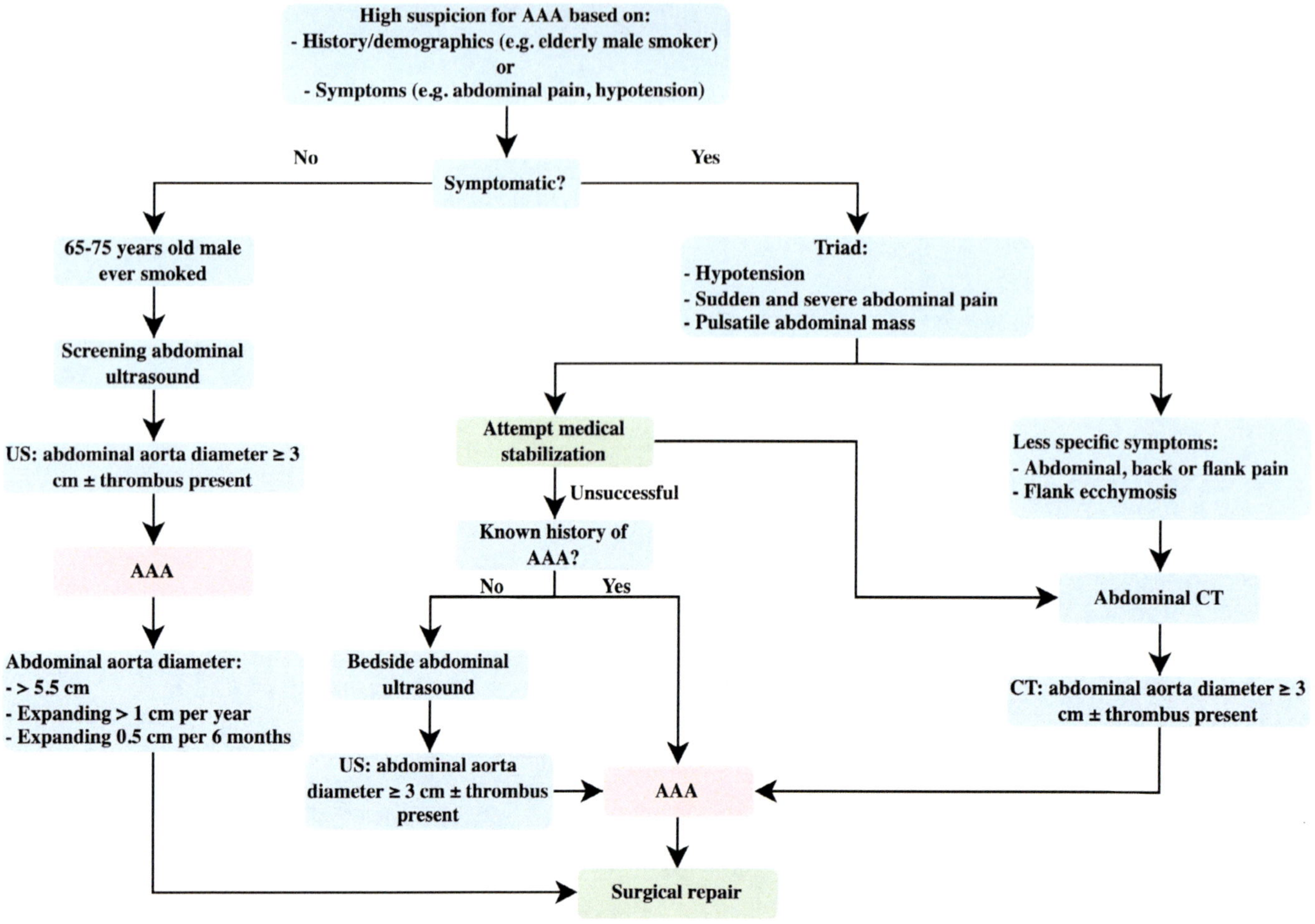

FIGURE 21.2.53 - Workup and Management of Abdominal Aortic Aneurysm

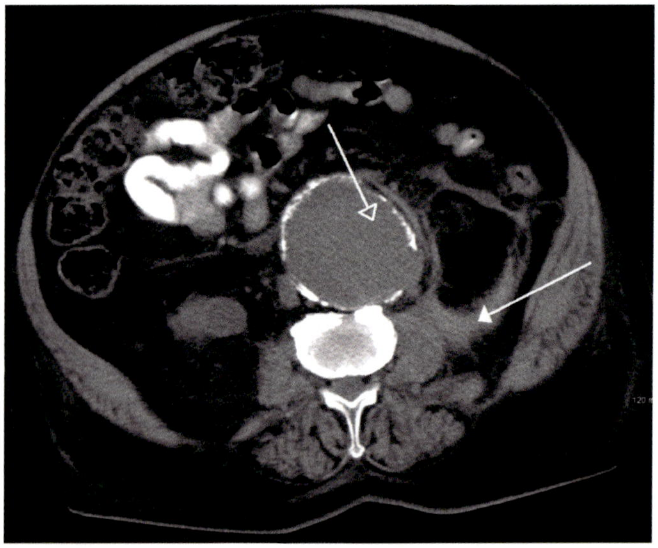

FIGURE 21.2.54 - CT Scan Showing a Ruptured Abdominal Aortic Aneurysm

VI. Treatment
   A. EVAR (endovascular aneurysm repair)
      1. Confirm with CT that patient is suitable for EVAR
      2. Requires space between the aneurysm and renal arteries for stent placement
   B. Open
      1. Hemodynamically unstable patients
      2. Stable patients with aneurysms too adjacent to renal arteries

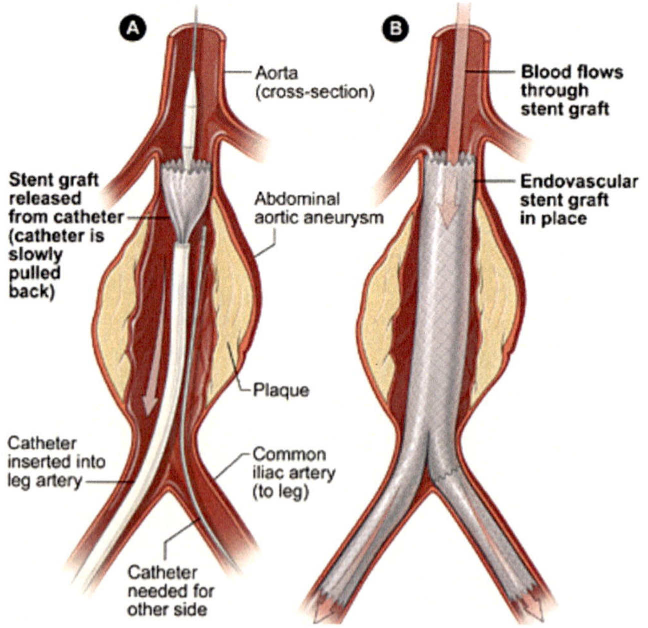

FIGURE 21.2.53 - The Procedure to Place a Endovascular Stent

REVIEW QUESTIONS

1. How are true and false aneurysms differentiated?

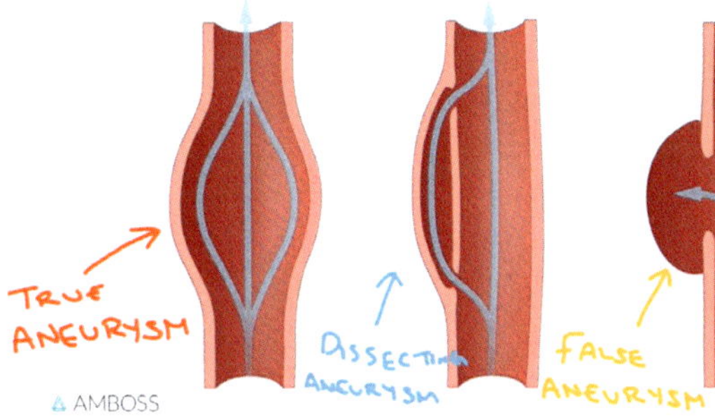

- **A true aneurysm is a full thickness dilatation of the vessel wall; whereas, a false aneurysm forms when there is a perforation of the vessel wall and accumulation of extravascular hematoma.**
- A true aneurysm involves the adventitia, media, and intima.
- In the image above, a dissecting aneurysm and a false aneurysm can also be seen.
- A dissecting aneurysm is found when there is an intimal tear in the vessel wall and formation of a second lumen, also called false lumen, is seen.

2. A 30-year-old Caucasian man comes to his primary care physician with concerns of his potential for developing an abdominal aortic dissection, which his father was recently diagnosed with. What are the key elements of the discussion to have with this patient?

- **The key elements to discuss with this patient would be risk factors for abdominal aortic aneurysm and smoking history.**
- One point of conversation would be his increased risk because he is male and has a positive family history.
- Being caucasian is also a risk factor.
- A key point for the physician is to obtain a smoking history, because it is a modifiable risk factor for the development of abdominal aortic aneurysms later in life.

3. A 57-year-old woman comes to the emergency department because of severe abdominal pain for 20 minutes. She was driving to work when the pain started, and describes it as the worst abdominal pain of her life. Her vital signs include blood pressure of 98/45 mmHg, pulse of 120 beats/min, respiratory rate of 18 breaths/min, oxygen saturations of 94%, and temperature of 37° C (98.6° F). An abdominal ultrasound shows a 5.1 cm abdominal aortic aneurysm just below the renal arteries and a negative FAST exam. The patient is sent for a CT scan to help in the diagnosis. In what way was the care of this patient mismanaged?

   A. A FAST exam should not have been performed
   B. A point-of-care glucose should have been obtained first
   C. Patient required urgent surgical consultation
   D. Blood cultures should have been obtained prior to CT

- **The correct answer is option C.**
- The resident was likely comforted by the lack of free fluid in the peritoneum, which is what the FAST exam was looking for.
- However, the absence of free fluid does not rule out a possible rupture.
- The aorta is retroperitoneal, so a ruptured abdominal aortic aneurysm would not show fluid in the peritoneal cavity.
- Only normotensive patients should go to the CT scanner.
- This patient was mismanaged in the way that the resident sent the patient for CT imaging.
- Instead, the surgeons should have been contacted immediately for a presumed ruptured abdominal aortic aneurysm.
- A is wrong because in a hypotensive patient with abdominal pain, a FAST exam is clinically indicated.
- B is wrong because while a point of care glucose is useful in resuscitation, this patient presentation is not consistent with hypoglycemia or a hyperglycemic state.
- D is wrong because blood cultures are not required prior to CT scans, but are indicated prior to antibiotics in critically ill patients.

Cardiology | Section 14: Acute Arterial Occlusion

I. Acute Arterial Occlusion: Definition
   A. Sudden decrease in blood flow to an extremity leading to ischemia

II. Acute Arterial Occlusion: Pathophysiology
   A. Embolism
      1. Clot from a proximal vessel or heart
   B. Atherosclerosis (thrombosis)
      1. Progressive narrowing
      2. Low flow and stasis
      3. Thrombosis

III. Acute Arterial Occlusion: Risk Factors
   A. Smoking
   B. Diabetes
   C. Hyperlipidemia
   D. Hypertension
   E. Atrial fibrillation

IV. Acute Arterial Occlusion: Clinical Features
   A. Pain
   B. Pallor
   C. Pulselessness
   D. Poikilothermia
   E. Paresthesias
   F. Paralysis

V. Acute Arterial Occlusion: Diagnosis
   A. Doppler ultrasound
   B. Angiography
      1. CT, MRI, or digital subtraction
   C. ECG
   D. Echocardiogram

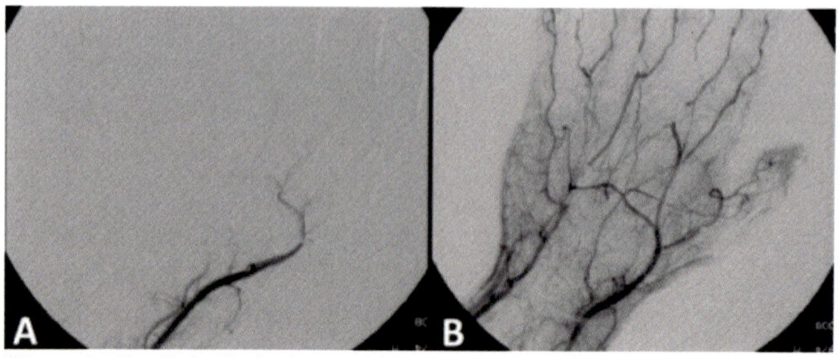

“Unrecognized hand ischemia after intraarterial drug injection: successful management of a “near miss” event” by Kyros Ipaktchi et al., Patient Safety in Surgery is licensed under CC BY 2.0

FIGURE 21.2.55 - Angiogram of Hand; A: Prior to Administering Thrombolytics; Hand B: After Administering Thrombolytics

VI. Acute Arterial Occlusion: Treatment
   A. Heparin
   B. Thrombolytics
   C. Embolectomy
      1. Catheter assisted with fogarty balloon or aspiration
      2. Surgical
   D. Amputation

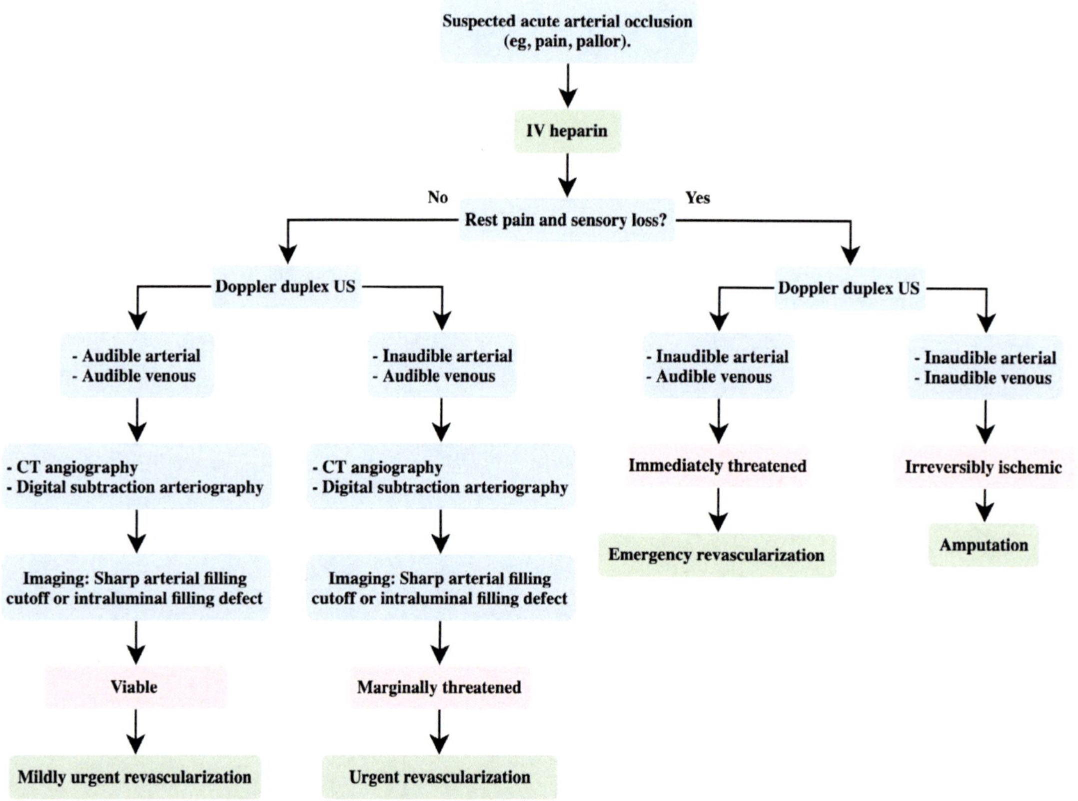

FIGURE 21.2.54 - Evaluation and Management of Acute Arterial Occlusion

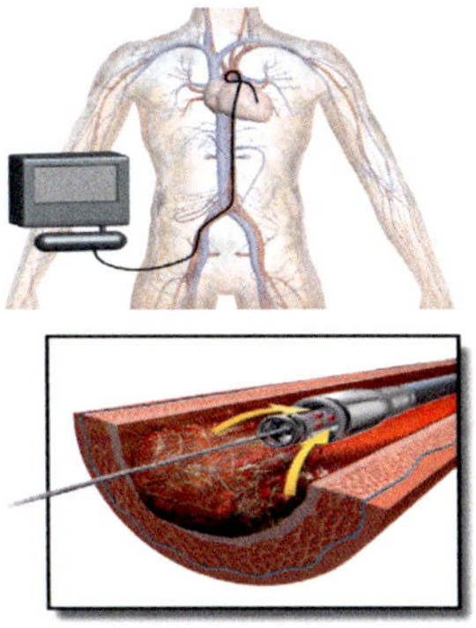

FIGURE 21.2.56 - Aspiration Embolectomy

REVIEW QUESTIONS

1. Why is diabetes a risk factor for acute arterial occlusion?
    - **Diabetes → hyperglycemia → endothelial cell dysfunction → vascular wall inflammation → increased release of cytokines and chemokines → monocyte recruitment → formation of lipid core → vessel occlusion**
    - Diabetes increases the development of atherosclerotic disease due to increased insulin resistance and subsequent hyperglycemia.
    - The hyperglycemia leads to endothelial cell dysfunction which results in the inflammation of the vascular wall.
    - The local inflammation in the vascular wall and the oxidative stress leads to increased release of cytokines and chemokines.
    - This leads to recruitment of monocytes which mature into macrophages and further release of cytokines.
    - When these inflammatory changes in the vessel wall are combined with hyperlipidemia, a common comorbidity, a lipid core is formed which can then embolize down to a small vessel leading to occlusion.

2. What are features of an acute arterial occlusion that are unlikely to occur in peripheral artery disease?
    - **Pulselessness, paralysis, and poikilothermia are features of an acute arterial occlusion that are unlikely to occur in peripheral artery disease.**
    - Both acute arterial occlusion and peripheral artery disease are states of impaired blood flow, but acute occlusion results in a complete lack of blood flow.
    - Both are likely to have pain and pallor, but unique features to acute occlusion would be pulselessness, paralysis, and poikilothermia

3. A 69-year-old man undergoes a procedure where a catheter is inserted into a vessel. Aspiration equipment is utilized and an embolized deposition of calcium and lipids are removed. What is required next as part of the work up for the likely etiology of this patient's diagnosis?

    A. CT head without contrast
    B. CT head with contrast
    C. Electrocardiogram
    D. Ankle-brachial indexes
    E. Echocardiogram

    - **The correct answer is option C.**
    - The procedure described is a catheter-assisted embolectomy where a clot was removed.
    - The most likely diagnosis is acute arterial occlusion.
    - According to the question stem, it was an embolized clot, not a thrombosis.
    - One of the most common causes of acute arterial occlusion secondary to an embolism is atrial fibrillation.
    - So an ECG should be done to evaluate for atrial fibrillation.
    - CT without contrast should always be done prior to CT with contrast to rule out hemorrhage, and the contrasted study will show if there is an occlusion. While this patient is at risk for a stroke, he is not currently demonstrating symptoms of stroke, so options A and B are incorrect.
    - Ankle-brachial indexes are used to diagnose peripheral artery disease, management of which would likely have started with conservative measures, and the surgery used is not an embolectomy, so option D is wrong.
    - The role of echocardiogram in the workup of atrial fibrillation is to evaluate for presence of thrombus, wall contractility, and valve disruption.
    - Echocardiogram wouldn't precede electrocardiogram so option E is wrong.

Cardiology | Section 15: Peripheral Artery Disease

I. Peripheral Artery Disease: Definition
   A. Narrowing of the arteries in the lower extremities leading to impaired blood flow and tissue ischemia

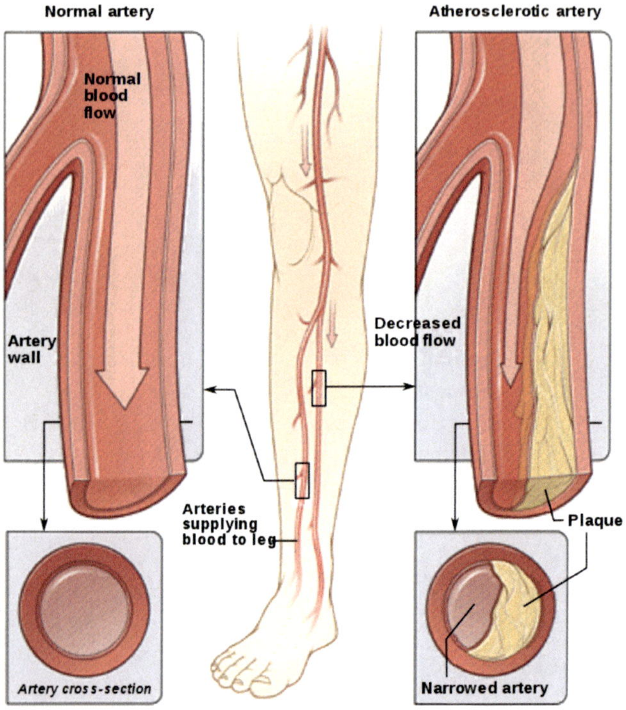

By Jmarchn - Own work, CC BY-SA 3.0, https://commons.wikimedia.org/w/index.php?curid=31200275

FIGURE 21.2.57 - Pathophysiology of Peripheral Artery Disease

II. Peripheral Artery Disease: Pathophysiology
   A. Atherosclerotic changes in the vessel walls
      1. Plaques (calcium, fat)
      2. Narrowing of the vessels
      3. Impaired ability to dilate
      4. Tissue ischemia

III. Peripheral Artery Disease: Risk Factors
   A. Smoking
   B. Diabetes
   C. Hyperlipidemia
   D. Hypertension

IV. Peripheral Artery Disease: Clinical Features
   A. Peripheral artery disease
      1. Intermittent claudication
      2. Pain after walking specific distances
      3. Aching
      4. Burning
      5. Night cramps
      6. Discoloration of the legs

V. Peripheral Artery Disease: Diagnosis
   A. Ankle brachial index
      1. Measure the difference in blood pressures between upper and lower extremities

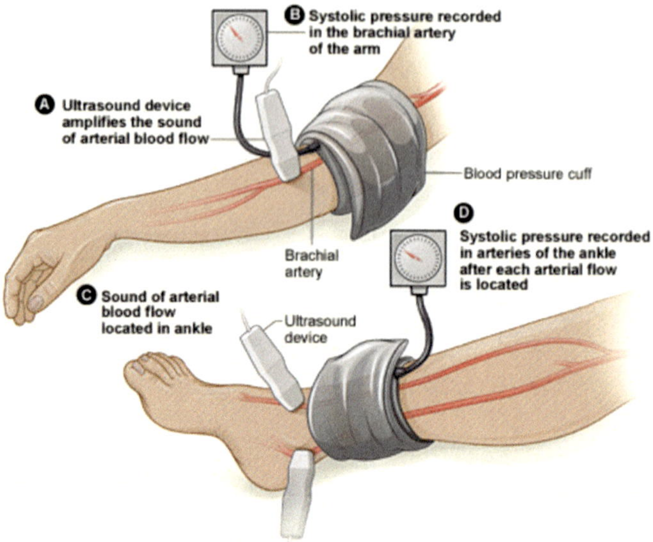

By National Heart Lung and Blood Institute (NIH) - https://www.nhlbi.nih.gov/health/health-topics/topics/pad/diagnosis, Public Domain, https://commons.wikimedia.org/w/index.php?curid=29587673

FIGURE 21.2.58 - Ankle-Brachial Index

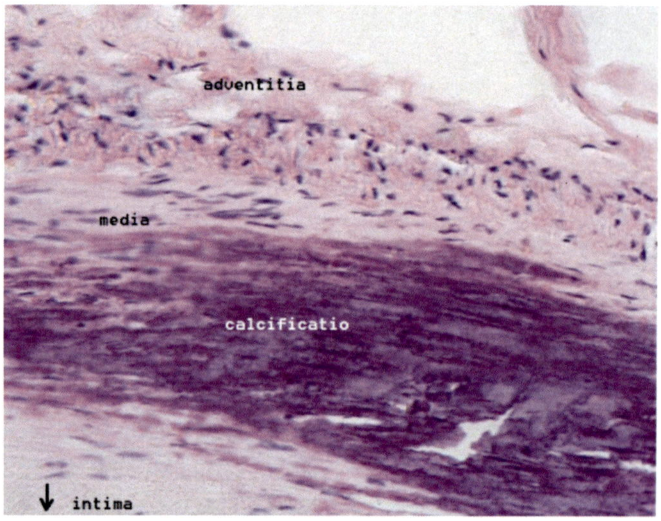

Public Domain, https://commons.wikimedia.org/w/index.php?curid=446171

FIGURE 21.2.59 - Monckeberg's Arteriosclerosis

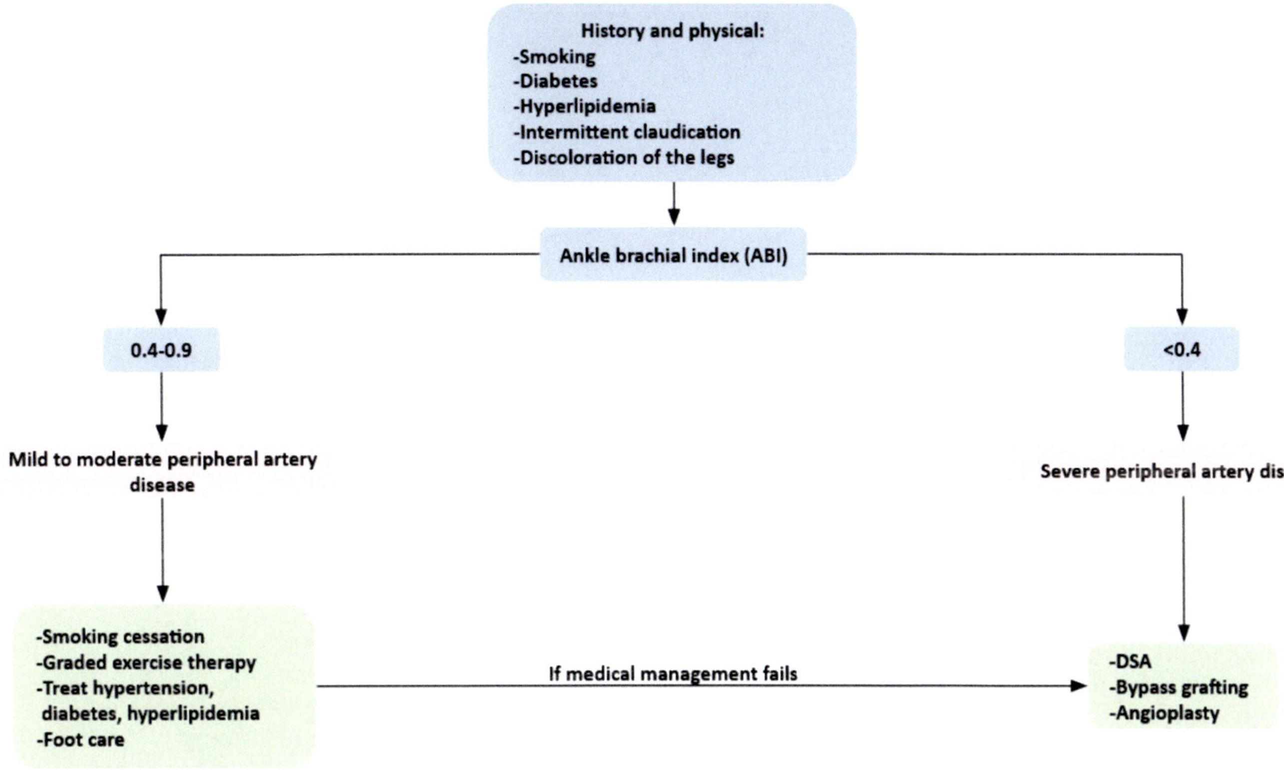

FIGURE 21.2.60 - Evaluation and Management of Peripheral Artery Disease

VI. Peripheral Artery Disease: Treatment
   A. Bypass grafting
      1. Creates alternate route
      2. High immediate success rate
   B. Angioplasty
      1. Balloon dilation ± stenting
      2. First line with multiple attempts prior to stenting
      3. Not used in lesions below knee

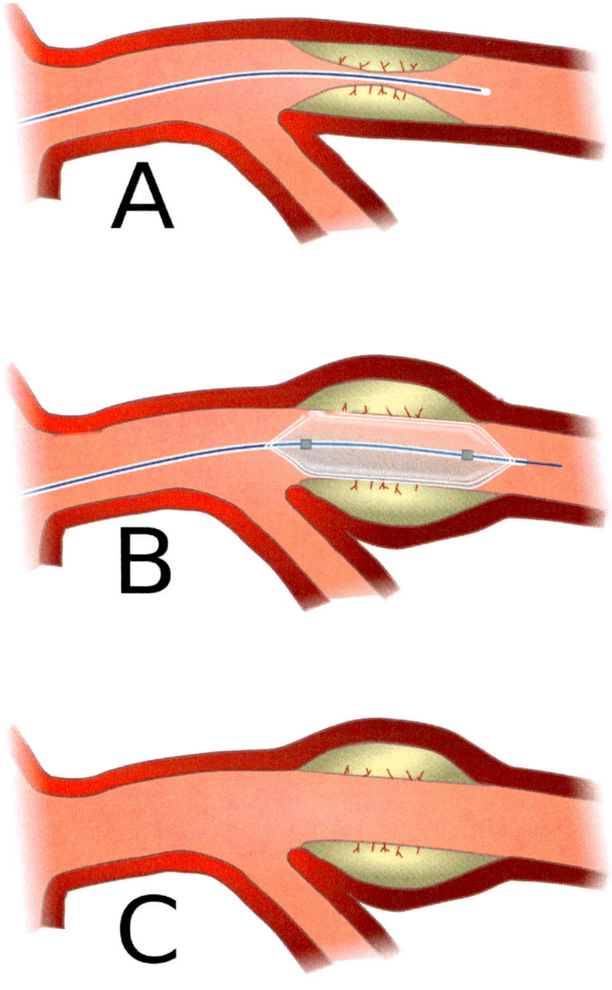

FIGURE 21.2.61 - Angioplasty

REVIEW QUESTIONS

1. Why is smoking a risk factor for peripheral artery disease?
    - **Nicotine → endothelial cell dysfunction → recruitment and activation of macrophages → necrotic core formation and development of atherosclerotic plaque → neovascularization, cell death, and plaque rupture.**
    - Nicotine results in oxidative stress which causes endothelial cell dysfunction and increased expression of adhesion molecules.
    - This results in increased macrophage recruitment.
    - The macrophages are then stimulated by the nicotine to secrete elevated levels of TNF-alpha, IL-1, and chemokines.
    - These inflammatory changes lead to necrotic core formation, which can contribute to the development of an atherosclerotic plaque.
    - The interaction of the vasa vasorum with the nicotine leads to plaque instability, evidenced by the expansion to intima, neovascularization, cell death, and plaque rupture.
    - This is how nicotine can lead to the formation and rupture of atherosclerotic plaques, which plays a very important role in the development of peripheral artery disease.

2. With what endocrine disorder would a patient likely have a falsely elevated ankle-brachial index score, and why?
    - **Diabetes, due to calcification and hardening of vessels.**
    - False elevations in the ankle brachial index come from calcification of the arteries which causes the ankle readings to be falsely elevated.
    - This is problematic because it can give the false impression that more blood is getting to the extremities than is in actuality.
    - Calcification and hardening of the vessels is a common complication of diabetes, which is why monckeberg sclerosis is more prevalent in this population.

3. A 69-year-old man is admitted to the hospital because of pain at rest in the lower extremities for the past 4 weeks. He was prescribed some medicines and advised to exercise but his symptoms failed to improve. Now, he is scheduled for a surgery. On the day of surgery, he undergoes a procedure where a catheter was inserted into a vessel in his left and right lower extremities, a balloon was inflated and meshwork was then placed. What is a medication this patient might have been started on to help manage the main risk factor for his disease process?

    A. Fluoxetine
    B. Rosuvastatin
    C. Metformin
    D. Bupropion
    E. Amiodarone

    - **The correct answer is option D.**
    - The procedure described is angioplasty with balloon dilatation and stent placement.
    - The most likely diagnosis in this patient is based on the procedure performed, which is peripheral artery disease in this case.
    - The most significant risk factor for peripheral artery disease is smoking.
    - A medication would have been started to try and help the patient quit smoking prior to surgical intervention.
    - Bupropion has been found to help people quit smoking.
    - Varenicline is another medication prescribed for smoking cessation.
    - Fluoxetine is an SSRI which is indicated in the treatment of anxiety and depression disorders, but has no direct impact on smoking cessation, so option A is wrong.
    - Rosuvastatin is a first line agent used in the treatment of hyperlipidemia.
    - Hyperlipidemia is a risk factor for peripheral artery disease, but its impact is not as significant as smoking, so option B is wrong.
    - Option C is wrong for the same reason; diabetes is not as much of a risk factor as smoking, which metformin is used to treat.
    - Amiodarone is an antiarrhythmic with a high side-effect profile and without utility in the treatment of smoking cessation, so option E is wrong.

Cardiology | Section 16: Cardiac Neoplasms

I. Definition
   A. Most common 1° cardiac tumor in adults
   B. Gelatinous tumor found most commonly in the left atrium

II. Clinical Presentation
   A. "Ball valve" obstruction of mitral valve annulus
      1. Multiple episodes of syncope
      2. Exercise intolerance
      3. Fatigue
      4. Shortness of breath due to pulmonary edema
   B. Embolization
      1. Ischemic stroke
         a) Dysarthria, dysphagia, vision abnormalities, weakness
      2. Prerenal acute kidney injury
         a) ↑ BUN, ↑ Cr, ↑ BUN/Cr ratio, ↓ urine output
      3. Acute mesenteric ischemia
         a) Severe abdominal pain, hematochezia, lactic acidosis
   C. IL-6 production by tumor
   D. Constitutional symptoms: fever, weight loss, night sweats

III. Diagnosis
   A. Heart auscultation
      1. Early diastolic "tumor plop" sound right after mitral valve opening
   B. Echocardiography
      1. Hyperechoic pedunculated mass in left atrium
   C. Biopsy
      1. Myxoma cells in glycosaminoglycan stroma

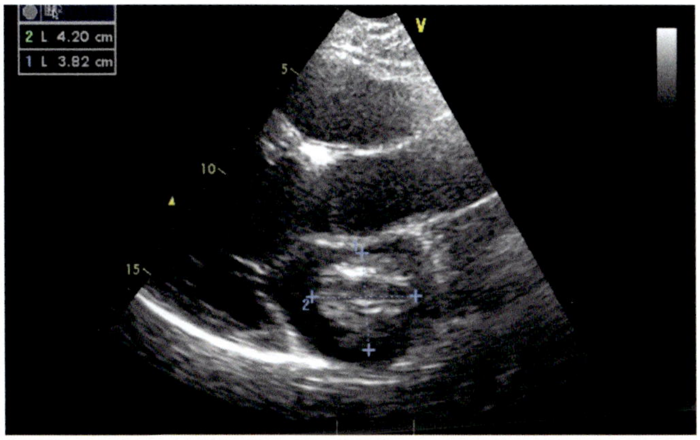

FIGURE 21.2.62 - Echocardiography of a Left Atrial Myxoma

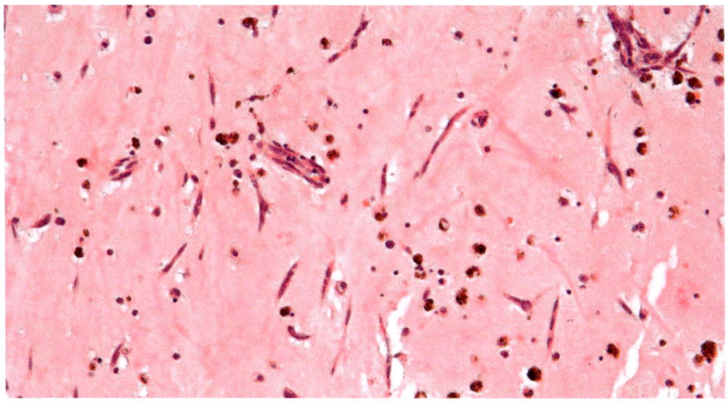

FIGURE 21.2.63 - Light Microscopy Showing Atrial Myxoma

IV. Management
   A. Surgical excision
   B. Heart transplantation in recurrent atrial myxoma

Cardiac Neoplasm	Key Features
Atrial myxoma	- Most common 1° cardiac tumor in adults - Multiple syncopal episodes and exercise intolerance (↓ CO) - Fever, night sweats, weight loss (↑ IL-6) - Early diastolic "tumor plop" sound on cardiac auscultation - Hyperechoic pedunculated mass in left atrium on echocardiography
Metastatic disease	- Most common cardiac tumor in adults - Commonly arises from breast cancer, lung cancer, and melanoma - Characteristic signs and symptoms of 1° cancer (e.g. breast lump, cough, hemoptysis, skin lesion) - Fever, night sweats, weight loss (↑ IL-6) - Multiple masses in the myocardium on echocardiography
Kaposi sarcoma	- Malignant vascular tumor caused by human herpesvirus-8 - Common in immunocompromised patients (e.g. HIV) - Vascular tumors in other locations (e.g. skin, GI tract, lungs) - Multiple vascular lesions in the myocardium on echocardiography
Cardiac rhabdomyoma	- Most common 1° cardiac tumor in children - Common in patients with tuberous sclerosis - Hamartomatous growth on biopsy - More common in ventricles than atria

TABLE 21.2.8 - Differential Diagnosis of Atrial Myxoma

REVIEW QUESTIONS

1. A 45-year-old man comes to the office because of 5 episodes of syncope over the last 4 months. He also complains of shortness of breath, fatigue, and exercise intolerance. Cardiac auscultation shows an early diastolic "plop" sound. Echocardiography shows a hyperechoic pedunculated mass in the left atrium. The biopsy of this mass will most likely reveal?

    - **The biopsy of the atrial myxoma typically shows the myxoma cells in glycosaminoglycan stroma.**
    - This patient comes to the office with 5 episodes of syncope over the last 4 months.
    - Cardiac auscultation shows an early diastolic plop sound.
    - Echocardiography shows a hyperechoic pedunculated mass in the left atrium.
    - All of these findings are consistent with the diagnosis of the left atrial myxoma.

2. A 50-year-old woman comes to the emergency department because of weakness, and difficulty speaking and swallowing for the last 3 hours. She has also had 6 episodes of syncope over the last 3 months. She had acute mesenteric ischemia 5 months ago. She has a family history of breast cancer in her mother and melanoma in her father. She has been smoking 3 packs of cigarettes per day for the last 30 years. Her vital signs include temperature of 37 °C (98.6 °F), blood pressure of 145/90 mmHg, heart rate of 84 beats/min, and respiratory rate of 15 breaths/min. Physical exam shows weakness in the left arm and the left lower face. Cardiac auscultation shows the plop sound shortly after S2. Echocardiography shows a single mass in the left atrium. Non-contrast head CT scan is performed. Which of the following is the best next step in the management of this patient?

    A. Surgical excision
    B. Chest X-ray
    C. Mammography
    D. Skin evaluation

- **The correct answer is option A.**
- This patient with weakness, dysarthria, and dysphagia likely has a stroke.
- She has had 6 episodes of syncope over the last 3 months.
- She also had an acute mesenteric ischemia 5 months ago.
- The cardiac auscultation shows the plop sound shortly after S2.
- Echocardiography shows a single mass in the left atrium.
- All of these findings are consistent with the diagnosis of an atrial myxoma.
- Embolization of the parts of atrial myxoma accounts for her current stroke and previous acute mesenteric ischemia.
- The best next step in the management of the patient with atrial myxoma is the surgical excision of the tumor.
- Option B, chest X-ray, is incorrect because it cannot confirm atrial myxoma. Additionally, although this patient has an extensive smoking history predisposing her to lung cancer, the metastatic lung malignancy cannot explain the single mass in the left atrium.
- Option C, mammography, is incorrect because it cannot confirm atrial myxoma. Furthermore, although this patient has a positive family history of breast cancer, metastatic breast cancer would present with multiple, rather than single, cardiac lesions.
- Option D, skin evaluation, is incorrect because it cannot confirm atrial myxoma. Although this patient has a positive family history of melanoma, metastatic melanoma would present with multiple, rather than single, cardiac lesions.

HEMATOLOGY & ONCOLOGY

HEM/ONC | Section 1: Principles of Cancer Therapy

I. Surgical Therapy
   A. Resection of the primary tumor with clear margins (e.g. Mohs surgery)
   B. Sampling of regional lymph nodes for TNM staging purposes
   C. Often used in conjunction with chemotherapy and radiotherapy

II. Mohs Surgery
   A. Commonly used to treat skin cancer on sensitive areas (e.g. face, ears)
   B. Procedure involves three basic steps
      1. Surgeon removes a thin layer of skin
      2. Pathologist inspects removed skin under a microscope
      3. First, two steps are repeated until the cancer is removed with clear margins
      4. Surgeon closes the skin

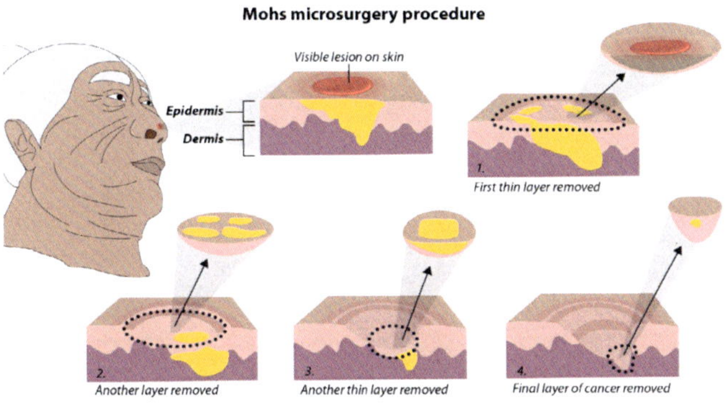

FIGURE 12.3.1 - Basic Steps of Mohs Surgery

III. Radiation Therapy
   A. Ionizing radiation is concentrated around cancer cells to induce DNA damage and subsequent cell death via
      1. Generation of reactive oxygen species
      2. Induction of double-strand breaks
   B. Can be used in combination with surgery to
      1. Shrink tumors in anticipation of surgery
      2. Prevent local tumor recurrence after surgery

IV. Medical Therapy
   A. Chemotherapy: kills all rapidly proliferating cells
   B. Targeted therapy: targets cells with specific oncogenic mutations
   C. Hormone therapy: treats hormone-dependent cancers
   D. Immunotherapy: primes the host immune system to kill cancer cells

V. Target Therapy
   A. Trastuzumab: HER2 inhibitor
      1. Causes cardiotoxicity (consider baseline echocardiography)
   B. Cetuximab: EGFR inhibitor
      1. Causes acneiform rash and serum sickness
   C. Imatinib: BCR-ABL tyrosine kinase inhibitor
      1. Treats chronic myeloid leukemia (9:22 translocation)

Type of Radiation Therapy	Key Feature(s)	Example(s) of Clinical Application
External beam radiation therapy	- Beams of high-energy X-rays are generated by a linear accelerator and delivered precisely to the tumor site	- Brain tumors - Breast tumors - Lung tumors
Brachytherapy	- A radioactive node is implanted at or near the tumor site	- Ocular cancer - Prostate cancer - Rectal cancer
Radioimmunotherapy	- A radioactive compound is conjugated to an antibody designed to target cancer cells and injected into the bloodstream	- Non-Hodgkin lymphoma

TABLE 21.3.1 - Radiation Therapy

Chemotherapy	Mechanism of Action	High-Yield Adverse Effects
Alkylating agents (e.g. cyclophosphamide, cisplatin, carboplatin)	- Damage DNA	- Cyclophosphamide: hemorrhagic cystitis, bladder carcinoma - Cisplatin, carboplatin: ototoxicity, peripheral neuropathy
Antimetabolites (e.g. methotrexate, fluorouracil)	- Methotrexate: interferes with folate and DNA synthesis - Fluorouracil: interferes with DNA replication	- Methotrexate: megaloblastic anemia, hepatotoxicity, stomatitis
Antimicrotubule agents (e.g. vinblastine, vincristine, paclitaxel)	- Interfere with cell division	- Peripheral neuropathy - Hair loss
Anthracyclines (e.g. bleomycin, doxorubicin, daunorubicin)	- Interfere with DNA replication and cause apoptosis	- Bleomycin: pulmonary fibrosis - Doxorubicin, daunorubicin: cardiotoxicity
Topoisomerase inhibitors (e.g. topotecan, irinotecan)	- Interfere with DNA replication	- Diarrhea

TABLE 21.3.2 - Important Chemotherapy Agents

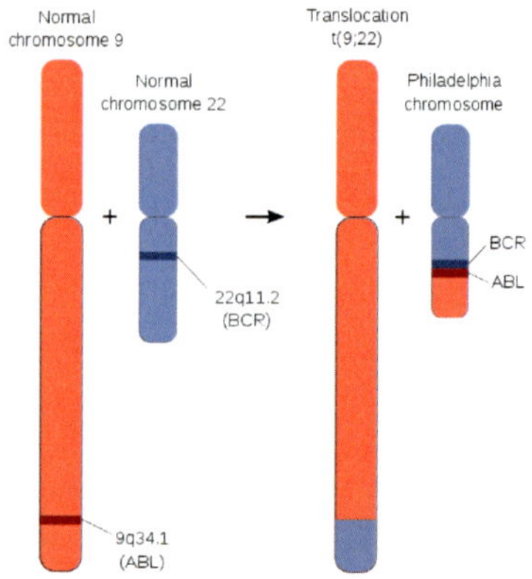

FIGURE 21.3.2 - Translocation Between Chromosome 9 and Chromosome 22

VI. Hormonal Therapy
   A. Tamoxifen: inhibits estrogen receptors in breast tissue
      1. Treats estrogen receptor-positive breast cancer
      2. Increases risk for endometrial carcinoma and uterine sarcoma
      3. Increases risk of blood clots
   B. Anastrozole: stops the conversion of androgens to estrogen by aromataseTreats estrogen
      1. receptor-positive breast cancer
      2. Increases risk of osteoporosis

VII. Immunotherapy
   A. PD-1 inhibitors (e.g. nivolumab, pembrolizumab)
   B. CTLA-4 inhibitors (e.g. ipilimumab)
   C. Both PD-1 and CTLA-4 are receptors that lead to inhibition of T cells
      1. Inhibition of these receptors primes the immune system to destroy cancer cells & host cells

Strategy	Description	Example
Adjuvant	- Treatment given in addition to or following the standard therapy	- Patient receives chemotherapy after breast cancer excision
Neoadjuvant	- Treatment given before the standard therapy	- Patient receives radiation therapy to shrink a tumor before surgical excision
Induction	- First therapy administered to patient - Designed to kill tumor cells quickly and potentially achieve remission	- High-dose initial chemotherapy given to a patient with acute leukemia
Medication	- Multidrug therapy that follows induction therapy - Designed to kill even more tumor cells	- Multidrug therapy given to a patient with acute leukemia
Maintenance	- Therapy given after consolidation chemotherapy - Designed to eradicate remaining tumor cells and/or keep the patient in remission	- Maintenance chemotherapy to prevent recurrence of lung cancer
Salvage	- Therapy offered following either cancer recurrence or when initial therapy fails - Designed to achieve remission again	- Multidrug therapies used in treatment of patients with diffuse large B-cell lymphoma

TABLE 21.3.3 - Primary Strategies of Cancer Therapy

REVIEW QUESTIONS

1. How can clinicians protect patients from developing hemorrhagic cystitis and bladder cancer that may be caused by prolonged use of cyclophosphamide?
    - **Clinicians can protect patients from developing hemorrhagic cystitis and bladder cancer by undertaking measures to flush acrolein (breakdown metabolite of cyclophosphamide) out of the patient's bladder.**
    - Cyclophosphamide produces a metabolite known as acrolein, which accumulates in the bladder and exerts significant toxicity.
    - If allowed to persist in the bladder for long periods of time, acrolein will inevitably lead to hemorrhagic cystitis and eventually bladder cancer.
    - To prevent this, clinicians should undertake measures to flush acrolein out of the patient's bladder.
    - This can be accomplished via frequent hydration and voiding, as well as use of a compound called mesna, which binds acrolein and promotes its urinary excretion.
    - Clinicians should always consider these measures whenever prescribing cyclophosphamide.

2. A 33-year-old male comes to the clinic because of worsening shortness of breath for the past few weeks. He has a known history of testicular cancer for which he underwent a prolonged course of multidrug chemotherapy. The patient states he has been in remission for about one year. His vitals signs include temperature of 37.2° C (98.96° F), blood pressure of 135/87 mmHg, pulse of 74 beats/minute, and respiratory rate of 19 breaths/minute. Physical examination shows fine inspiratory crackles at lung bases. A chest X-ray is obtained and shows reticulonodular opacities. A follow-up CT scan of the chest shows interlobular septal thickening and honeycombing. These pulmonary findings can most likely be attributed to one of the following chemotherapeutic agents?

    A. Cyclophosphamide
    B. Carboplatin
    C. Vincristine
    D. Bleomycin
    E. Irinotecan

    - **The correct answer is option D.**
    - This is a case of a 33-year-old male with a known history of testicular cancer who now presents with worsening shortness of breath.
    - Importantly, his cancer is now in remission after a prolonged course of multidrug chemotherapy.
    - The findings of fine inspiratory crackles on physical examination, reticulonodular opacities on chest X-ray, and interlobular septal thickening and honeycombing on chest CT are all consistent with a diagnosis of pulmonary fibrosis.
    - Among the listed chemotherapeutic agents, only bleomycin can lead to pulmonary fibrosis after prolonged use.
    - Option A is incorrect because cyclophosphamide is associated with hemorrhagic cystitis and bladder cancer.
    - Option B is incorrect because carboplatin is associated with ototoxicity and peripheral neuropathy.
    - Option C is incorrect because vincristine is associated with hair loss and peripheral neuropathy.
    - Option E is incorrect because irinotecan is mostly associated with diarrhea.

HEM/ONC | Section 2: Oncologic Emergencies

I. Tumor Lysis Syndrome: General Characteristics
   A. Rapid lysis of tumor cells causes rapid release of intracellular contents into the bloodstream, leading to life-threatening consequences
      1. Electrolyte derangements
      2. Metabolic abnormalities
   B. Occurs following initiation of chemotherapy for tumors with high burden or rapid cell turnover

II. Tumor Lysis Syndrome: Clinical Features
   A. Constitutional symptoms (e.g. malaise, nausea)
   B. Release of potassium → hyperkalemia, ECG changes
   C. Release of phosphate → hypocalcemia, tetany, seizures, acute kidney injury from calcium phosphate crystals
   D. Release of uric acid → hyperuricemia, gout, acute kidney injury from uric acid crystals

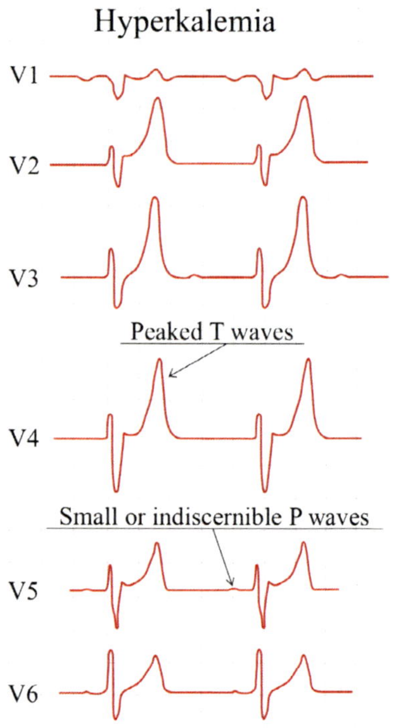

FIGURE 21.3.3 - ECG Findings in Hyperkalemia

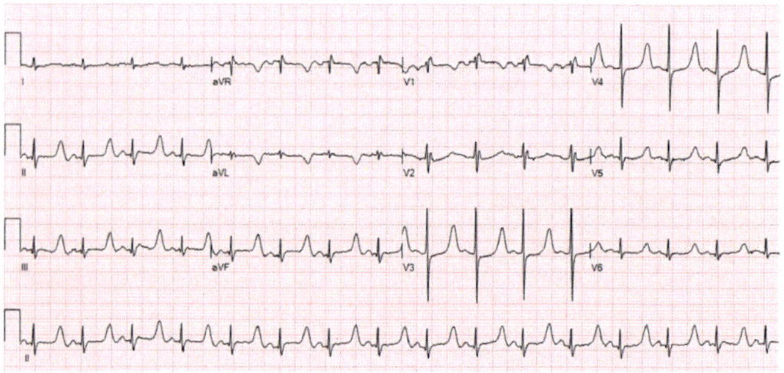

FIGURE 21.3.4 - ECG with Prolonged QT Interval in Hypocalcemia

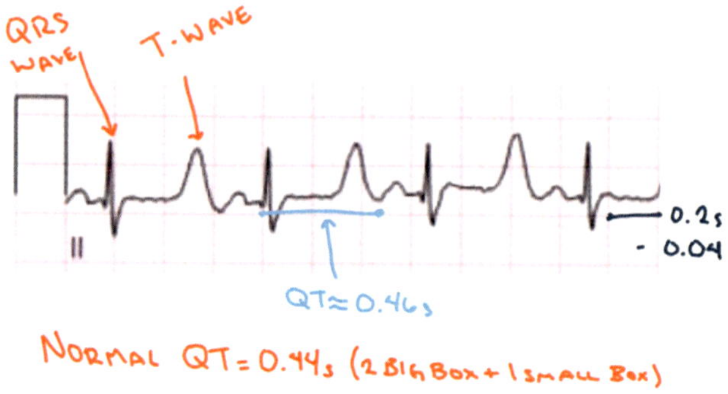

FIGURE 21.3.5 - QT Interval Explained

III. Tumor Lysis Syndrome: Treatment
   A. Prophylaxis: IV normal saline
   B. Treatment
      1. IV calcium gluconate (to stabilize cardiac membranes)
      2. Reduce potassium levels: insulin and glucose
      3. IV fluids
      4. Continuous telemetry
      5. Reduce uric acid levels: allopurinol, rasburicase, or febuxostat

IV. Hypercalcemia: General Characteristics
   A. Elevated serum calcium in the setting of an associated malignancy
   B. Common scenarios
      1. Multiple myeloma: hypercalcemia + pancytopenia
      2. Squamous cell carcinoma of the lung (paraneoplastic PTHrP)
      3. Breast cancer metastases to the bone

V. Hypercalcemia: Clinical Features
   A. Stones (kidney stones)
   B. Groans (abdominal pain)
   C. Bones (bone pain)
   D. Psychiatric overtones (neuropsychiatric symptoms)

VI. Hypercalcemia: Treatment
   A. Immediate treatment warranted in the setting of
      1. Severe hypercalcemia (serum Ca^{2+} > 14 mg/dL)
      2. Symptomatic hypercalcemia
   B. Aggressive normal saline hydration + calcitonin
   C. Loop diuretics for volume overloaded patients (e.g. cirrhosis)
   D. Bisphosphonates (e.g. alendronate)
      1. Inhibit osteoclasts

VII. Spinal Cord Compression: General Characteristics
   A. Compression of spinal nerve roots secondary to epidural tumors
   B. Common associated cancers
      1. Multiple myeloma
      2. Breast cancer
      3. Lung cancer
      4. Prostate cancer

VIII. Spinal Cord Compressions: Clinical Features
   A. Progressive back pain, worse at night
   B. Constitutional symptoms (e.g. weight loss, fatigue)
   C. Lower motor neuron symptoms (e.g. lower extremity weakness)
   D. Upper motor neuron symptoms (e.g. muscle spasticity)

IX. Spinal Cord Compressions: Diagnosis and Treatment
   A. Emergency MRI
   B. Treatment
      1. Intravenous high-dose steroids
      2. Radiation therapy
      3. Surgical decompression with neurosurgery

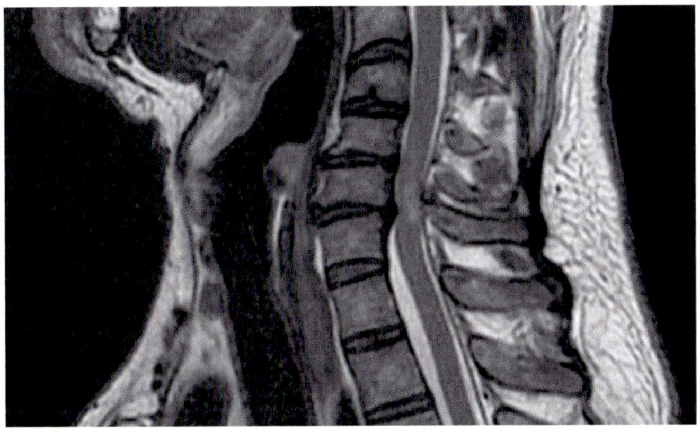

FIGURE 21.3.6 - MRI Showing Spinal Cord Compression

X. Cardiac Tamponade: General Characteristics
   A. A life-threatening emergency that arises following build up of fluid in the pericardial cavity
      1. Accumulating fluid increases intrapericardial pressure above the diastolic ventricular pressure
      2. This restricts ventricular expansion and filling, leading to an acute drop in preload, stroke volume, and cardiac output

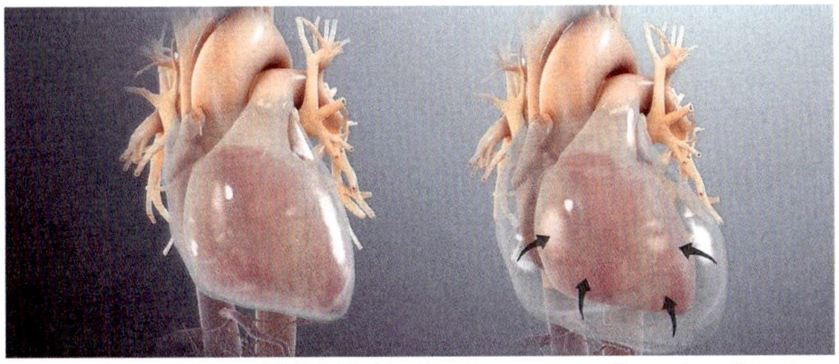

FIGURE 21.3.7 - Cardiac Tamponade

XI. Cardiac Tamponade: Clinical Features
   A. Distended neck veins
   B. Hypotension
   C. Muffled heart sounds
   D. Pulsus paradoxus

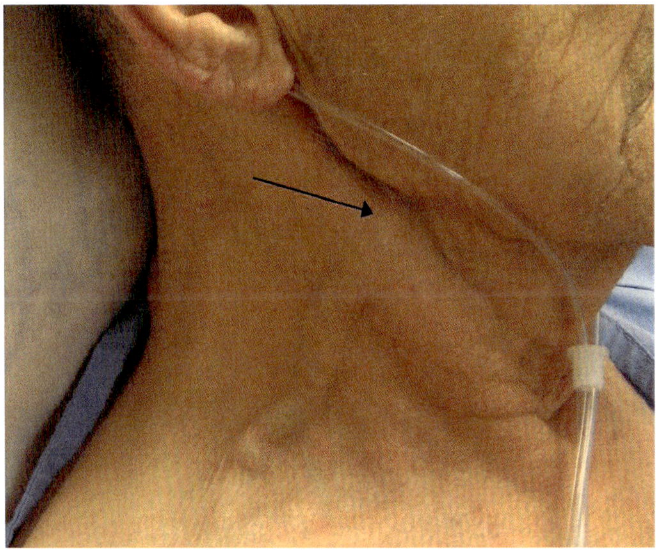

FIGURE 21.3.8 - Jugular Venous Distension

XII. Cardiac Tamponade: Diagnosis and Treatment
   A. Diagnosis
      1. ECG
      2. Echocardiography
   B. Treatment
      1. Urgent pericardiocentesis or pericardial window

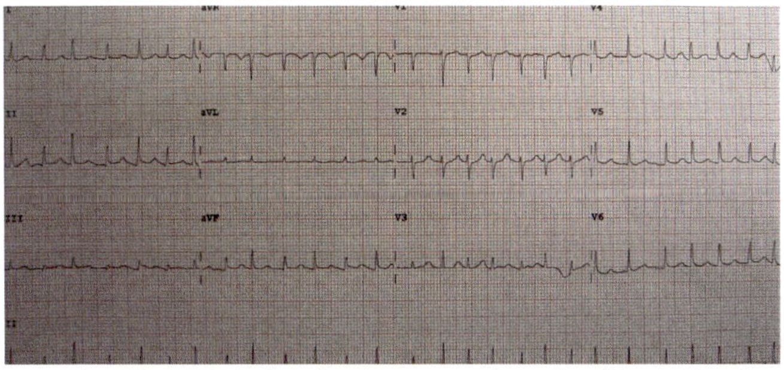

FIGURE 21.3.9 - ECG Showing Electrical Alternans

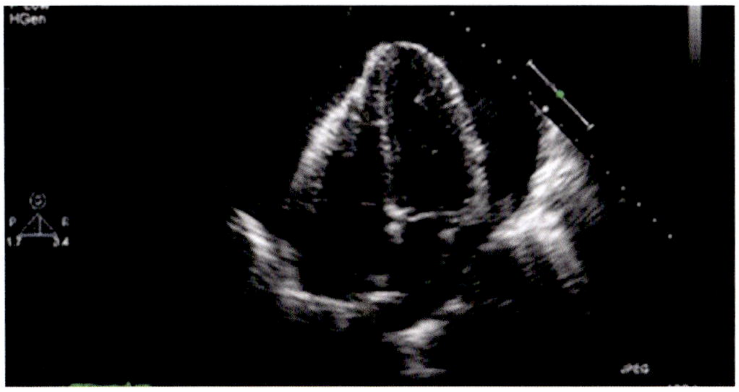

FIGURE 21.3.10 - Echocardiogram Showing Increased Pericardial Fluid

REVIEW QUESTIONS

1. How will the levels of serum potassium, phosphate, and calcium change in patients with tumor lysis syndrome?
    - **In patients with tumor lysis syndrome, serum potassium and phosphate will increase, while serum calcium will decrease.**
    - This is because potassium and phosphate will be released from cancer cells upon their death from chemotherapy.
    - The released phosphate will sequester calcium and therefore reduce its levels in the serum.

2. In patients with hypercalcemia of malignancy, will serum parathyroid hormone (PTH) be low or high relative to normal?
    - **In patients with hypercalcemia of malignancy, serum parathyroid hormone will be low.**
    - This is due to negative feedback that is exerted on the parathyroid glands by serum calcium.
    - This is in contrast to hypercalcemia that occurs as a result of primary hyperparathyroidism, in which it is the excessive production of PTH that drives the spike in serum calcium.

3. A 68-year-old woman is brought to the emergency department due to acute shortness of breath that started 1 hour ago. She has a past medical history of metastatic breast cancer for which she receives chemotherapy. Her vital signs include temperature of 37 °C (98.6 °F), blood pressure of 65/50 mmHg, heart rate of 150 beats/min, and respiratory rate of 17 breaths/min. The physical examination shows a jugular venous pressure of 11 cm and diminished heart sounds. ECG shows QRS complexes with varying amplitude. There are no ST segment changes or T wave abnormalities. Which of the following is the best next step in the diagnosis of this patient?

    A. Echocardiography
    B. Chest CT scan
    C. Serum CK-MB measurement
    D. Serum troponin measurement

    - **The correct answer is option A.**
    - This patient with a past medical history of metastatic breast cancer presents with Beck's triad.
    - The triad consists of severe hypotension, jugular venous distension, and diminished heart sounds. All these findings suggest the diagnosis of pericardial tamponade, possibly due to metastatic cancer.
    - Pericardial tamponade is further supported by the finding of electrical alternans, which refers to the alternating QRS amplitudes on ECG.
    - The best next step in the diagnosis of a patient suspected of having pericardial tamponade is echocardiography to assess for fluid in the pericardial space.
    - Option B is incorrect because a chest CT scan is time-consuming and the patient is hemodynamically unstable.
    - Options C and D are incorrect because serum CK-MB and troponin are measured when acute coronary syndrome is suspected.
    - This patient has no ST segment changes or T wave abnormalities on ECG. Additionally, the presence of Beck's triad indicates pericardial tamponade rather than acute coronary syndrome.

RENAL & GENITOURINARY

Renal/GU | Section 1: Renal Cystic Disease

I. ADPKD: Introduction
   A. Characterized by progressive cystic dilatation of the renal tubules
   B. Inherited as an autosomal dominant trait
   C. Mutation in *PKD1* and *PKD2* genes
   D. Can progress to Chronic Kidney Disease

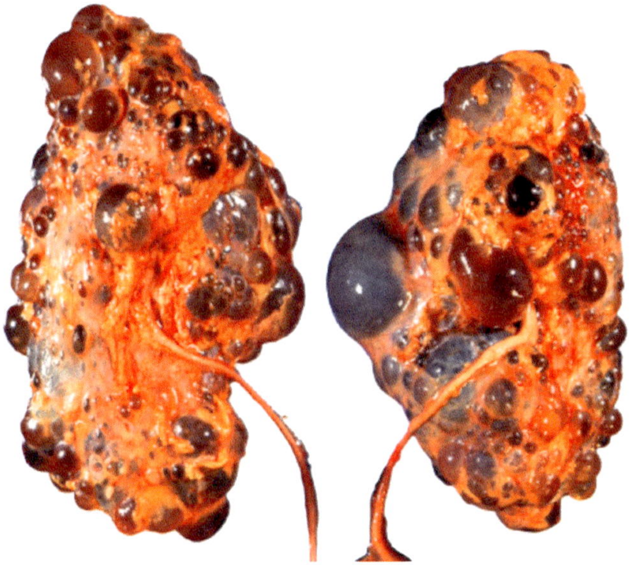

Credit: Centers for Disease Control and Prevention's Public Health Image Library (PHIL)

FIGURE 21.4.1 - Gross Image of Multiple Bilateral Cysts in the Kidneys

II. ADPKD: Clinical Features
   A. Usually asymptomatic until > 30 years
   B. Hematuria (due to rupture of cysts into the collecting system)
   C. Flank pain (sharp, localized pain)
   D. Hypertension
   E. Palpable kidneys

III. ADPKD: Associated Findings
   A. Intracerebral berry aneurysm (5-20% of cases)
   B. Cysts in liver, spleen, pancreas
   C. Kidney stones
   D. Infection of renal cyst
   E. Diverticula, hernia
   F. Mitral valve prolapse, aortic regurgitation

IV. ADPKD: Diagnosis
   A. Ultrasound - confirmatory, multiple bilateral cysts throughout the renal parenchyma
   B. CT scan, MRI
   C. Genetic testing

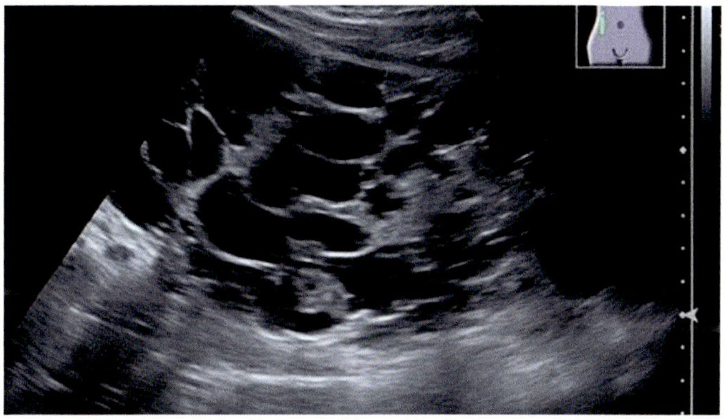

Kristoffer Lindskov Hansen, Michael Bachmann Nielsen and Caroline Ewertsen, CC BY 4.0 <https://creativecommons.org/licenses/by/4.0>, via Wikimedia Commons

FIGURE 21.4.2 - Ultrasound Image Showing Multiple Cysts in Polycystic Kidney Disease

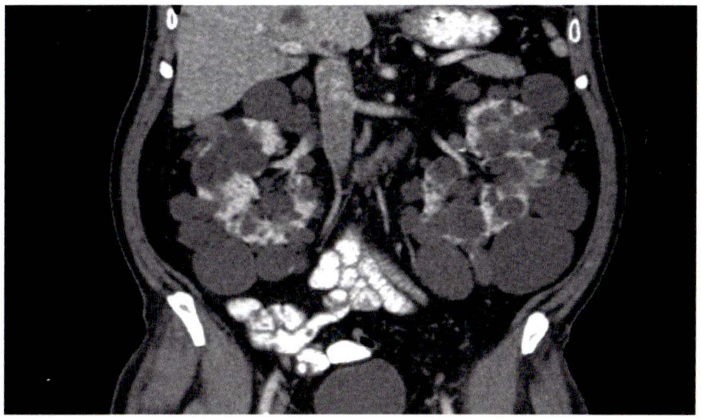

Own work, author: Steven Fruitsmaak

FIGURE 21.4.3 - CT Scan Showing Multiple Bilateral Cysts in Kidney

V. ADPKD: Treatment
   A. Anti-hypertensives: ACEIs, ARBs
   B. Infection: antibiotics
   C. ESRD: renal replacement therapy
   D. High fluid intake (unless GFR < 30ml/min/1.73m^2)

VI. ARPKD: Introduction
   A. Characterized by cystic dilatation of the renal collecting ducts
   B. Less common but more severe
   C. Autosomal recessive inheritance
   D. Mutations in *PKHD1 gene*

VII. ARPKD: Clinical features
   A. Hypertension (increased renin)
   B. Flank mass and distended abdomen
   C. Biliary dysgenesis (Caroli's disease, hepatic fibrosis, portal hypertension)
   D. Pulmonary insufficiency (secondary to lung hypoplasia)
   E. Death within first few days of life if associated with oligohydramnios (Potter's sequence)

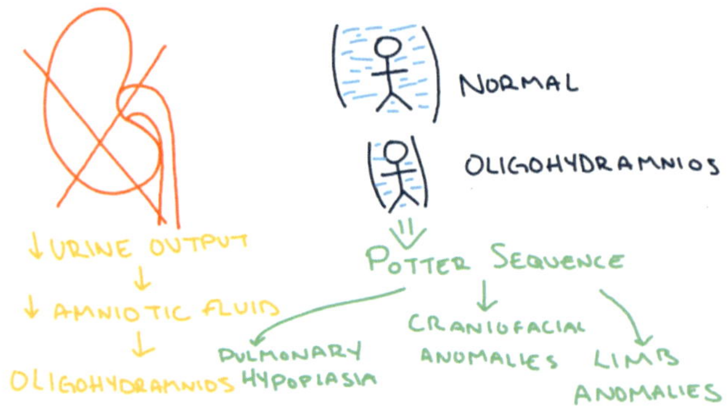

FIGURE 21.4.4 - Pathophysiology Behind Potter Sequence

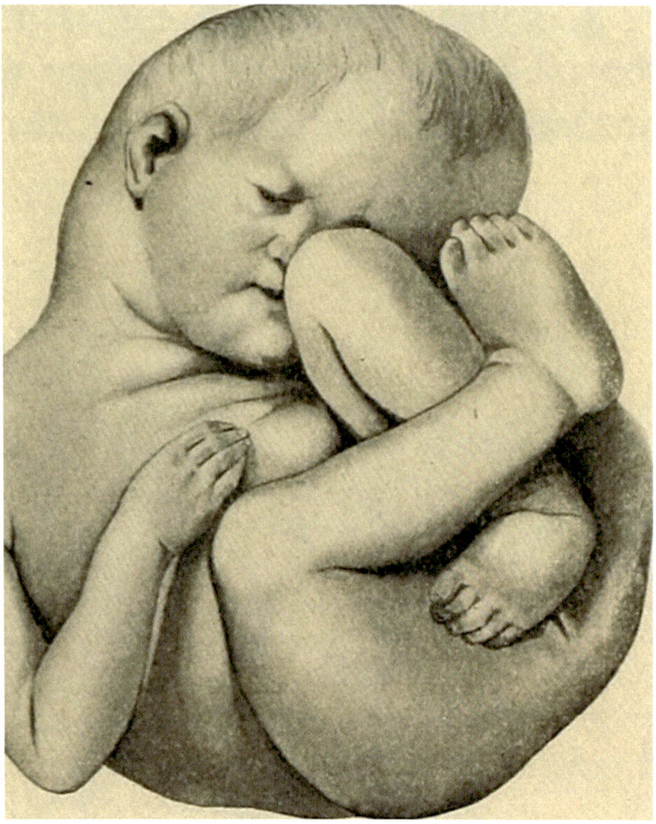

Public domain

FIGURE 21.4.5 - Potter Sequence

VIII. ARPKD: Diagnosis
- A. Ultrasound
  1. Prenatal renal and liver changes, oligohydramnios
  2. Bilateral enlarged kidneys with multiple renal cysts, hepatomegaly, dilated bile ducts, hepatic fibrosis
- B. CT scan, MRI
- C. Genetic testing

IX. ARPKD: Treatment
- A. No definite therapy
- B. Supportive respiratory care and mechanical ventilation
- C. Antihypertensive drugs (e.g. ACE inhibitors)
  1. Renal replacement therapy

X. Medullary Sponge Kidney: Introduction
- A. Congenital disorder
- B. Cystic dilatation of terminal collecting ducts
- C. Associated with Beckwith-Wiedemann Syndrome (WT2)

XI. Medullary Sponge Kidney: Clinical Features
- A. Asymptomatic
- B. Hematuria, flank pain
- C. Type 1 RTA, Nephrocalcinosis and recurrent nephrolithiasis
- D. Urinary tract infections

XII. Medullary Sponge Kidney: Diagnosis
- A. Intravenous pyelography
  1. "Bouquets of flowers" like appearance
- B. Others: CT scan, Ultrasound

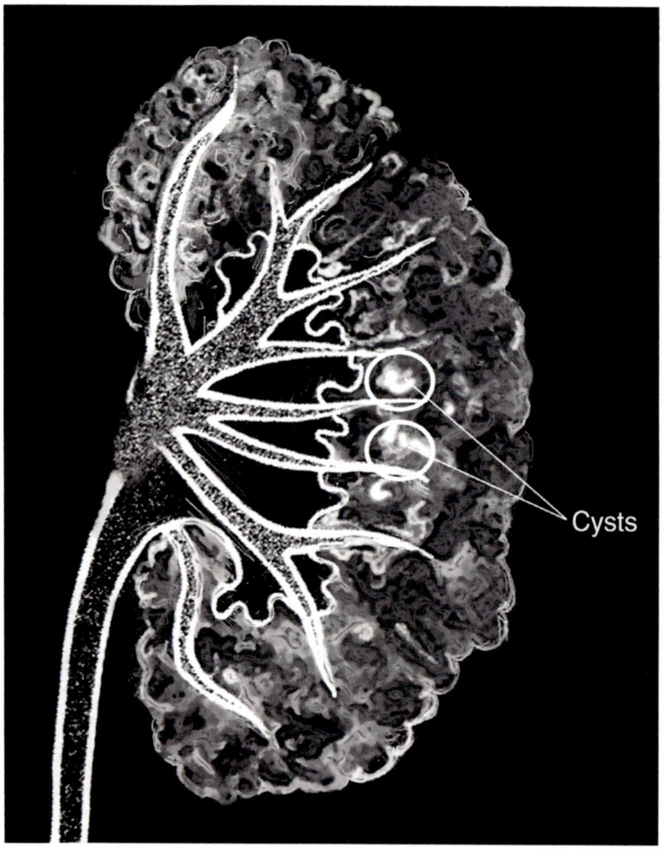

NIDDK, Public domain, via Wikimedia Commons

FIGURE 21.4.6 - "Bouquet of Flowers" Presentation in Medullary Sponge Kidney

XIII. Medullary Sponge Kidney: Treatment
- A. Antibiotics to treat UTI
- B. Prevention of stone formation
- C. Drugs
  1. Thiazides
  2. Potassium citrate

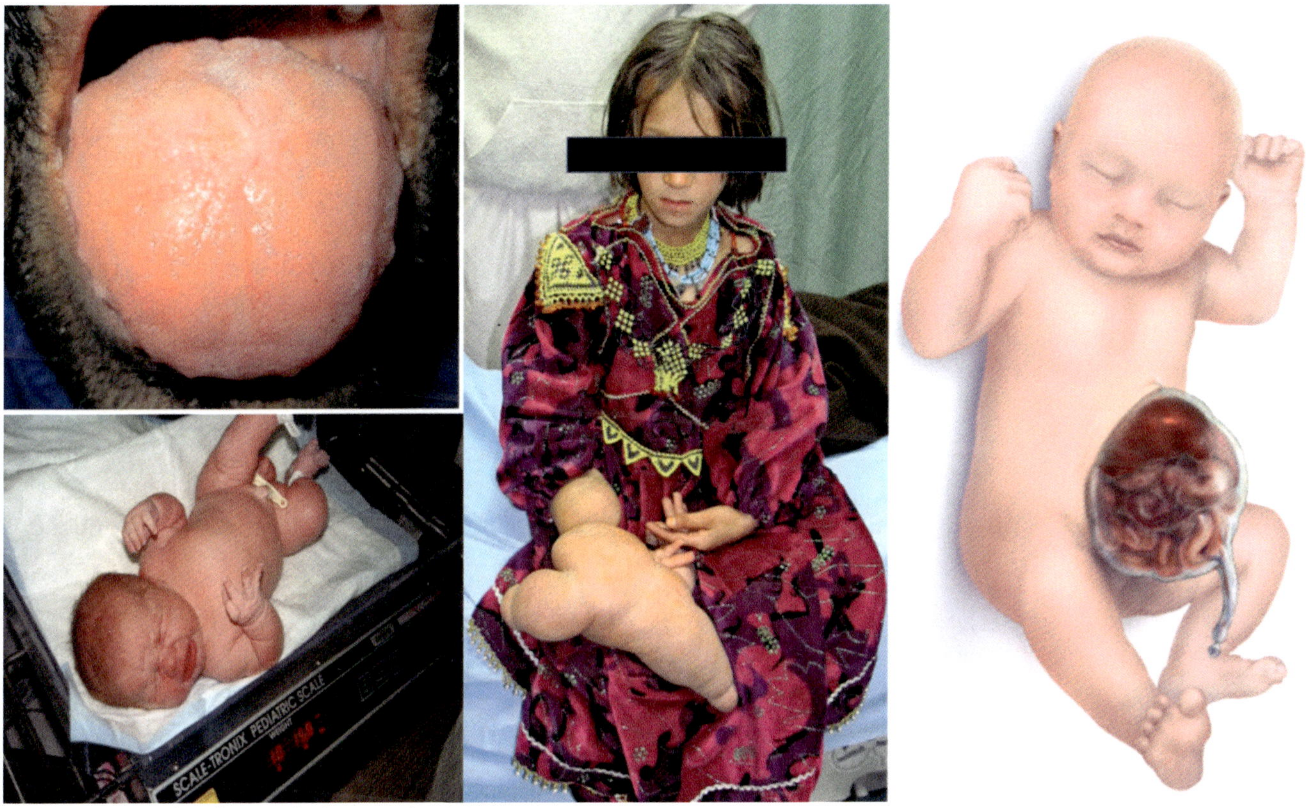

FIGURE 21.4.7 - Major Findings in Beckwith-Wiedemann Syndrome Patients

XIV. Simple Renal Cysts: Introduction

A. Most common
B. Incidence increases with age
C. Single or multiple and bilateral

XV. Simple Renal Cysts: Clinical Features

A. Asymptomatic
B. Hematuria, flank pain
C. Hypertension
D. Infection

XVI. Simple Renal Cysts: Diagnosis

A. Diagnosis: incidental
   1. Ultrasonography: round, well demarcated, anechoic mass
   2. CT scan

XVII. Simple Renal Cysts: Treatment

A. Not required unless symptomatic
B. Pain management by NSAIDs
C. Antibiotics

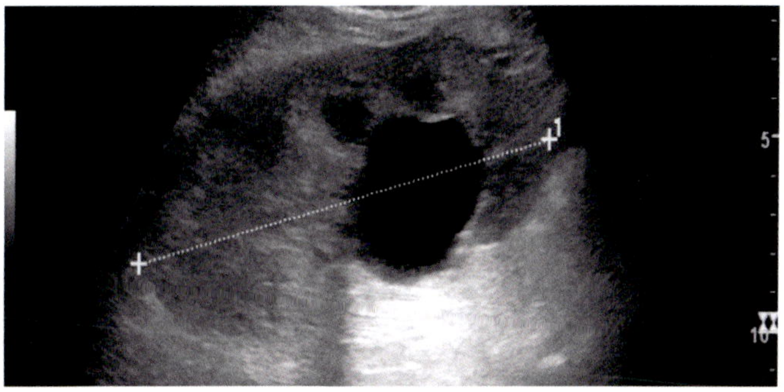

FIGURE 21.4.8 - Ultrasound Showing Simple Renal Cyst and a Well Demarcated Round Anechoic Mass

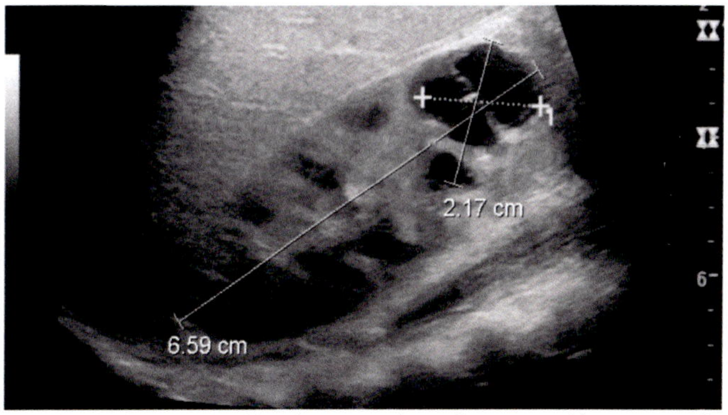

FIGURE 21.4.9 - Ultrasound Showing a Complex Renal Cyst with Thicker Walls with Septations

REVIEW QUESTIONS

1. A 45-year-old man comes to the emergency department because of a severe headache that started 2 hours ago. He describes it as the worst headache of his life. His past history is significant for polycystic kidney disease which was diagnosed 10 years ago. What is the best next step in management?
   - **The next best step would be to obtain a non-contrast CT of the brain to evaluate this patient for a potential subarachnoid hemorrhage.**
   - Patients with ADKPK are at risk of developing berry aneurysms.
   - Berry aneurysms are aneurysms that can develop in any part of the circle of Willis in the brain.
   - An aneurysm can rupture, leading to hemorrhage in the subarachnoid space.

2. What is the mechanism that leads to hypertension in patients with autosomal dominant polycystic kidney disease?
   - **The mechanism of hypertension in patients with ADPKD is as follows: Cysts → focal ischemia → decreased renal perfusion → RAAS upregulated → HTN**
   - Hypertension in patients with ADPKD is treated with either ACE-inhibitors or ARBs.
   - Both of these classes of medications inhibit the renin-angiotensin-aldosterone system, which is significantly revved up in patients with ADPKD.
   - The multiple cysts that form in the kidneys lead to focal ischemia and thus poor perfusion.
   - This process stimulates the RAAS to increase the blood pressure with a goal of increasing perfusion.
   - The resultant high blood pressure can be very deleterious and even speed up the rate of disease progression in patients with ADPKD.
   - Clinicians utilize ACE-inhibitors and ARBs to inhibit the RAAS and decrease the blood pressure.

3. A 28-year-old primigravida woman at her 38th week of gestation is brought to the emergency department by her husband because of labor pains for the past hour. An obstetric ultrasound shows oligohydramnios, clubbed feet, and multiple cysts in the kidneys bilaterally. What complication is anticipated in the newborn after delivery?
   - **The fetus will likely experience respiratory distress soon after delivery.**
   - The ultrasound findings described in the question stem suggest polycystic kidney disease based on the presence of multiple renal cysts and oligohydramnios.
   - Since this happened in utero, this is a case of autosomal recessive polycystic kidney disease (ARPKD) rather than autosomal dominant polycystic kidney disease (ADPKD), which typically presents in adulthood.
   - ARPKD significantly impairs renal function and thus significantly decreases the amount of urine produced by the fetus.
   - Since amniotic fluid is mostly made up of the baby's urine, ARPKD will lead to oligohydramnios or insufficient amniotic fluid in utero.
   - This can lead to fetal compression and pulmonary hypoplasia.
   - Fetal compression occurs because there is not enough amniotic fluid to cushion the fetus against the uterine wall.
   - Pulmonary hypoplasia occurs because amniotic fluid is necessary for proper development of the fetal lungs.

REVIEW QUESTIONS

4. A 12-year-old boy is brought to the clinic for an evaluation. His mom says he experienced five urinary tract infections over the past year. Physical examination is notable for macroglossia and hemihypertrophy with the boy's left arm and leg larger than his right arm and leg. Laboratory evaluation is notable for microscopic hematuria on urinalysis. Intravenous pyelography is obtained and it shows a "bouquets of flowers" appearance of kidneys. What is the most likely underlying diagnosis?

   - **This boy's macroglossia and hemihypertrophy, in conjunction with a likely diagnosis of medullary sponge kidney, are strongly suggestive of Beckwith-Wiedemann Syndrome as the underlying diagnosis.**
   - This boy likely has medullary sponge kidney disease.
   - The notable clues are recurrent urinary tract infections in a male, finding of microscopic hematuria on urinalysis, as well as the classic "bouquets of flowers" appearance of kidneys seen on intravenous pyelography.
   - Medullary sponge kidney disease is not the only diagnosis in this boy as it does not explain his macroglossia and notable hemihypertrophy.

5. A 34-year-old man comes to the emergency department because of bilateral flank pain and hematuria for the past 2 weeks. Past medical history is significant for multiple episodes of urinary tract infections which were treated with antibiotics. His father died at the age of 60 years due to an intracranial bleed. Vitals include temperature of 37.7° C (100° F), heart rate of 98 beats/minute and blood pressure of 150/90 mmHg in both arms. Physical examination shows non-tender flank masses which are palpable bilaterally. Ultrasound abdomen shows bilaterally enlarged kidneys with multiple anechoic masses. Microscopic urinalysis reveals RBCs at 8-10/hpf. What is the most likely diagnosis?

   A. Autosomal recessive polycystic kidney disease
   B. Autosomal dominant polycystic kidney disease
   C. Medullary sponge kidney
   D. Simple renal cyst
   E. Renal cell carcinoma
   F. Pheochromocytoma

- **The correct answer is option B.**
- This patient presented with bilateral flank pain and hematuria.
- His past history revealed multiple urinary tract infections and a positive family history as his father had an intracranial bleed which is suspicious of an intracranial aneurysm.
- Ultrasound findings further revealed bilateral enlarged kidneys with multiple anechoic masses.
- Microscopic urinalysis exam showed 8-10 RBCs/hpf suggestive of microscopic hematuria.
- This directs the diagnosis of this patient towards autosomal dominant polycystic kidney disease.
- Option A is incorrect because autosomal recessive polycystic kidney disease presents in infancy, not in adulthood.
- Option C is incorrect because ultrasound of medullary sponge kidney would reveal echogenic medullary pyramids, rather than bilaterally enlarged kidneys with multiple anechoic masses.
- Option D is incorrect because simple renal cysts are typically asymptomatic and unilateral. Additionally, ultrasound findings would show a single mass, rather than multiple masses.
- Option E is incorrect because it typically presents as painless hematuria and does not have the ultrasound findings described in the vignette. Furthermore, this patient does not have any risk factors to suggest renal cell carcinoma, such as smoking or exposure to azo dyes.
- Option F is incorrect because pheochromocytomas typically do not cause flank pain and hematuria. Rather, they present as cases of periodic extreme elevations in blood pressure or resistant hypertension.

Renal/GU | Section 2: Neoplasms: Renal Cell Carcinoma

I. Renal Cell Carcinoma: Definition
   A. Adenocarcinoma arising from proximal convoluted tubule (PCT)
   B. Most common 1° renal cancer
   C. Most commonly sporadic
   D. Can be part of von-Hippel-Lindau syndrome

II. Renal Cell Carcinoma: Risk Factors
   A. Male gender
   B. Age 50-70 years
   C. Smoking
   D. Obesity

III. Renal Cell Carcinoma: Clinical Presentation
   A. Classic triad
      1. Flank pain
      2. Palpable flank mass
      3. Hematuria
   B. Renal vein invasion and thrombosis
      1. Acute exacerbation of flank pain
      2. Hematuria
      3. Varicocele if left renal vein invasion
   C. Hematogenous metastasis to
      1. Lungs: cough, hemoptysis, SOB
      2. Bones: diffuse bone pain and tenderness
   D. Signs of hypercalcemia due to PTHrP production
      1. Kidney stones, bone pain, increased urinary frequency, abdominal pain, altered mental status
   E. Signs of polycythemia due to EPO production
      1. Headache
      2. Blurred vision
      3. Venous and arterial thrombosis
   F. Signs of Cushing syndrome due to ectopic ACTH production
      1. Truncal obesity, purple striae, thin extremities, “buffalo hump”, “moon facies”
   G. Refractory hypertension due to renin production

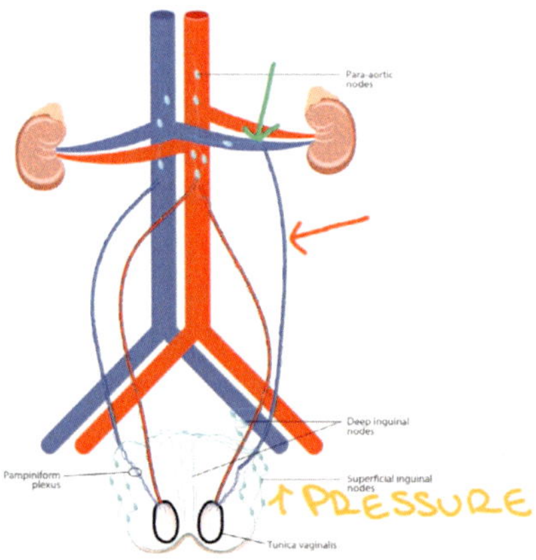

FIGURE 21.4.10 - Drainage of the Left and Right Spermatic Veins

IV. Renal Cell Carcinoma: Diagnosis
   A. Abdominal CT scan
      1. Irregular renal mass with internal septations
   B. Gross examination of surgically excised tumor
      1. Golden-yellow mass with internal septations
   C. Histological examination of surgically excised tumor
      1. Polygonal clear cells filled with carbohydrates and lipids

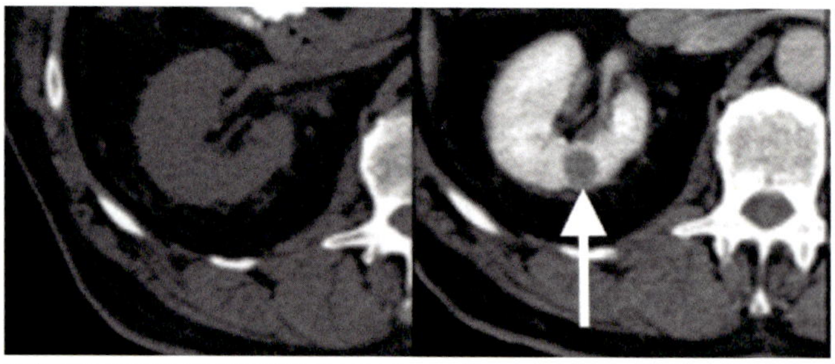

FIGURE 21.4.11 - Abdominal CT Scan With and Without Contrast Showing Renal Cell Carcinoma

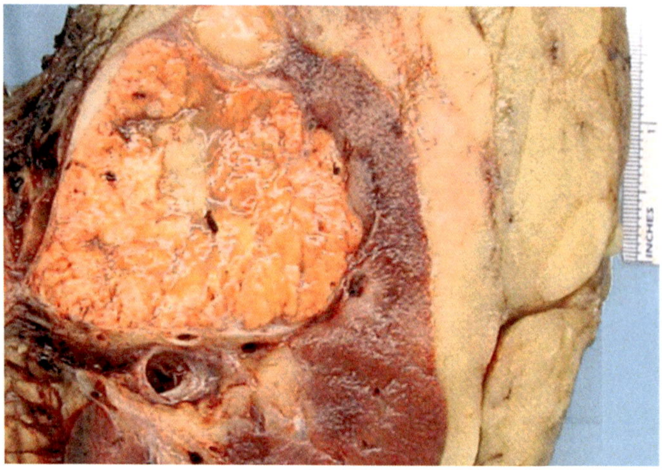

FIGURE 21.4.12 - Gross Morphological Image of Renal Cell Carcinoma

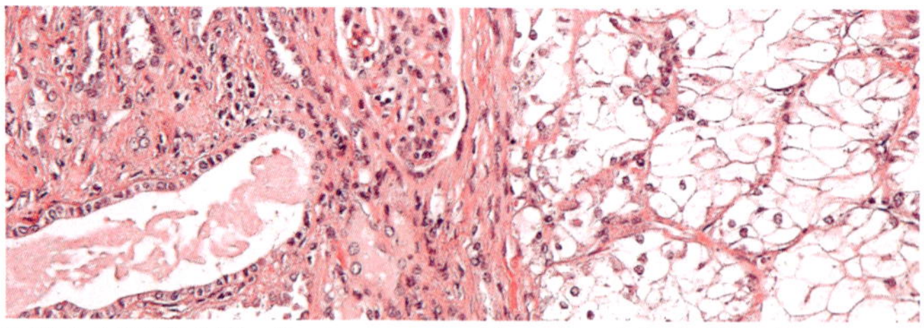

FIGURE 21.4.13 - Light Microscopy Showing Renal Cell Carcinoma

V. Renal Cell Carcinoma: Management
   A. Ipsilateral nephrectomy for early-stage disease
   B. Immunotherapy
      1. Aldesleukin (IL-2 analog)
      2. IFN-α
      3. Ipilimumab (CTLA-4 inhibitor)
   C. Resistant to chemotherapy and radiotherapy

REVIEW QUESTIONS

1. An 80-year-old woman is brought to the physician because of left flank pain, hematuria, and 20 kg of unintentional weight loss over the past 4 months. She has been smoking 3 packs of cigarettes per day for the last 40 years. Her BMI is normal. Abdominal CT scan with contrast shows an irregular mass in the left kidney with internal septations. What is the most likely risk factor for this patient's condition?

   - **Considering that she has been smoking 3 packs of cigarettes per day for the last 40 years, the most likely risk factor for her condition is her long-term smoking history.**
   - This patient presents with left flank pain, hematuria, and 20 kg of unintentional weight loss over the past 4 months.
   - Abdominal CT scan shows an irregular mass in the left kidney with internal septations.
   - This presentation is consistent with the diagnosis of renal cell carcinoma.

2. A 55-year-old man is brought to the emergency department because of increased urinary frequency, abdominal pain, constipation and confusion over the past 1 month. He has been smoking 2 packs of cigarettes per day for the last 40 years. His BMI is 40 kg/m^2. The patient was diagnosed with renal cell carcinoma 3 months ago. What is the most likely underlying mechanism of this patient's current symptoms?

   - **This patient's cancer likely produces parathyroid hormone related peptide (PTHrP) as a paraneoplastic syndrome which causes symptomatic hypercalcemia.**
   - This patient presents with increased urinary frequency, abdominal pain, constipation, and confusion.
   - These are consistent with the signs and symptoms of hypercalcemia.
   - He was diagnosed with renal cell carcinoma 3 months ago.

3. A 69-year-old man comes to the physician due to an unintentional weight loss of 25 kg and flank pain for the past 6 months. He has been smoking 2 packs of cigarettes per day for the last 50 years. His vital signs include temperature of 36° C (98.6° F), blood pressure of 170/95 mmHg, and heart rate of 79 beats/min. The physical examination shows no abnormalities. Urinalysis shows 30 red blood cells/hpf (Ref: < 3 RBCs/hpf) with no casts. An abdominal CT scan with contrast shows a complex left renal mass with irregular borders, internal septations, and calcifications. Which of the following parts of the nephron most likely gave rise to this patient's renal mass?

   A. Proximal convoluted tubule
   B. Loop of Henle
   C. Distal convoluted tubule
   D. Collecting tubule

   - **The correct answer is option A.**
   - This elderly man with a 100 pack-year smoking history reports an unintentional weight loss of 25 kg and flank pain for the past 6 months.
   - These clues increase suspicion for an underlying malignancy.
   - Urinalysis reveals 30 red blood cells/hpf with no casts.
   - The absence of casts indicates a non-glomerular hematuria.
   - An abdominal CT scan shows a complex left renal mass with irregular borders, internal septations, and calcifications.
   - All these malignant features suggest the diagnosis of renal cell carcinoma in this patient.
   - Renal cell carcinoma arises from the proximal convoluted tubule.
   - Option B and option C are incorrect because renal tumors do not arise from these segments of the nephron.
   - Option D is incorrect because this segment gives rise to a benign renal tumor known as oncocytoma. Oncocytoma is characterized by a benign-looking mass with regular borders and without internal septations on CT scan.

Renal/GU | Section 3: Prostate and Bladder Cancer

I. Prostate Cancer: Definition
   A. Adenocarcinoma most commonly arising from posterior lobe of prostate (vs. BPH)

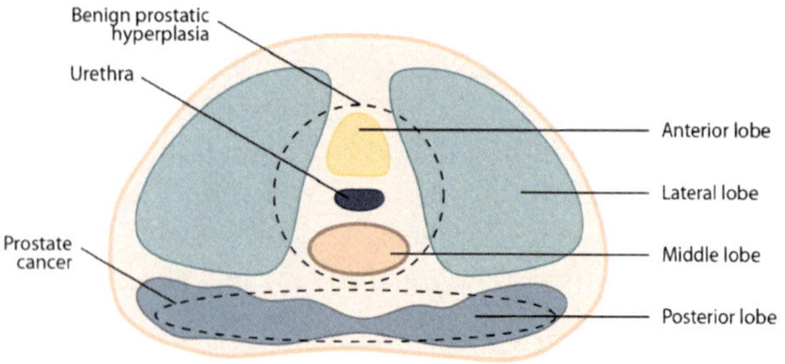

FIGURE 21.4.14 - Cross-Section of the Prostate Gland

II. Prostate Cancer: Risk Factors
   A. Age > 50 years
   B. African-American descent
   C. Positive family history

III. Prostate Cancer: Clinical Presentation
   A. Nonspecific
      1. Weight loss
      2. Fatigue, low-grade fever
   B. Symptoms due to local expansion
      1. Difficulty initiating urination
      2. Weak urine flow
      3. Hematuria
   C. Symptoms due to metastasis
      1. Lower back pain (vertebral metastasis via Batson plexus)
      2. Diffuse bone pain

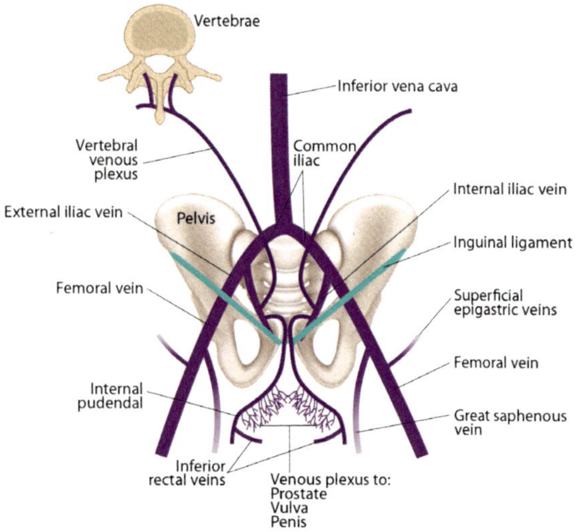

FIGURE 21.4.15 - Batson or Vertebral Venous Plexus

IV. Prostate Cancer: Diagnosis
   A. Initial laboratory investigations
      1. ↑ Total PSA with ↓ fraction of free PSA (vs. BPH)
      2. ↑ Prostatic acid phosphatase (PAP)
   B. Confirmatory investigation
      1. Ultrasound-guided transrectal core needle biopsy
      2. Histologically graded via Gleason grade
      3. Mucin positive cells arranged in tubules
   C. Studies for metastatic disease
      1. ↑ Alkaline phosphatase (ALP)
      2. Normal gamma-glutamyl transferase (GGT)
   D. Bone scan
      1. Metabolically active osteoblastic metastasis with increased radiotracer uptake

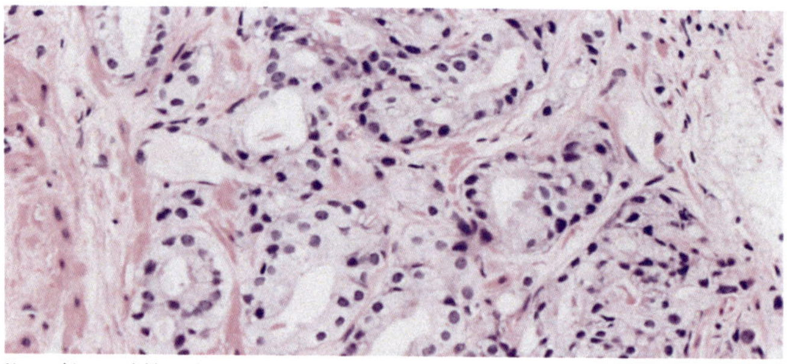

FIGURE 21.4.16 - Light Microscopy Showing Prostate Cancer

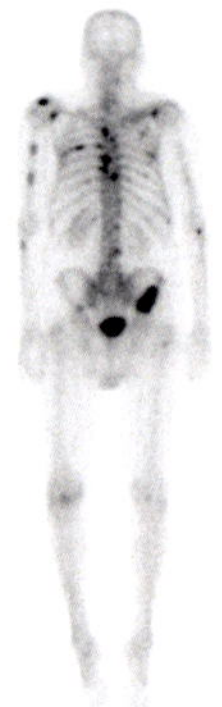

FIGURE 21.4.17 - Bone Scan Showing Metastatic Osteoblastic Lesions of Prostate Cancer

V. Prostate Cancer: Management
   A. Prostatectomy for early-stage disease
   B. Chemotherapy
   C. Radiation therapy
      1. External radiation therapy
         a) External device sends radiation beam to prostate cancer
      2. Brachytherapy
         a) Surgical insertion of radioactive material in the prostate

VI. Bladder Cancer: Definition
   A. Malignancy of bladder epithelium
   B. Two histological subtypes
      1. Most common: transitional cell (urothelial) carcinoma
      2. Squamous cell carcinoma

VII. Bladder Cancer: Risk Factors
   A. Transitional cell carcinoma ("**P**ee **SAC**")
      1. **P**henacetin
      2. **S**moking
      3. **A**niline dyes (industrial exposure)
      4. **C**yclophosphamide
   B. Squamous cell carcinoma (4 S's)
      1. ***S**chistosoma haematobium* (Middle Eastern water sources)
      2. Chronic "**S**ystitis" (cystitis)
      3. **S**moking
      4. Chronic kidney **S**tones

VIII. Bladder Cancer: Clinical Presentation
   A. Non-specific symptoms
      1. Fever
      2. Weight loss
      3. Fatigue
   B. Urinary symptoms
      1. Painless hematuria

IX. Bladder Cancer: Diagnosis
   A. Urinalysis
      1. ≥ 3 RBCs/hpf
   B. Urine microscopy
      1. No casts (non-glomerular bleeding)
   C. Renal function tests (e.g. BUN, creatinine)
      1. Normal unless bilateral ureter obstruction from tumor
      2. Bilateral ureter obstruction: postrenal AKI
   D. Cystoscopy
      1. Fungating mass with possible ulceration and necrosis
   E. Biopsy
      1. Transitional cell carcinoma
   F. Papillae with dysplastic urothelium and fibrovascular core
      1. Squamous cell carcinoma
   G. Keratin pearls and intercellular bridges (desmosomes)

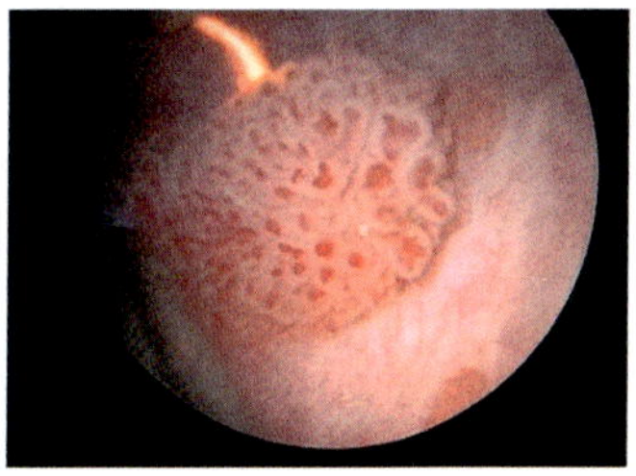

FIGURE 21.4.18 - Cystoscopy Showing Bladder Cancer

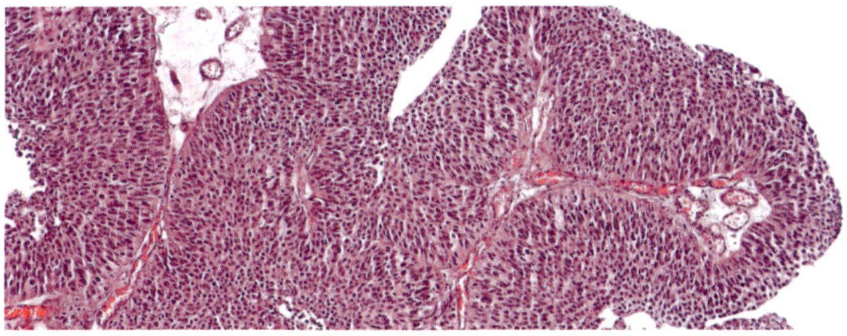

FIGURE 21.4.19 - Histological Image of Transitional Cell Carcinoma of Bladder

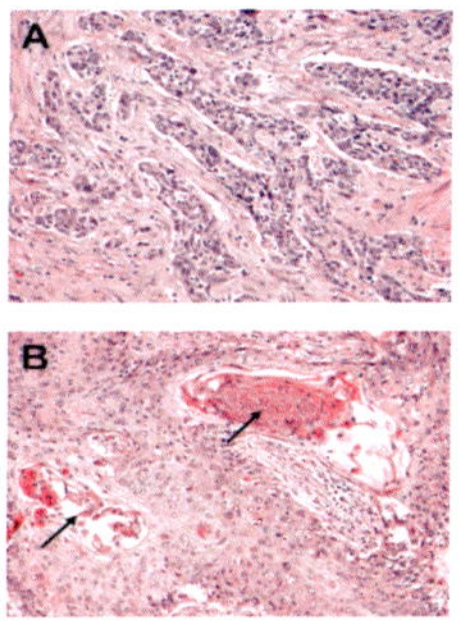

FIGURE 21.4.20 - Light Microscopy Showing Squamous Cell Carcinoma of Bladder

X. Bladder Cancer: Management
   A. Surgical excision for early-stage disease
   B. Chemotherapy
   C. Radiation therapy

Condition	Key Features	Management
Prostate cancer	- Arises from posterior lobe of prostate - ↑ PAP and protein-bound PSA - Risk factors: age > 50 years, African-American descent	- Prostatectomy - Chemotherapy - External radiation therapy - Brachytherapy
Bladder cancer	- Transitional cell carcinoma (most common): phenacetin, smoking, aniline dyes, cyclophosphamide - Squamous cell carcinoma: *Schistosoma haematobium*, chronic cystitis, smoking, chronic kidney stones	- Surgical excision - Chemotherapy - Radiotherapy
Renal cell carcinoma	- Most common 1° renal cancer - Most commonly sporadic - Rarely associated with von-Hippel-Lindau syndrome - Risk factors: male at 50-70 years, smoking	- Ipsilateral nephrectomy - Immunotherapy (e.g. aldesleukin, ipilimumab) - Resistant to chemotherapy and radiotherapy

TABLE 21.4.1 - Summary of Genitourinary Neoplasms

REVIEW QUESTIONS

1. A 70-year-old African American man comes to the physician because of hematuria, difficulty initiating urine stream, and weight loss of 15 kgs over the past 3 months. A digital rectal exam reveals nodularity of the prostate gland. His total PSA is 20 ng/mL (0-4 ng/mL). What is the next best step in the management of this patient?

- **The next best step in the management of the patient with suspected prostate cancer is transrectal, ultrasound-guided core needle biopsy of the prostate gland.**
- This patient presents with hematuria, difficulty initiating urine stream, and weight loss of 15 kg over the past 3 months.
- The digital rectal exam reveals nodularity of the prostate gland.
- His total PSA is 20 ng/mL.
- All these findings point towards the diagnosis of prostate cancer.

2. A 55-year-old woman comes to the physician because of painless hematuria and unintentional weight loss of 12 kg over the last 3 months. She has worked as a hair stylist for the last 35 years. She is a lifetime nonsmoker. She takes no medications. Cystoscopy reveals a fungating mass in the bladder mucosa with central ulceration and necrosis. What is the most likely risk factor for this patient's current condition?

- **The most likely risk factor for this patient is aniline dyes which predisposed her to the development of bladder cancer.**
- This patient presents with painless hematuria and unintentional weight loss of 12 kg over the last 3 months.
- Cystoscopy reveals a fungating mass in the bladder mucosa with central ulceration and necrosis.
- This presentation is consistent with the diagnosis of bladder cancer.
- Considering that she has worked as a hair stylist for the last 35 years, she has likely been exposed to aniline dyes.

3. A 57-year-old man comes to the physician reporting red urine for the past 4 weeks. He is a businessman and he frequently travels to the Middle East. He is a lifetime nonsmoker. His vital signs include temperature of 37° C (98.6° F), blood pressure of 130/85 mmHg, and heart rate of 81 beats/min. The physical examination shows no abnormalities. Urinalysis is significant for 100 red blood cells/hpf without RBC casts (Ref: < 3 RBCs/hpf). Cystoscopy reveals an exophytic mass in the bladder with central ulceration. Biopsy of the mass is taken and it shows keratin pearls and intercellular bridges under microscopy. Which of the following microbes is most likely responsible for this patient's current condition?

   A. Schistosoma mansoni
   B. Schistosoma haematobium
   C. Clonorchis sinensis
   D. Diphyllobothrium latum

- **The correct answer is option B.**
- This man with a past history of frequent travels to the Middle East presents with red urine.
- He has a non-glomerular hematuria confirmed by urinalysis findings of 100 red blood cells/hpf without RBC casts.
- Cystoscopy reveals an exophytic mass in the bladder with central ulceration.
- Biopsy shows keratin pearls and intercellular bridges.
- All these clues indicate the diagnosis of squamous cell carcinoma of the bladder.
- The microbe most likely responsible for this patient's bladder cancer is *Schistosoma haematobium*.
- *Schistosoma haematobium* is a trematode transmitted by skin exposure to contaminated water. This infection is prevalent in Middle Eastern countries.
- Option A, *Schistosoma mansoni*, is incorrect because this trematode is known to cause hepatic fibrosis and portal hypertension rather than bladder cancer.
- Option C, *Clonorchis sinensis*, is incorrect because this trematode causes biliary tract diseases such as cholangiocarcinoma rather than bladder cancer.
- Option D, *Diphyllobothrium latum*, is incorrect because this cestode causes B_{12} deficiency anemia, not bladder cancer.

Renal/GU | Section 4: Neoplasms: Testicular Cancer & Penile Cancer

I. Testicular Cancer: Definition
   A. Malignancy of testicular cells
   B. Two groups
      1. Germ cell tumors
      2. Non-germ cell tumors
         a) Sex cord stromal tumors
         b) Lymphoma
   C. Most common in young men

II. Testicular Cancer: Risk Factors
   A. Cryptorchidism
      1. ↑ temperature → malignant degeneration of germ cells, Leydig cells, or Sertoli cells
   B. Klinefelter syndrome
      1. Dysgenesis of seminiferous tubules → germ cell tumors
      2. Leydig cell dysfunction → sex cord stromal tumors

III. Testicular Cancer: Clinical Presentation
   A. Painless swelling in the testicle that does not transilluminate (vs. hydrocele)
   B. Dull ache in groin and lower abdomen
   C. Sensation of heaviness in the scrotum

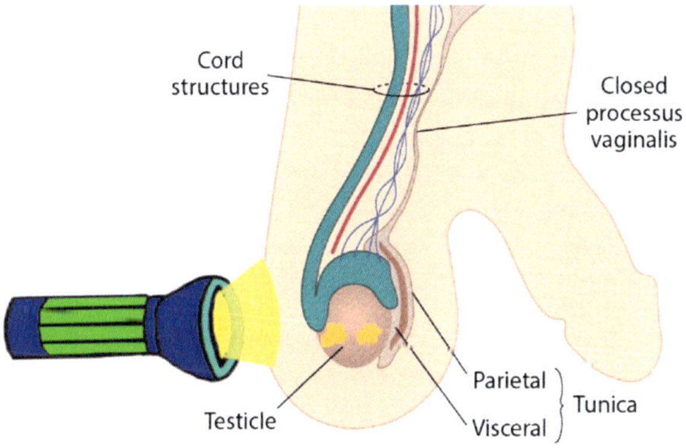

FIGURE 21.4.21 - Transillumination Test in Testicular Cancer

IV. Testicular Cancer: Diagnosis
   A. Testicular ultrasound
      1. Ultrasound features depend on the specific subtype of testicular cancer
   B. Abdominal CT scan
      1. Looks for metastasis to para-aortic lymph nodes
   C. Biopsy avoided due to risk of scrotal seeding during procedure
   D. Testicle completely excised and microscopically examined
   E. Histological exam of surgically excised testicle
      1. Germ cell tumors
         a) Seminoma, embryonal carcinoma, teratoma, yolk sac tumor, choriocarcinoma
      2. Sex cord stromal tumors
         a) Leydig cell tumor, Sertoli cell tumor
      3. Testicular lymphoma (common in elderly men)
   F. Seminoma
      1. Most common testicular germ cell tumor
      2. Malignant, homogenous mass analogous to ovarian dysgerminoma
      3. Large cells with watery cytoplasm and "fried egg" appearance
      4. ↑ placental ALP (PALP)
      5. Late metastasis: good prognosis
   G. Embryonal carcinoma
      1. Painful hemorrhagic mass with necrosis
      2. ↑ hCG and normal AFP if pure embryonal carcinoma (rare)
      3. ↑ hCG and ↑ AFP if mixed with other tumor types (common)
   H. Teratoma
      1. Malignant in adult males; benign in boys
      2. Derivatives of ectoderm, mesoderm, and endoderm
   I. Yolk sac tumor (endodermal sinus tumor)
      1. Most common testicular tumor in boys < 3 years old
      2. Malignant, yellow, mucinous tumor
      3. Schiller-Duval bodies: glomeruloid structures
      4. ↑↑ AFP
   J. Choriocarcinoma
      1. Malignant tumor of syncytiotrophoblasts and cytotrophoblasts
      2. No villi
      3. Hematogenous spread to lungs and brain
      4. ↑↑ hCG
         a) Gynecomastia (hCG similar to LH)
         b) Hyperthyroidism (hCG similar to TSH)
   K. Leydig cell tumor
      1. Benign golden-colored tumor with Reinke crystals (eosinophilic cytoplasmic inclusions)
      2. Produces androgens or estrogens → precocious puberty or gynecomastia
   L. Sertoli cell tumor (androblastoma): benign
   M. Testicular lymphoma: elderly men; diffuse large B-cell lymphoma

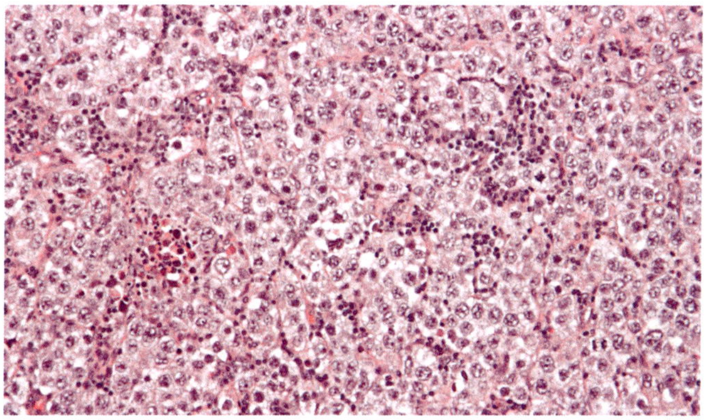

FIGURE 21.4.22 - Light Microscopy of Seminoma

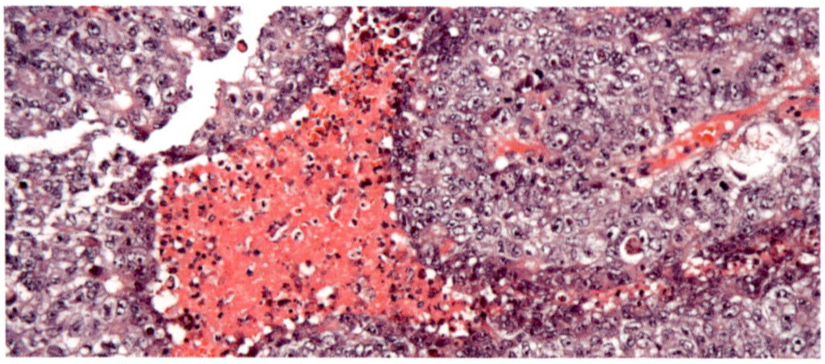

FIGURE 21.4.23 - Light Microscopy of Embryonal Carcinoma

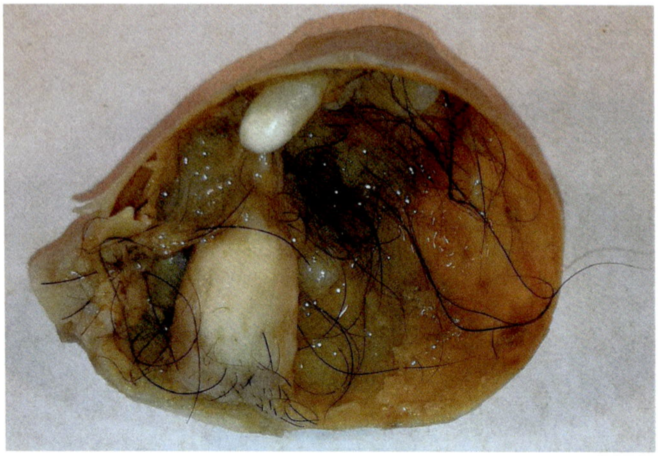

FIGURE 21.4.24 - Gross Picture of a Teratoma

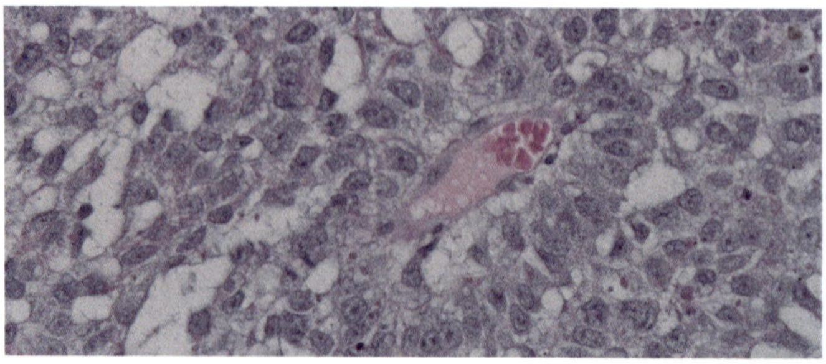

FIGURE 21.4.25 - Light Microscopy Showing Schiller-Duval Bodies in Yolk Sac Tumor

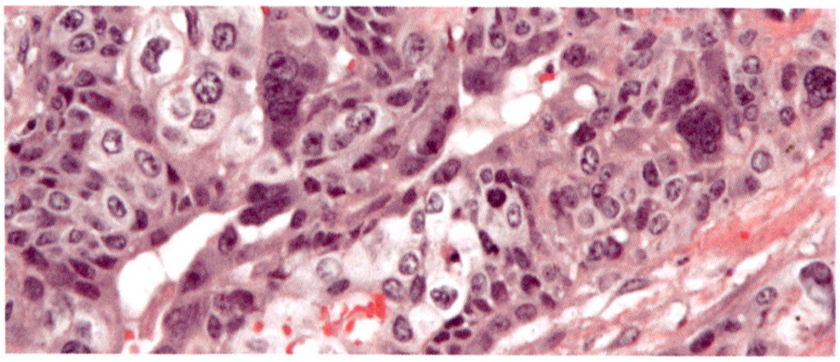

FIGURE 21.4.26 - Light Microscopy of Choriocarcinoma

V. Testicular Cancer: Management
   A. Radical orchiectomy before histologic diagnosis
   B. Chemotherapy
   C. Radiation therapy

Testicular Cancer	Key Features
Seminoma	- Most common testicular germ cell tumor - Large cells with watery cytoplasm and “fried egg” appearance - ↑ Placental alkaline phosphatase (PALP) - Excellent prognosis due to late metastasis
Embryonal carcinoma	- Painful hemorrhagic mass with necrosis - ↑ hCG and normal AFP if pure embryonal carcinoma (rare) - ↑ hCG and ↑ AFP if mixed with other tumor types (common)
Teratoma	- Malignant in adult males - Benign in boys - Derivatives of ectoderm, mesoderm, and endoderm
Yolk sac tumor	- Most common testicular tumor in boys < 3 years - Schiller-Duval bodies: glomeruloid structures - ↑↑ AFP
Choriocarcinoma	- Malignant tumor of syncytiotrophoblasts and cytotrophoblasts - Hematogenous spread to lungs and brain - ↑↑ hCG - Gynecomastia - Hyperthyroidism
Leydig cell tumor	- Benign golden-colored tumor - Reinke crystals (eosinophilic cytoplasmic inclusions) - Gynecomastia (estrogen) - Precocious puberty (androgen)
Sertoli cell tumor	- Androblastoma - Benign
Testicular lymphoma	- Common in elderly men - Diffuse large B-cell lymphoma

TABLE 21.4.2 - Testicular Cancer Types

VI. Penile Cancer: Definition
   A. Squamous cell carcinoma of penile epithelium
   B. Prevalent in Africa, Asia, and South America

VII. Penile Cancer: Risk Factors
   A. Lack of circumcision
   B. High risk human papillomavirus (HPV 16 & 18) infection

VIII. Penile Cancer: Clinical Presentation
   A. Plaque on glans penis or penile shaft
   B. +/- enlarged superficial inguinal lymph nodes
   C. Precursor in situ lesions
      1. Bowen disease
      2. Erythroplasia of Queyrat
      3. Bowenoid papulosis
   D. Bowen disease
      1. Leukoplakia (white plaque) on penile shaft
   E. Erythroplasia of Queyrat
      1. Erythroplakia (red plaque) on glans penis
   F. Bowenoid papulosis
      1. Dark red or brown papules on penile shaft and groin
      2. Unclear malignant potential

IX. Penile Cancer: Diagnosis
   A. Biopsy of penile plaque and superficial inguinal lymph nodes
      1. Keratin pearls and intercellular bridges

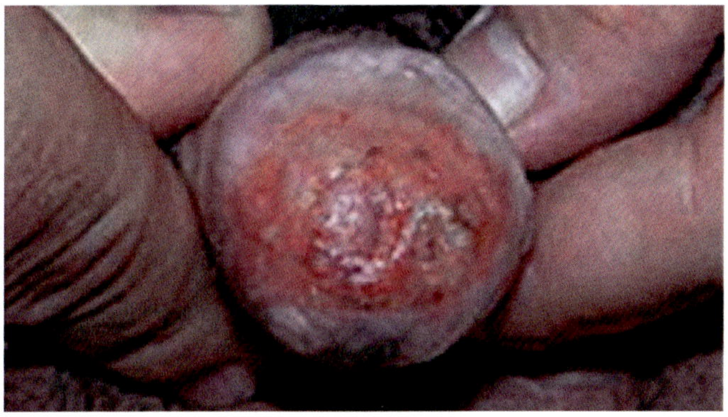

FIGURE 21.4.27 - Erythroplasia of Queyrat

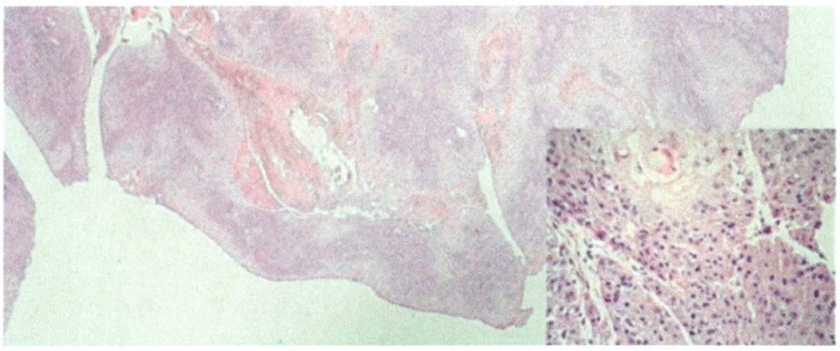

FIGURE 21.4.28 - Light Microscopy Showing Keratin Pearls in Squamous Cell Carcinoma

X. Penile Cancer: Management
   A. Surgical excision of penile lesion +/- superficial inguinal lymph nodes
   B. Chemotherapy
   C. Radiation therapy

Condition	Key Features	Management
Prostate cancer	- Arises from posterior lobe of prostate - ↑ PAP and protein-bound PSA - Risk factors: age > 50 years, African-American descent	- Prostatectomy - Chemotherapy - External radiation therapy - Brachytherapy
Bladder cancer	- Transitional cell carcinoma (most common): phenacetin smoking, aniline dyes, cyclophosphamide - Squamous cell carcinoma: *Schistosoma haematobium*, chronic cystitis, smoking, chronic kidney stones	- Surgical excision - Chemotherapy - Radiotherapy
Renal cell carcinoma	- Most common 1° renal cancer - Most commonly sporadic - Rarely associated with von-Hippel-Lindau syndrome - Risk factors: male at 50-70 years, smoking	- Ipsilateral nephrectomy - Immunotherapy (e.g. aldesleukin, ipilimumab) - Resistant to chemotherapy and radiotherapy
Testicular cancer	- Germ cell tumors - Sex cord stromal tumors - Lymphoma - Risk factors: Cryptorchidism, Klinefelter syndrome	- Radical orchiectomy - Chemotherapy - Radiotherapy
Penile cancer	- Carcinoma in situ lesions: Bowen disease, Erythroplasia of Queyrat, Bowenoid papulosis - Risk factors: Lack of circumcision, HPV 16 & 18	- Surgical excision of penile plaque +/- superficial inguinal lymph nodes - Chemotherapy - Radiotherapy

TABLE 21.4.3 - Summary of Genitourinary Neoplasms

REVIEW QUESTIONS

1. A 35-year-old man comes to the office because of a left testicular mass, scrotal heaviness, and weight loss for the past 3 months. The physical examination shows a left testicular mass that does not transilluminate with the penlight. He has high placental alkaline phosphatase (PALP) levels. A radical orchiectomy is performed. Gross examination shows a homogenous mass. Histological exam of the mass shows large cells with watery cytoplasm. What is the most likely histological type of testicular tumor in this patient?
   - **All these findings are consistent with the diagnosis of seminoma, the most common germ cell tumor of the testicle.**
   - This patient presents with a left testicular mass, scrotal heaviness, and weight loss.
   - He has high placental alkaline phosphatase (PALP) levels.
   - Gross exam of the surgical specimen reveals a homogenous mass.
   - Histological exam, on the other hand, shows large cells with watery cytoplasm.

2. A 46-year-old man underwent a radical orchiectomy for testicular cancer. Histological examination of the surgical specimen shows intracellular eosinophilic inclusions. The physical exam reveals bilateral gynecomastia. What is the most likely pathophysiologic mechanism of this patient's physical exam finding?
   - **Leydig cell tumors can produce estrogens resulting in breast tissue hyperplasia and gynecomastia.**
   - This patient underwent a radical orchiectomy for testicular cancer.
   - The physical exam reveals bilateral gynecomastia.
   - The histological exam of the surgical specimen reveals intracellular eosinophilic inclusions.
   - This description is consistent with Reinke crystals in Leydig cell tumors.

3. A 55-year-old man comes to the physician due to a penile lesion that he first noticed 6 months ago. He has lost 15 kg over the last 3 months. He is uncircumcised. He engages in unprotected sexual intercourse with both men and women. His past medical history is significant for genital warts treated with topical therapy. Vital signs include temperature of 37° C (98.6° F), blood pressure of 135/75 mmHg, heart rate of 86 beats/min, and respiratory rate of 14 breaths/min. The physical examination shows a white plaque on the penile shaft. Which of the following is the best next step in the management of this patient?

   A. Topical podophyllin
   B. Topical salicylic acid
   C. Pelvic ultrasound
   D. Biopsy

   - **The correct answer is option D.**
   - This patient presents with a penile lesion and 15 kg weight loss.
   - He is uncircumcised.
   - He engages in unprotected sexual intercourse with both men and women.
   - The physical exam reveals a white plaque on the penile shaft.
   - This presentation is concerning penile cancer.
   - The best next step in the management of the patient with suspected penile cancer is to biopsy the penile lesion.
   - Option A, topical podophyllin, and option B, topical salicylic acid, are incorrect because they are used in the treatment of genital warts.
   - Before starting the treatment, it should be determined whether this lesion is a cancer or a genital wart by performing a biopsy.
   - Option C, pelvic ultrasound, is incorrect because it is not used to diagnose penile cancer.

Renal/GU | Section 5: Scrotal Swelling

I. Testicular Torsion: Introduction
   A. Acute condition
   B. Sudden onset scrotal pain and swelling
   C. Twisting of the spermatic cord and obstruction of blood flow
   D. Defect in processus vaginalis

II. Testicular Torsion: Pathophysiology
   A. Congenital defect of the processus vaginalis
      1. Twisting of the spermatic cord along its axis
      2. Upward and transverse displacement of the testis
      3. Diminished or absent blood flow to the affected testis
   B. Physical exertion or trauma

III. Testicular Torsion: Risk Factors
   A. Neonates, young male (12-18 years commonly)
   B. Bell-clapper deformity
   C. Blunt trauma
   D. Previous history of testicular torsion
   E. Undescended testis
   F. Iatrogenic

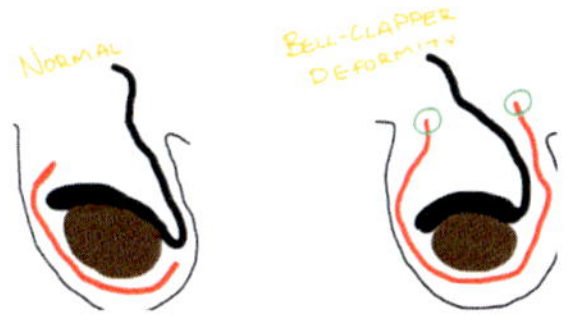

FIGURE 21.4.29 - Normal Testis vs. Bell-Clapper Deformity

IV. Testicular Torsion: Clinical Presentation
   A. Testicular pain (within 24 hours)
   B. Nausea/vomiting
   C. Upward displaced testis
   D. Cremasteric reflex: absent
   E. Prehn's sign: negative

V. Testicular Torsion: Diagnosis
   A. Clinical diagnosis (emergency)
   B. Doppler ultrasound (confirmatory)
      1. Diminished or absent blood flow to affected testes
      2. Twisting of spermatic cord
   C. Urinalysis: to rule out UTI and epididymo-orchitis

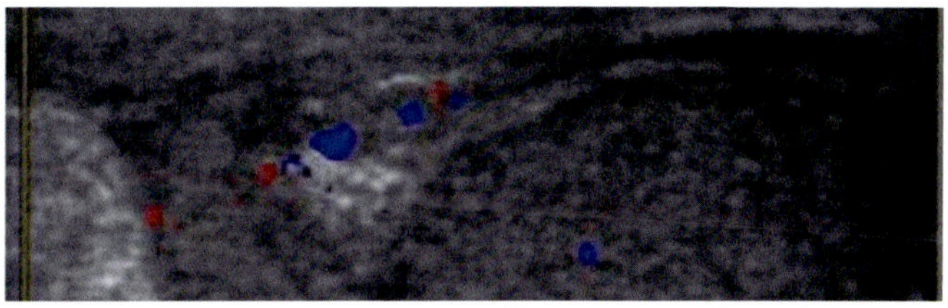

FIGURE 21.4.31 - Doppler Image Showing Testicular Torsion Impeding the Normal Blood Flow

VI. Testicular Torsion: Treatment
   A. Emergency
      1. Manual detorsion and bilateral elective orchiopexy (< 2 hours)
      2. Surgical detorsion
      3. Orchiectomy

VII. Epididymitis: Introduction
   A. Infection of the epididymis
   B. Most common cause of scrotal pain in adults
   C. Acute
   D. Chronic (> 6 weeks)

VIII. Epididymitis: Etiology
   A. Infectious
      1. UTI: *E.coli* (most common), *Pseudomonas*, other coliforms
      2. Commonly seen in children and elderly

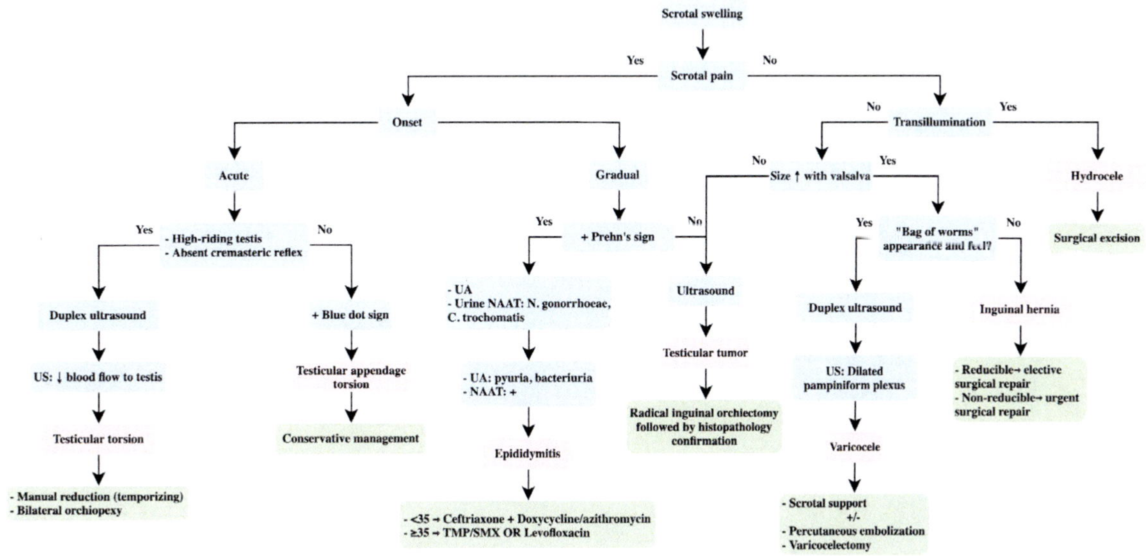

FIGURE 21.4.30 - Clinical Process of Testicular Torsion

3. STDs: *N. gonorrhoeae*, *C. trachomatis* (age < 35, sexually active)

B. Non-infectious: trauma, auto-immune

IX. Epididymitis: Risk Factors
- A. Sexually active males (STDs)
- B. Obstructive uropathy
- C. Trauma

X. Epididymitis: Clinical Presentation
- A. Gradual testicular pain and swelling
- B. Scrotal erythema/cellulitis
- C. Prehn's sign: positive
- D. Cremasteric reflex: present
- E. Fever, dysuria, frequency, urgency

XI. Epididymitis: Diagnosis
- A. History and clinical examination
- B. Urinalysis and urine culture
- C. Urine nucleic acid amplification test (NAAT): *N. gonorrhoeae*, *C. trachomatis*
- D. Scrotal ultrasound: to rule out other conditions

XII. Epididymitis: Treatment
- A. Antibiotics (oral or parenteral)
    1. < 35 years: ceftriaxone, doxycycline/ azithromycin
    2. ≥ 35 years: levofloxacin, TMP-SMX
- B. NSAIDs
- C. Scrotal support

XIII. Hydrocele: Introduction
- A. Painless scrotal swelling
- B. Fluid accumulation between parietal and visceral layers of the tunica vaginalis

XIV. Hydrocele: Etiology
- A. Idiopathic (most common)
- B. Congenital
    1. Communicating
    2. Non-communicating
- C. Acquired
    1. Infection, trauma

XV. Hydrocele: Pathophysiology
- A. Communicating hydrocele
    1. Failure of processus vaginalis to close
    2. Accumulation of peritoneal fluid in the scrotal sac
- B. Non-communicating hydrocele
    1. Fluid accumulation from the mesothelium of the tunica vaginalis

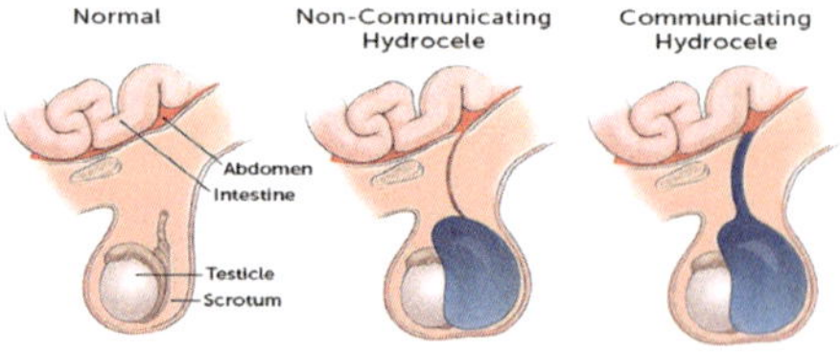

FIGURE 21.4.32 - Non-Communicating Hydrocele and Communicating Hydrocele Compared to the Normal Scrotum

XVI. Hydrocele: Clinical Presentation
- A. Painless scrotal swelling
- B. Reducible/non-reducible
- C. Positive transillumination test
- D. Size increases with Valsalva test (communicating hydrocele)
- E. Resolves spontaneously within first year of life

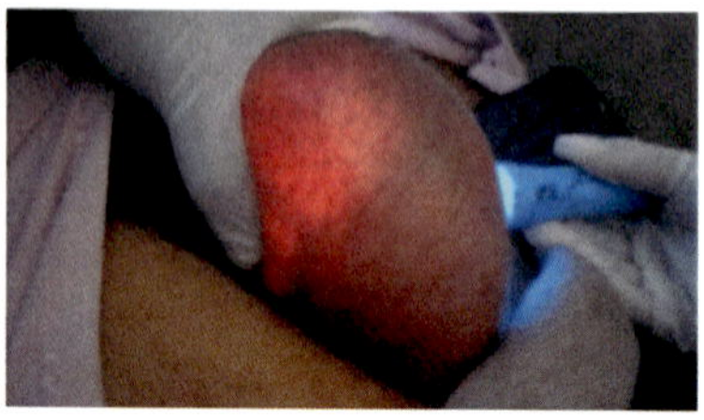

FIGURE 21.4.33 - Transillumination Test

XVII. Hydrocele: Diagnosis
- A. Clinical diagnosis
- B. Positive transillumination: cystic fluid collection
- C. Scrotal ultrasound (if diagnosis uncertain)

XVIII. Hydrocele: Treatment
- A. Congenital
    1. Spontaneous resolvement within the first year of life
- B. Surgical repair
    1. Excision of hydrocele sac
    2. Indications: symptomatic, failure of spontaneous resolution, risk of infertility

XIX. Varicocele: Introduction
- A. Abnormal dilatation and tortuosity of the pampiniform plexus of spermatic veins
- B. Most common cause of scrotal swelling
- C. Can lead to infertility

XX. Varicocele: Pathophysiology
- A. Incompetent venous valves or venous obstruction → increased intravenous pressure → dilation and tortuosity of pampiniform plexus
- B. Left spermatic vein (common)
    1. Longer course
    2. Inserts at a 90° angle into left renal vein
    3. Nutcracker phenomenon (compression of left spermatic vein)

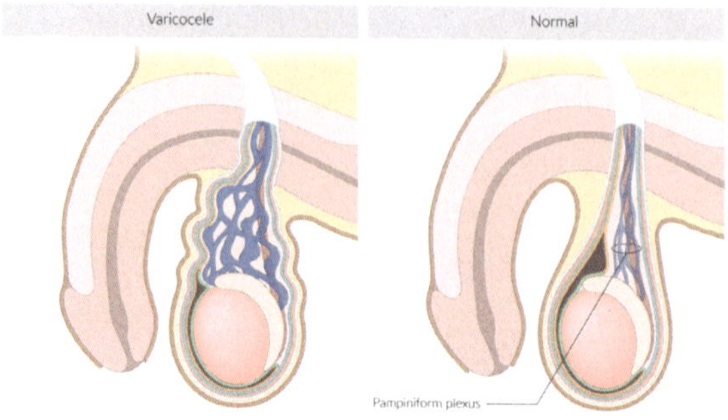

FIGURE 21.4.34 - Varicocele Showing Tortuosity of Pampiniform Plexus

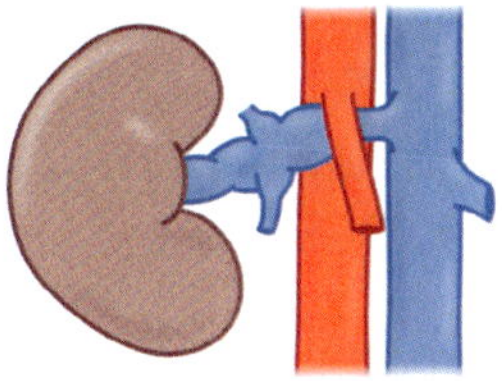

FIGURE 21.4.35 - Nutcracker Phenomenon

XXI. Varicocele: Clinical Presentation
- A. Painless scrotal swelling
- B. Dull ache in the scrotal (when standing)
- C. Fullness of the scrotum
- D. "Bag of worms" texture on palpation
- E. Reduced fertility
- F. Negative transillumination

XXII. Varicocele: Diagnosis
- A. Clinical examination
- B. Doppler ultrasound
    1. Dilated pampiniform plexus (> 2 mm)
    2. To rule out IVC obstruction
- C. Abdominal CT scan (unilateral right-sided varicocele)
1. Varicocele: Treatment
- D. Conservative management
    1. Commonly in elderly
    2. Scrotal support, NSAIDs
- E. Surgical management
    1. Preferred in young individuals to preserve fertility
    2. Varicocelectomy: surgical ligation of dilated testicular veins
- F. Percutaneous venous embolization

REVIEW QUESTIONS

1. A 15-year-old boy is admitted to the hospital due to severe right scrotal pain that started 2 hours ago during a football match. He says that the ball accidentally hit his scrotum shortly after which the pain began. The physical exam shows an elevated, swollen, and erythematous right testicle with an absent cremasteric reflex. What is the most likely pathophysiology for this patient's current condition?
    - **The pathophysiology of testicular torsion includes twisting of the spermatic cord along its axis, superior and transverse displacement of the testis, and diminished arterial blood flow.**
    - This patient presents with severe right scrotal pain after trauma during a football match.
    - The physical exam shows elevated, swollen, and erythematous right testicle with absent cremasteric reflex.
    - This is a classic presentation for testicular torsion.

2. How do you confirm a successful manual detorsion?
    - **A successful manual detorsion can be confirmed if there is a decrease in pain intensity, the high-riding testis comes to the bottom of the scrotum with a horizontal lie, and there is a return of the arterial blood flow on color doppler ultrasound.**

3. How can we differentiate epididymitis from testicular torsion according to the Prehn's sign and cremasteric reflex?
    - **In epididymitis both Prehn's sign and cremasteric reflex are present. In testicular torsion both Prehn's sign and cremasteric reflex are absent.**

4. A 16-year-old boy is admitted to the emergency department due to severe scrotal pain. Six hours ago he was playing football while he suddenly felt pain in his right groin. He is in acute distress. His physical exam shows a right erythematous, swollen scrotum with a right testicle in a horizontal position. Stroking along the patient's right inner thigh does not elicit ipsilateral testicular elevation. Manual elevation of the testicle does not relieve the pain either. Which of the following is the next best step in the management of this patient?
    - A. Surgical detorsion and ipsilateral orchiopexy
    - B. Surgical detorsion and bilateral orchiopexy
    - C. Ipsilateral orchiectomy and contralateral orchiopexy
    - D. Bilateral orchiectomy

    - **The correct answer is option B.**
    - This patient is admitted to the emergency department with 6 hours of right scrotal pain, red, swollen scrotum, testicle in a horizontal position, and an absent cremasteric reflex.
    - This presentation is most consistent with testicular torsion.
    - The ideal treatment for testicular torsion, especially 6 hours after symptom onset, is surgical detorsion.
    - The physician needs to examine both the affected testicle to the scrotal wall and the unaffected testicle because of the high risk for torsion in the future.
    - Option A is incorrect because this patient needs bilateral orchiopexy to prevent future torsion of the unaffected testicle.
    - Options C and D are incorrect because unless there is clear evidence of tissue necrosis, we try to preserve the testicle and not perform orchiectomy either unilaterally or bilaterally.

GASTROENTEROLOGY

Gastroenterology | Section 1: Colonic Polyps & Colorectal Cancer

I. Colonic Polyps
   A. Neoplastic polyps
      1. Adenomatous polyps, serrated polyps
   B. Non-neoplastic polyps
      1. Hyperplastic, hamartomatous, inflammatory pseudopolyps, mucosal and submucosal polyps

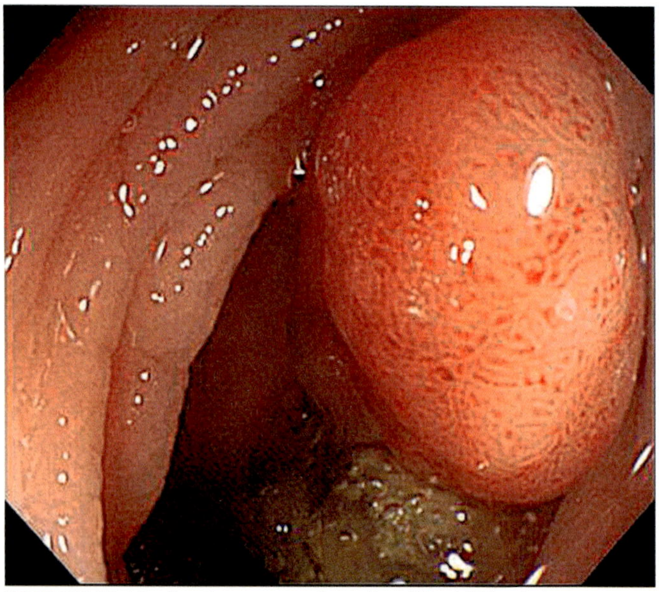

FIGURE 21.5.1 - Endoscopic Image of an Adenomatous Polyp

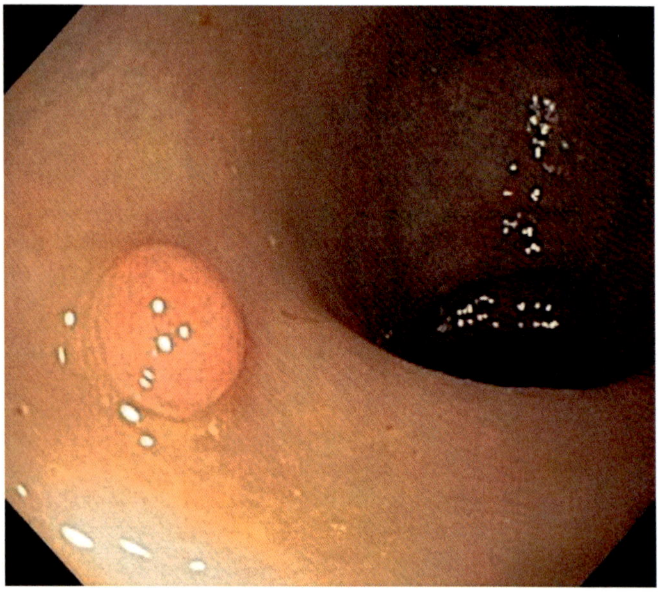

FIGURE 21.5.2 - Endoscopic Image Showing a Serrated Polyp

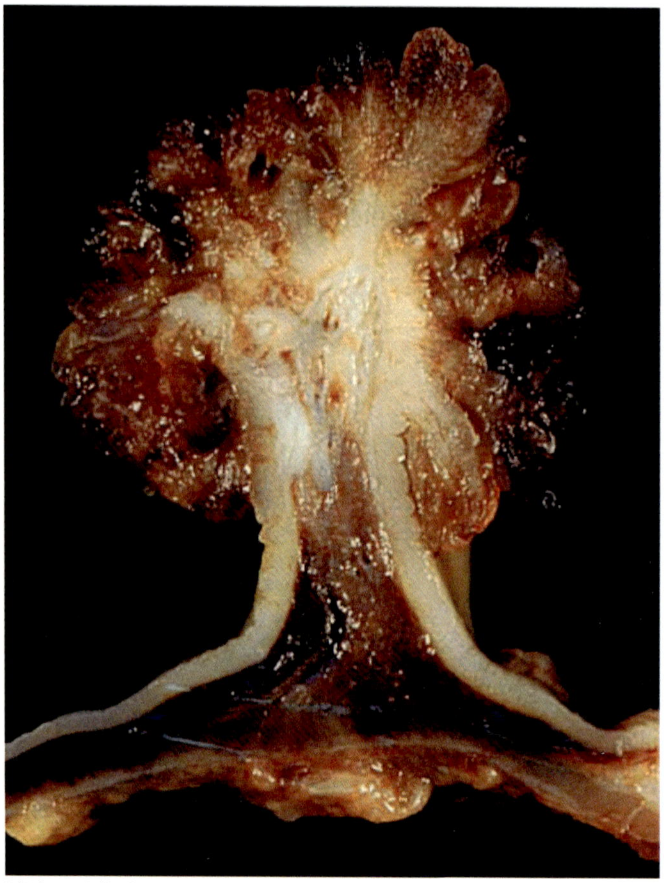

FIGURE 21.5.3 - Gross Image of Tubulovillous Polyp

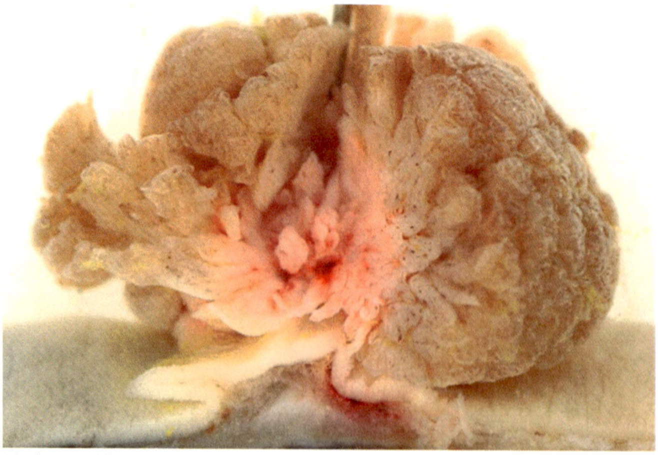

FIGURE 21.5.4 - Gross Image of a Villous Polyp

II. Colonic Polyps
   A. In adenomatous polyps, ↑ risk of developing colorectal cancer if
      1. Large size (≥ 1cm)
      2. Large number (≥ 3 concurrent adenomas)
      3. Villous > tubular
      4. Sessile > pedunculated

III. Colorectal Cancer: Epidemiology
   A. Third most common cancer of adults in the US
   B. Second leading cause of cancer deaths among adults in the US
   C. Peak age of incidence is 70-80 years

IV. Colorectal Cancer: Risk Factors
   A. Age ≥ 50 years
   B. Personal history of prior colorectal cancer or adenomatous polyps
   C. Family history of colorectal cancer or adenomatous polyps
   D. Familial colorectal cancer syndromes
   E. Inflammatory bowel disease
   F. Dietary factors (↓ fiber, ↑ fat and red meat)

V. Colorectal Cancer: Subtypes
   A. IBD-associated CRC
   B. Familial CRC syndromes
      1. Familial adenomatous polyposis
      2. Lynch syndrome
      3. Peutz-Jeghers syndrome
      4. Familial juvenile polyposis coli
   C. *S. gallolyticus* and *C. septicum* bacteremia-associated CRC

VI. Subtypes: IBD-Associated CRC
   A. Ulcerative colitis > Crohn's disease
   B. Risk associated with duration and extent of the disease
   C. Risk is present even in the absence of symptomatic disease
   D. Colonoscopy with mucosal sampling every 1-3 years, starting 8-10 years after the initial diagnosis
      1. Colectomy if dysplasia detected

VII. Subtypes: Familial Adenomatous Polyposis
   A. Autosomal dominant *APC* tumor suppressor gene mutation
   B. Hundreds of adenomatous polyps develop in colon, starting at puberty
   C. 100% progression to colorectal cancer by age 40
   D. Gardner syndrome (FAP + osteomas and desmoid tumors)
   E. Turcot syndrome (FAP + brain tumors)
   F. Annual colonoscopy starting at age 10-12 years
      1. Urgent proctocolectomy if colorectal cancer or high-grade adenoma detected
   G. Screening for upper GI tumors recommended
   H. Genetic testing for *APC* mutations

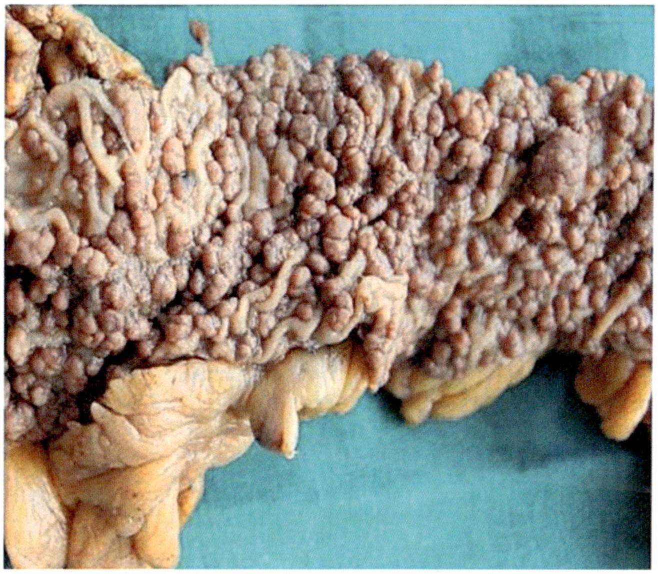

FIGURE 21.5.5 - Gross image of Colon in Familial Adenomatous Polyposis

VIII. Subtypes: Lynch Syndrome
   A. Also called hereditary nonpolyposis colorectal cancer (HNPCC)
   B. Autosomal dominant mutation in DNA repair genes (*MSH, MLH*)
      1. ↑ risk of colorectal, skin, endometrial and ovarian cancers
   C. Absence of adenomatous polyposis
   D. Colonoscopy every 1-2 years, starting at age 20-25 years
   E. Annual endometrial biopsies starting at age 30-35 years

IX. Subtypes: Peutz-Jeghers Syndrome
   A. Hamartomatous polyps throughout the gastrointestinal tract
   B. ↑ Risk of colorectal and other gastrointestinal cancers
   C. Hyperpigmented macules on the lips, hands, and genitalia

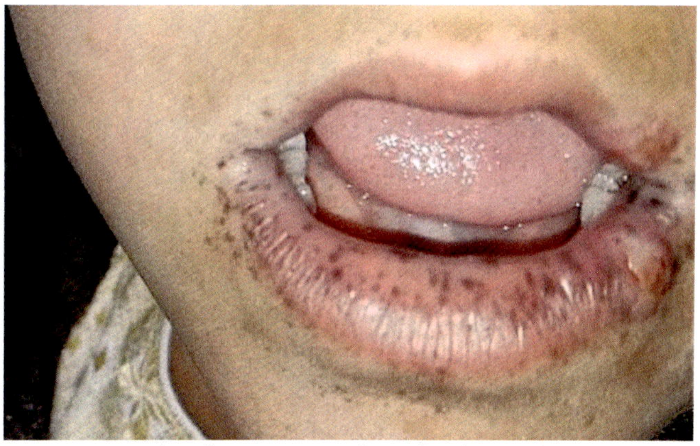

FIGURE 21.5.6 - Hyperpigmented Macules on the Lips in Peutz-Jeghers Syndrome

X. Subtypes: Familial Juvenile Polyposis Coli
   A. Numerous hamartomatous polyps in the colon before 5 years of age
   B. Slightly increased risk of colorectal cancer

XI. Subtypes: *S. gallolyticus* and *C. septicum* bacteremia-associated CRC
   A. Strong association with colorectal cancer
   B. Colonoscopy is indicated in all patients with *Streptococcus gallolyticus* (*S. bovis* type 1) or *Clostridium septicum* bacteremia and/or endocarditis, in the absence of a prior or current history of colorectal cancer

XII. Colorectal Cancer: Clinical Presentation
   A. Asymptomatic at early stages
   B. Symptoms develop during advanced disease
   C. Right-sided cancer
      1. Bulky, exophytic mass (large caliber of right colon)
      2. Occult bleeding, melena, iron deficiency anemia, weight loss
      3. Iron deficiency anemia in an elderly male is colon cancer unless proven otherwise
   D. Left-sided cancer
      1. Infiltrating mass, obstructive symptoms (small caliber of left colon)
      2. Large bowel obstruction (apple-core lesion), altered bowel habits (diarrhea, constipation), pencil stools, hematochezia
   E. Rectal cancer
      1. Hematochezia, tenesmus, pain

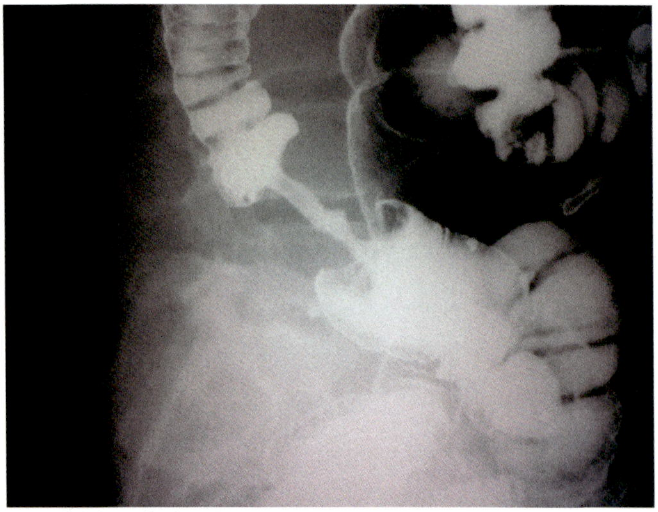

FIGURE 21.5.7 - Barium Enema in Colorectal Cancer Showing Apple-core Sign

XIII. Colorectal Cancer: Workup
   A. Colonoscopy with biopsy
   B. CT chest, abdomen, pelvis, LFTs
   C. CEA tumor marker

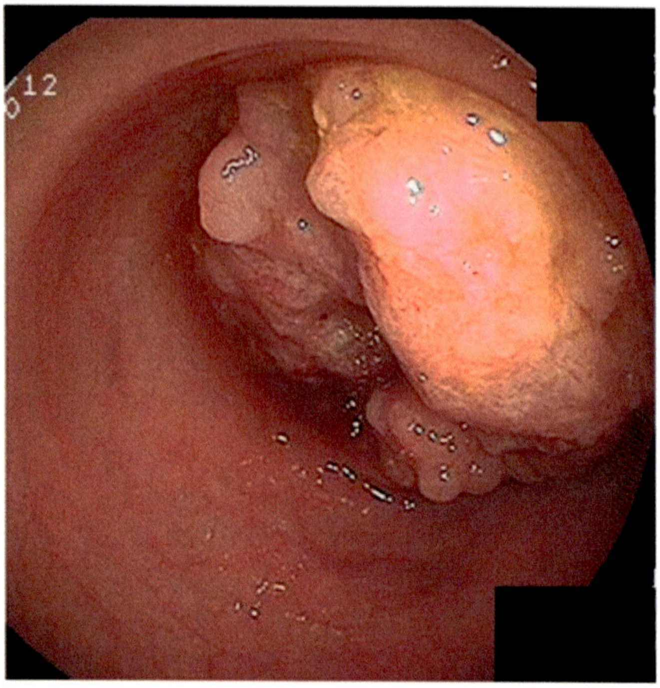

FIGURE 21.5.8 - Colonoscopy Showing Colon Cancer

XIV. Colorectal Cancer: Management
   A. Surgical resection of the affected bowel segment + lymph node dissection
   B. Adjuvant chemotherapy, radiotherapy
   C. CEA tumor marker to monitor recurrence
   D. Follow up colonoscopy at 1 year and then every 3 years

XV. Colorectal Cancer: Screening
   A. Virtually all colorectal cancers arise from adenomas
      1. Progression from adenoma to invasive cancer takes ~ 10 years
   B. Colonoscopy is the investigation of choice
   C. Alternatives: flexible sigmoidoscopy, fecal occult blood testing (FOBT), fecal immunochemical testing (FIT), CT colonography
   D. All individuals
      1. Screening started at age 50
      2. Colonoscopy every 10 years
      3. Alternatives: flexible sigmoidoscopy every 5 years, fecal occult blood testing annually, or a combination of these (if abnormal → perform colonoscopy)
   E. Positive family history
      1. ≥ 1 1st degree relative affected before age 60
      2. ≥ 2 1st degree relatives affected at any age
      3. Colonoscopy every 5 years, starting at age 40, or 10 years before the age of diagnosis of their relative, whichever comes first

REVIEW QUESTIONS

?

1. An 8-year-old boy is brought to the physician by his parents for an annual well-child visit. His father and uncle were diagnosed with colon cancer at the age of 30 and 28 respectively. Genetic testing of the patient's father shows a mutated *APC* gene. The patient's mother is healthy. What is the appropriate screening recommendation for colorectal cancer in this boy?

   - **Colon cancer screening recommendations for this patient would be to have a colonoscopy every year starting at the age of 10-12 years old, due to his family history of FAP.**
   - The father and uncle of this patient were diagnosed with colon cancer at the age of 30 and 28, respectively.
   - This is a very young age for colorectal cancer to be sporadic.
   - Genetic testing of the patient's father reveals a mutated *APC* gene.
   - This finding confirms the diagnosis of familial adenomatous polyposis, or FAP.
   - Familial adenomatous polyposis is an autosomal dominant disease.
   - Therefore, the patient has at least a 50% chance of having inherited the mutated gene.

2. A 25-year-old woman comes to the physician for a regular check-up. She has no specific complaints. Vital signs and physical examination are unremarkable. The patient's father was diagnosed with colon cancer at the age of 45. When should colonoscopy screening be started in this patient?

   - **The correct screening age for this patient would be 35 years.**
   - A colonoscopy should be performed at age 40, or 10 years prior to the age of diagnosis of their first-degree relative, whichever comes first.
   - 35 years is 10 years before the age of diagnosis of their father.

3. A 69-year-old man comes to the physician due to fever and shortness of breath for the past 3 weeks. He has no cough. He has been smoking 2-packs of cigarettes per day for the past 50 years but he does not drink alcohol or use illicit drugs. His vital signs are significant for a temperature of 39° C (102.2° F), blood pressure of 135/80 mmHg, heart rate of 110 beats/min, and respiratory rate of 15 breaths/min. Physical examination shows a pansystolic murmur at the apex radiating to the left axilla, as well as linear hemorrhages under the fingernails. A transesophageal ultrasound shows large vegetations on the mitral valve along with mitral regurgitation. Blood cultures are positive for *Clostridium septicum*. Which of the following is the best next step in the management of this patient?

   A. Chest CT
   B. Abdominal X-ray
   C. Colonoscopy
   D. Sigmoidoscopy

   - **The correct answer is option C.**
   - This man presents with fever and shortness of breath for the past 3 weeks.
   - The physical examination shows a pansystolic murmur at the apex radiating to the left axilla.
   - There are linear hemorrhages under the fingernails.
   - A transesophageal ultrasound shows large vegetations on the mitral valve along with mitral regurgitation.
   - All these findings suggest subacute bacterial endocarditis.
   - Blood cultures are positive for *Clostridium septicum*.
   - When bacterial endocarditis is caused by either *Clostridium septicum* or *Streptococcus gallolyticus*, one should suspect an underlying colorectal cancer.
   - This is because invasion of cancer deep into the colonic mucosa can introduce these bacteria into the bloodstream causing sepsis and endocarditis.
   - In order to screen for colorectal cancer, one should order a colonoscopy in this patient.
   - Options A and B are incorrect because chest CT and abdominal X-ray are not helpful for detecting colorectal cancer.
   - Option D is incorrect because sigmoidoscopy allows for inspection of only the sigmoid colon. The colorectal cancer in this patient may be anywhere along the colon which is why colonoscopy is a better option.

Gastroenterology | Section 2: Diverticular Disease, Angiodysplasia of the Colon, Acute Mesenteric Ischemia, Chronic Mesenteric Ischemia, Ischemic Colitis

I. Diverticular Disease: Diverticulosis
   A. A condition in which many false diverticula form in the colon
      1. False diverticula are outpouchings of the mucosa and submucosa through focal areas of weakness in muscularis
   B. Most common in sigmoid colon
   C. Risk factors
      1. Older adults, constipation, low fiber, high fat and red meat consumption
   D. Uncomplicated disease is usually asymptomatic
      1. Complications: diverticulitis, diverticular bleeding
   E. Diagnosis
      1. Barium enema, colonoscopy
      2. X-ray usually normal
   F. Management
      1. High fiber diet

II. Diverticular Disease: Diverticulitis
   A. Fecal/food impaction → microperforation → inflammation or infection of the diverticula
   B. Left lower quadrant pain, fever, leukocytosis
   C. Complicated diverticulitis
      1. Intestinal obstruction, fistulas, perforation, abscess formation
   D. Diagnosis
      1. CT scan (focal thickening of colonic wall, pericolic fat stranding)
      2. Barium enema or colonoscopy contraindicated in acute case
   E. Conservative management for uncomplicated cases
      1. IV antibiotics, IV fluids, bowel rest
      2. Colonoscopy after resolution of acute episode
   F. Surgical management is indicated for complicated diverticulitis, diverticulitis unresponsive to medical management or recurrent diverticulitis

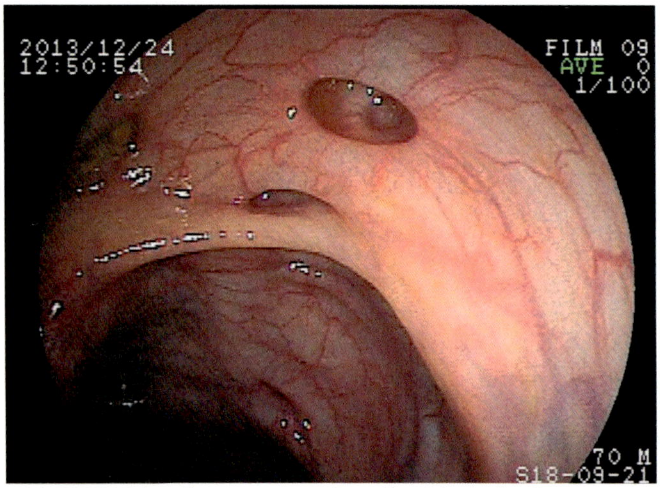

FIGURE 21.5.9 - Endoscopic Image of Two Diverticula

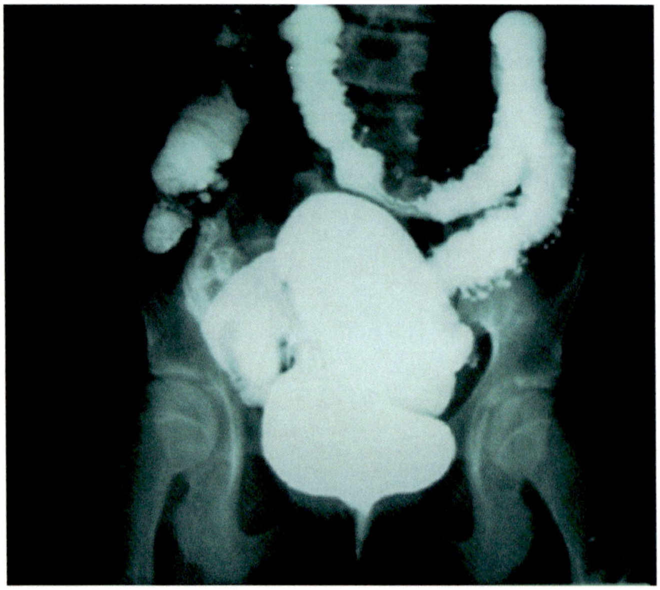

FIGURE 21.5.10 - Barium Enema Showing Diverticulosis

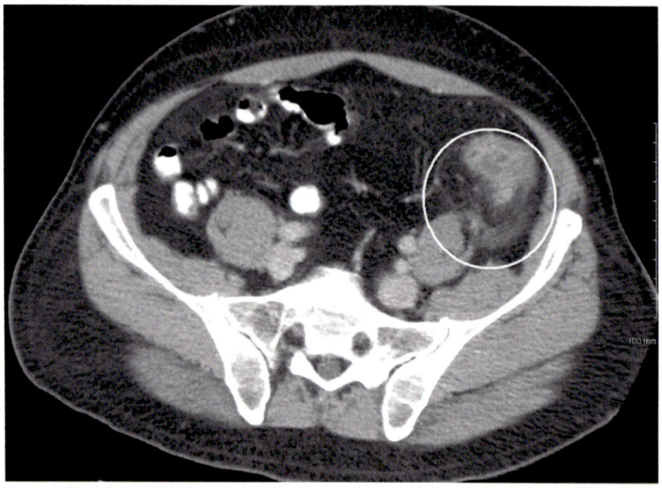

FIGURE 21.5.11 - CT Scan Showing Diverticulitis

III. Diverticular Disease: Diverticular Bleeding
   A. Painless hematochezia
      1. Weakened vasa recta in diverticular wall
      2. May cause hemodynamic instability
   B. Most common cause of gross lower GI bleeding in adults > 40 years
   C. Confirmed on colonoscopy
   D. Usually resolves spontaneously

IV. Angiodysplasia
   A. Tortuous dilation of submucosal veins, usually in the right colon
   B. Most commonly affects elderly
      1. Associated with aortic stenosis, von Willebrand disease, end-stage renal disease
   C. Painless, intermittent lower GI bleeding, usually small volume
   D. Diagnosed on colonoscopy
      1. Most resolve spontaneously

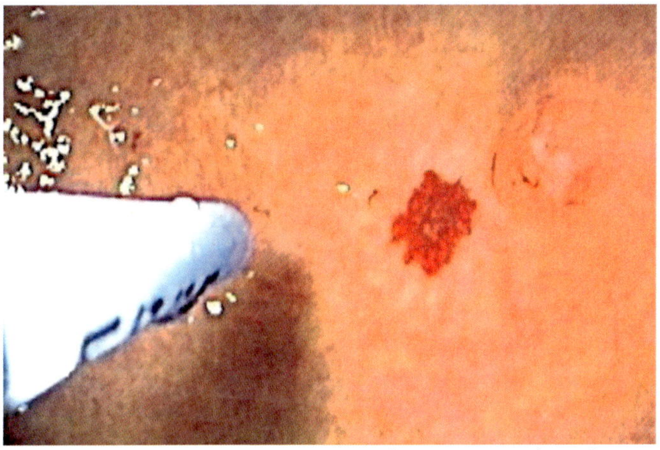

FIGURE 21.5.12 - Angiodysplastic Lesion on Endoscopy

V. Acute Mesenteric Ischemia
  A. Acute blockage of mesenteric vessels
    1. Emboli (e.g. atrial fibrillation), arterial thrombosis (e.g. atherosclerotic lesions)
    2. Superior mesenteric vessels most commonly affected
  B. Acute abdominal pain, ‘out of proportion’ to physical findings
  C. Diagnosed on CT angiography
  D. IV fluids, antibiotics, underlying cause (e.g. heparin, embolectomy)

VI. Chronic Mesenteric Ischemia
  A. ‘Intestinal angina’
    1. Atherosclerosis of mesenteric arteries
    2. Recurrent, postprandial, crampy abdominal pain
    3. Food aversion, weight loss
  B. Diagnosed via CT angiography
  C. Management includes risk reduction (e.g. statins, antihypertensive drugs), revascularization, nutritional support

VII. Ischemic Colitis
  A. Nonocclusive ischemia
    1. Acute hypotension, hypovolemia, cardiovascular surgery, shock, trauma
  B. ‘Watershed areas’: splenic flexure, rectosigmoid junction
  C. Most common in older adults
  D. Crampy abdominal pain, followed by bloody diarrhea
  E. CT scan (segmental bowel wall thickening), colonoscopy (edematous, friable mucosa), barium enema (thumbprinting)
  F. Management
    1. Supportive care (bowel rest, fluids, antibiotics)
    2. Surgical intervention and resection of necrotic bowel

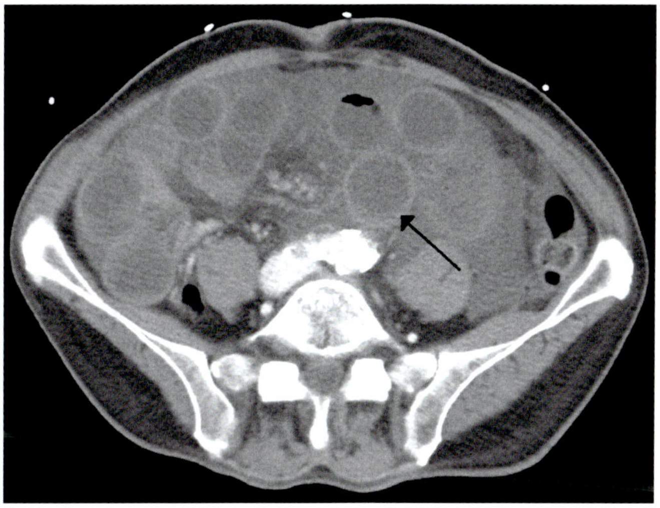

FIGURE 21.5.13 - CT Scan of Ischemic Colitis

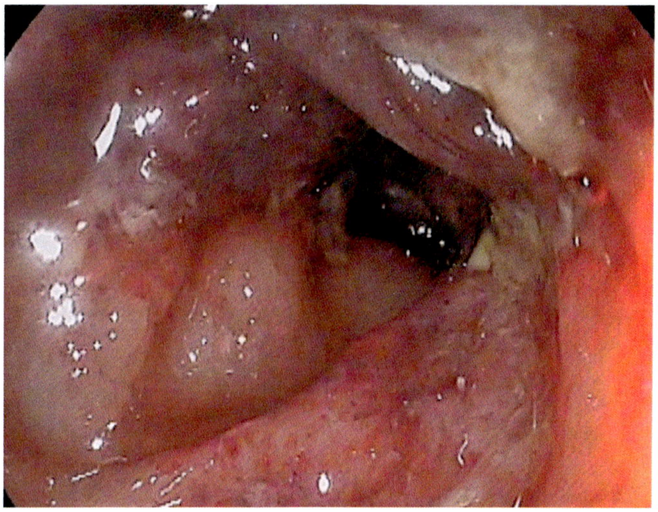

FIGURE 21.5.14 - Endoscopic Image of Ischemic Colitis

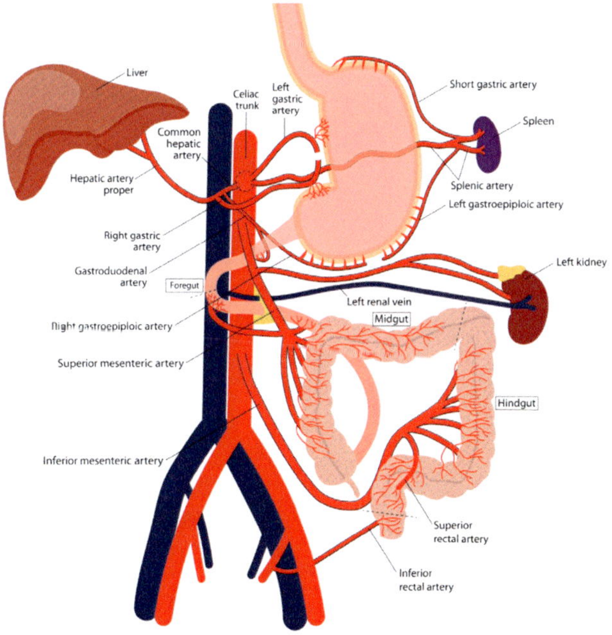

FIGURE 21.5.15 - Anatomy of Gastro-Intestinal System

REVIEW QUESTIONS

1. A 69-year-old man is brought to the emergency department due to severe left lower quadrant pain for the past day. He has a long history of constipation. Vital signs are significant for a temperature of 39° C (102.2° F). What is the best initial step in the evaluation of this patient?

   - **The best initial step in the evaluation of the patient with suspected diverticulitis is abdominal CT scan.**
   - This elderly man presents with a fever of 39° C and left lower quadrant pain for the past day.
   - He has a long history of constipation.
   - These clues point to the diagnosis of acute diverticulitis.
   - CT scan typically shows focal thickening of the colonic wall and pericolic fat stranding.
   - Enema and colonoscopy are contraindicated in case of acute diverticulitis due to risk of colonic rupture.

2. A 72-year-old woman comes to the physician due to 20 kg weight loss over the past 2 years. She experiences dull abdominal pain while eating every meal causing her to limit her oral intake. Past medical history is significant for peripheral artery disease and myocardial infarction. What is the best diagnostic test for this patient's current condition?

   - **The best diagnostic test for this patient's current condition is a CT angiography.**
   - This elderly woman with 20 kg weight loss experiences dull abdominal pain during every meal causing her to eat less.
   - This is a classic sign of chronic mesenteric ischemia, also known as "intestinal angina".
   - Chronic mesenteric ischemia is even more likely given her history of peripheral artery disease and myocardial infarction.
   - Chronic mesenteric ischemia is definitively diagnosed with CT angiography which shows atherosclerotic narrowing of the mesenteric vessels

3. A 58-year-old woman is currently being evaluated because of worsening abdominal pain. She underwent a coronary artery bypass graft procedure 4 hours ago, which was complicated by significant blood loss. Vital signs include temperature of 36° C (96.8° F), blood pressure of 100/80 mmHg, heart rate of 84 beats/min, and respiratory rate of 16 breaths/min. Physical examination shows diffuse abdominal tenderness with no rigidity or guarding. Abdominal CT scan shows segmental bowel wall thickening while colonoscopy shows edematous, friable mucosa. Which of the following bowel segments is most likely affected by this patient's current condition?

   A. Ileocecal junction
   B. Rectosigmoid junction
   C. Hepatic flexure
   D. Cecum

   - **The correct answer is option B.**
   - This woman complains of severe abdominal pain after losing a lot of blood during coronary artery bypass graft procedure.
   - The physical exam reveals diffuse abdominal tenderness with no rigidity or guarding.
   - Abdominal CT scan shows segmental bowel wall thickening while colonoscopy shows edematous, friable mucosa.
   - All these findings point towards the diagnosis of ischemic colitis.
   - Ischemic colitis affects the watershed regions of the colon, which are supplied by the most distal branches of major arteries.
   - These watershed regions involve the splenic flexure and the rectosigmoid junction.
   - Options A, C, and D are incorrect because the ileocecal junction, hepatic flexure, and cecum are not watershed areas. They are supplied intensively by the major branches of the superior mesenteric artery.

Gastroenterology | Section 3: Large Bowel Obstruction, Ogilvie Syndrome, Colonic Volvulus & Pilonidal Disease

I. Large Bowel Obstruction
   A. Crampy abdominal pain, constipation, abdominal distention
   B. Vomiting less pronounced; contains fecal matter
   C. Colon cancer is the most common cause in adults
      1. Other causes: volvulus, diverticulitis, postoperative adhesions
   D. Diagnosis
      1. Plain radiography
      2. Abdominal CT scan
   E. Management
      1. Treatment of the underlying cause
      2. Decompression
      3. Surgical intervention if complications suspected (e.g. ischemia, perforation)

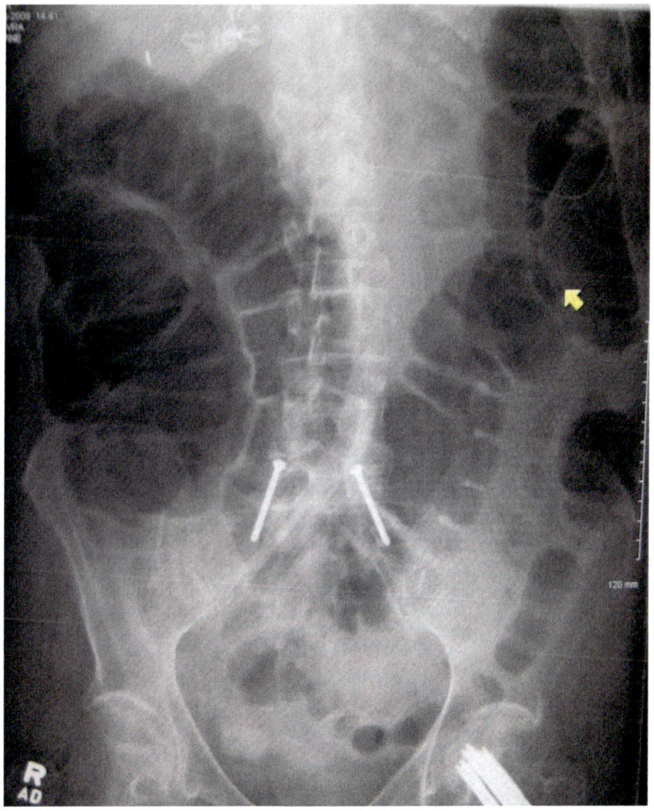

FIGURE 21.5.16 - Abdominal X-Ray: Large Bowel Obstruction

II. Ogilvie Syndrome
   A. Clinical features and radiologic evidence of large bowel obstruction, in the absence of any mechanical obstruction
   B. Recent surgery, medical illness (e.g. sepsis), electrolyte imbalance, and medications (e.g. anticholinergic agents, narcotics)
   C. Management: supportive (e.g. withdrawal of offending agent, correction of electrolyte imbalance, NPO, IVF, NG suction) → neostigmine if no response → colonic decompression

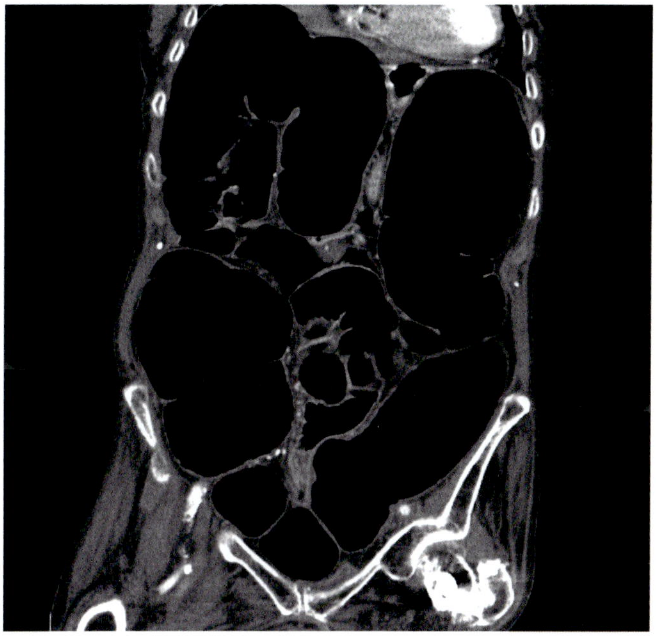

FIGURE 21.5.17 - CT Scan of Abdomen: Ogilvie Syndrome

III. Colonic Volvulus
   A. Twisting of a loop of colon around its mesentery
   B. Most commonly affects sigmoid colon
   C. Obstruction, strangulation, infarction, perforation
   D. Abdominal X-ray (e.g. coffee-bean sign of sigmoid volvulus)
   E. Management
      1. Sigmoidoscopy for sigmoid volvulus (diagnostic and therapeutic)
      2. Surgical untwisting for cecal volvulus

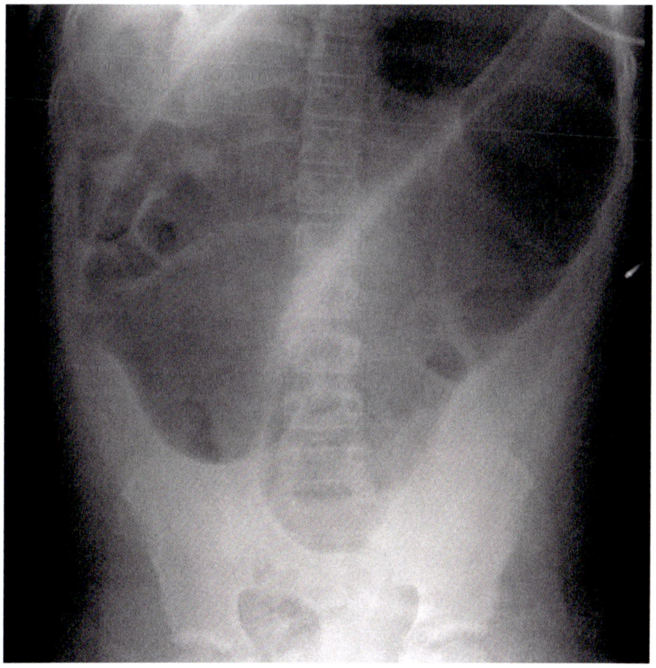

FIGURE 21.5.18 - Abdominal X-Ray: Sigmoid Volvulus

IV. Pilonidal Disease
   A. Infected hair follicle in the intergluteal cleft → pushed inward through movements of the buttocks → sinus tract → recurrent local inflammation and/or infection
   B. Painful, red swelling in the intergluteal cleft
   C. Risk factors include obesity and prolonged sitting
   D. Clinical diagnosis
   E. Treatment
      1. Incision and drainage of acute abscess
      2. Removal of pilonidal tract

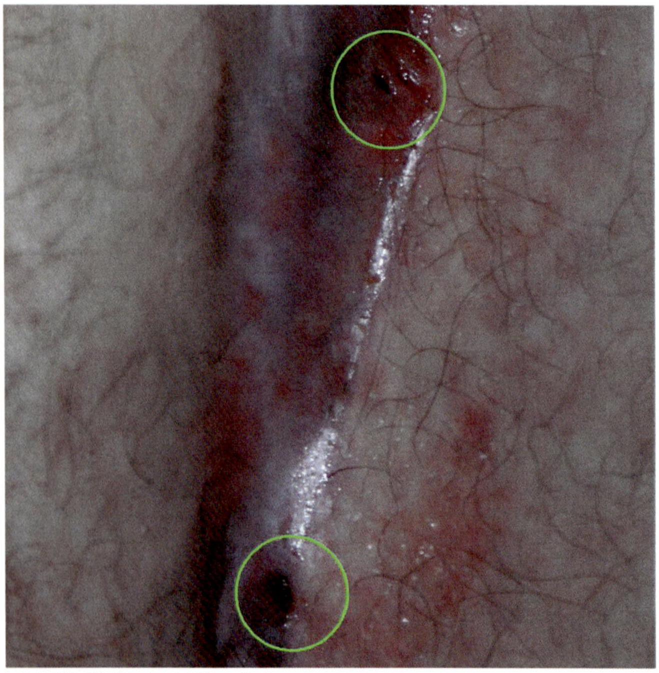

JerryTahl, Public domain, via Wikimedia Commons

FIGURE 21.5.19 - Pilonidal Disease

REVIEW QUESTIONS ?

1. An 81-year-old man is brought to the emergency department because of severe abdominal pain and vomiting for 4 hours. Past medical history includes osteoarthritis and chronic constipation. Vital signs include temperature of 36° C (96.8° F), blood pressure of 135/80 mmHg, heart rate of 84 beats/min, and respiratory rate of 15 breaths/min. Physical examination shows left lower quadrant pain with no rebound tenderness or rigidity. Abdominal X-ray shows twisting of the sigmoid colon around its mesentery. Laboratory studies are unremarkable. Which of the following is the best next step in the management of this patient?
   A. Laparoscopy
   B. Laparotomy
   C. Sigmoidoscopy
   D. Air enema

- **The correct answer is option C.**
- This elderly man presents with vomiting and severe abdominal pain.
- The physical examination shows left lower quadrant pain with no rebound tenderness or rigidity.
- Abdominal X-ray shows twisting of the sigmoid colon around its mesentery.
- These are the classic signs and symptoms of sigmoid volvulus.
- The patient's vital signs are unremarkable indicating that he is hemodynamically stable.
- Laboratory studies are also unremarkable making bowel ischemia and necrosis unlikely.
- Therefore, this patient needs sigmoidoscopy with detorsion.
- Options A and B are incorrect because laparoscopy and laparotomy are reserved for hemodynamically unstable patients with bowel ischemia and necrosis.
- Option D is avoided in sigmoid volvulus because air enema can cause colonic rupture.

Gastroenterology | Section 4: Liver Cysts and Malignancies: Hydatid Liver Cysts & Hepatocellular Carcinoma

I. Hydatid Liver Cyst: Definition
   A. Parasitic disease caused by *Echinococcus granulosus*

II. Hydatid Liver Cyst: Risk Factors
   A. Ingestion of food contaminated with dog feces

III. Hydatid Liver Cyst: Clinical Presentation
   A. Hepatic manifestations
      1. Hepatomegaly
      2. Nausea, vomiting
      3. Right upper quadrant pain
   B. Extrahepatic manifestations
      1. Cyst rupture may result in anaphylaxis
      2. Lung and brain involvement

IV. Hydatid Liver Cyst: Diagnosis
   A. Complete blood count
      1. Eosinophilia
   B. Serology
      1. Positive anti-*Echinococcus* IgG or IgM antibody

V. Imaging
      1. Ultrasonography: hepatic cysts with eggshell calcifications and internal septations

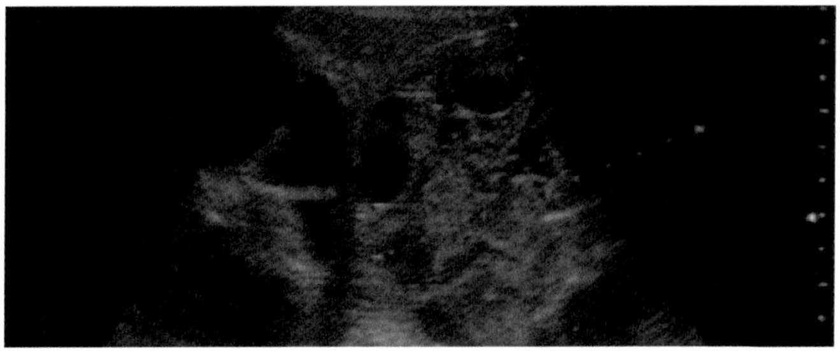

FIGURE 21.5.20 - Ultrasound Image Showing Hydatid Liver Cysts

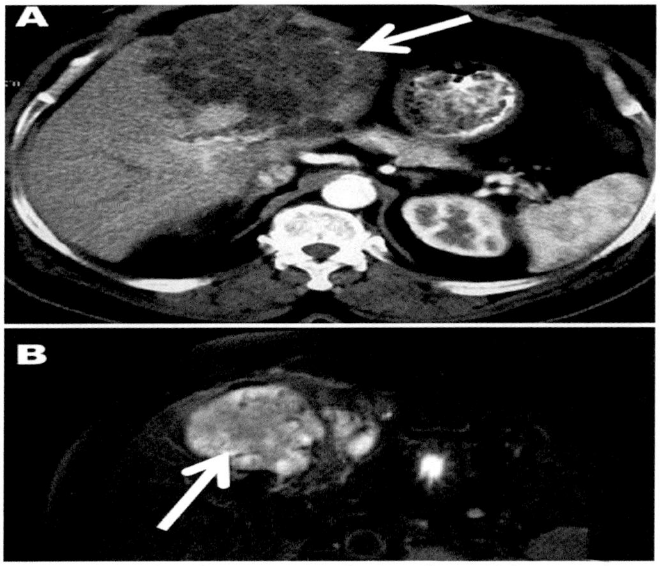

FIGURE 21.5.21 - CT Scan Showing Hydatid Liver Cysts

VI. Hydatid Liver Cyst: Management
   A. Small cysts (< 5 cm)
      1. Albendazole
   B. Large cysts
      1. Imaging-guided percutaneous drainage in combination with albendazole
   C. Complicated cysts
      1. Surgery and albendazole

VII. Hepatocellular Carcinoma: Definition
   A. Primary malignant tumor of the liver

VIII. Hepatocellular Carcinoma: Risk Factors
   A. Cirrhosis (e.g. NAFLD, Wilson disease, hemochromatosis, HCV)
   B. Alcohol
   C. Hepatitis B
   D. Aflatoxins produced by aspergillus

IX. Hepatocellular Carcinoma: Clinical Presentation
   A. Asymptomatic
   B. Weight loss, mild fever
   C. Symptoms of decompensated cirrhosis:
      1. Jaundice, ascites, coagulopathy, hepatosplenomegaly
   D. Metastasis-related symptoms (e.g. bone pain)
   E. Inappropriate absolute polycythemia
      1. Thrombosis
   F. Budd-Chiari syndrome
      1. Hepatic vein thrombosis due to blood hyperviscosity or direct cancer spread
      2. Acute exacerbation of abdominal pain, ascites, and hepatosplenomegaly

X. Hepatocellular Carcinoma: Diagnosis
   A. High-risk patients (e.g. cirrhotics) screened for HCC with AFP and abdominal ultrasound every 6 months
   B. Imaging
      1. Ultrasonography (best initial step): mass with irregular borders
      2. Triple phase contrast CT: hypodense, irregular mass
   C. Ultrasound-guided liver biopsy
      1. Needed for definitive diagnosis

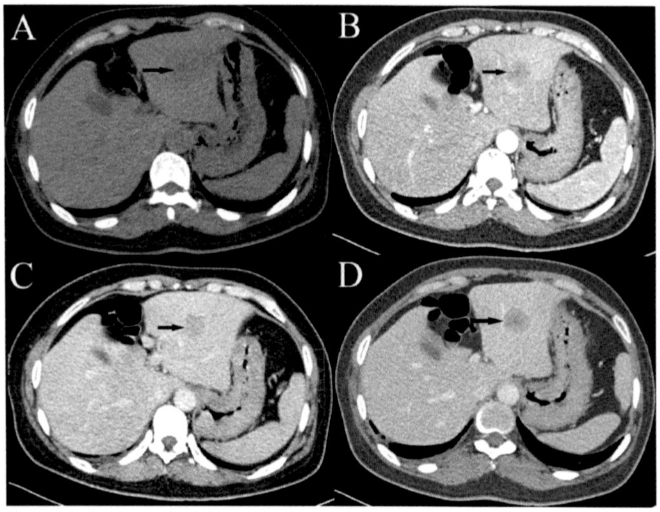

FIGURE 21.5.22 - Triple Phase CT Scan of Hepatocellular Carcinoma

XI. Hepatocellular Carcinoma: Management
   A. Surgical resection
   B. Ablative therapy
   C. Chemotherapy
   D. Liver transplantation
   E. Prevention
      1. Hepatitis B vaccination
      2. Avoid alcohol

Condition	Key Features	Imaging Findings	Management
Cavernous hemangioma	- Most common benign liver tumor - ↑ risk with pregnancy and OCPs - Biopsy contraindicated due to risk of bleeding	- US: hyperechoic homogeneous mass	- If asymptomatic or small: - Observation with serial ultrasound - If symptomatic or large: - Surgical resection, arterial embolization
Hepatic adenoma	- Women of reproductive age - ↑ risk with OCPs and anabolic steroids - Risk of malignant transformation to HCC - Biopsy contraindicated due to risk of bleeding	- US: well-demarcated hyperechoic lesion(s) - Contrast CT: early peripheral enhancement	- If asymptomatic or small: - Stop OCPs or anabolic steroids - Repeat imaging in 6 months - If symptomatic or large: - Surgical resection - Follow up with CT or MRI with 6-12 months intervals
Focal nodular hyperplasia	- Second most common benign liver tumor - Not associated with OCPs	- US: central arteries with spoke-wheel appearance - Contrast CT: central stellate scar	- If asymptomatic: - Observation with serial ultrasound - If symptomatic: - Surgical resection
Hydatid liver cysts	- Infection with *Echinococcus* species - Ingestion of food contaminated with dog feces - Cyst rupture can cause anaphylaxis	- US: smooth liver cysts with peripheral eggshell calcifications and internal septations	- Small cysts (< 5 cm): - Albendazole - Large cysts: - Percutaneous drainage with albendazole
Hepatocellular carcinoma	- Cirrhosis - Alcohol - Chronic HBV - Aflatoxins	- US: mass with irregular borders - Triple phase contrast CT: hypodense irregular mass	- Surgical resection - Ablative therapy - Chemotherapy - Liver transplantation - Prevention: HBV vaccination, alcohol avoidance

TABLE 21.5.1 - Summary of Liver Cysts and Malignancies

REVIEW QUESTIONS

1. How can a hydatid liver cyst and hepatic adenoma be distinguished on imaging?
   - **On ultrasound, the hydatid liver cyst presents as a smooth cyst with peripheral calcifications. There may also be septations present. In contrast, a hepatic adenoma presents as a solid mass on the ultrasound.**

2. A 62-year-old man with a 30-year history of alcoholic cirrhosis comes to the physician with unintentional 15 kg of weight loss over the past 4 months. He states that the jaundice and right upper quadrant discomfort have worsened. Urine color also seems to be darker than before. Physical examination shows a positive abdominal fluid wave and muscle atrophy of the extremities. What is the best initial imaging modality?
   - **The best initial imaging modality in the diagnosis of suspected hepatocellular carcinoma is a right upper quadrant ultrasound.**
   - This patient with a 30-year history of alcoholic cirrhosis comes to the physician with an unintentional 15 kg of weight loss over the past 4 months.
   - His jaundice and right upper quadrant discomfort have worsened since then.
   - His urine color is darker than before.
   - These changes suggest an obstructive jaundice due to the hepatic mass.
   - Clinical deterioration of the patient with long-standing cirrhosis raises suspicion for hepatocellular carcinoma.

3. A 36-year-old woman presents to her primary care physician because of dull right upper quadrant pain for the past 6 months. She works as a farmer. Currently is taking no medications and states stopped her OCPs 1 year ago. Denies alcohol consumption and drug use. Viral hepatitis panel is negative. Vital signs include temperature of 36° C (96.8° F), blood pressure of 125/85 mmHg, heart rate of 70 beats/min, and respiratory rate of 14 breaths/min. Right upper quadrant ultrasound shows a 3 cm hepatic mass with a hypoechoic center, internal septations, and a hyperechoic calcified rim. Which of the following is the most likely diagnosis?

   A. Hepatic adenoma
   B. Hydatid liver cyst
   C. Cavernous hemangioma
   D. Focal nodular hyperplasia

   - **The correct answer is option B.**
   - This woman presents with right upper quadrant pain for the past 6 months.
   - Right upper quadrant ultrasound shows a 3 cm hepatic mass with a hypoechoic center, internal septations, and a hyperechoic calcified rim.
   - This description is consistent with a hepatic cyst accompanied by peripheral eggshell calcifications.
   - Considering that she is a farmer with possible exposure to dog and sheep, her mass is most likely a hydatid liver cyst caused by *Echinococcus granulosus* infection.
   - Option A is incorrect because hepatic adenoma presents as a well-demarcated hyperechoic lesion on hepatic ultrasound.
   - Option C is incorrect because the ultrasound typically shows a hyperechoic homogeneous mass in patients with cavernous hemangioma.
   - Option D is incorrect because focal nodular hyperplasia presents as a mass with central arteries and a spoke-wheel appearance.

Gastroenterology | Section 5: Gallstone Related Disease

I. Cholelithiasis: Definition
   A. Cholelithiasis: calculi present in the gallbladder
   B. Calculi can be of many types in the gallbladder
   C. Asymptomatic cholelithiasis: no clinical symptoms
   D. Symptomatic cholelithiasis: symptoms such as biliary colic

II. Cholelithiasis: Pathophysiology
   A. Cholesterol stones: most common
      1. Dysregulated cholesterol metabolism → ↑ cholesterol saturation in bile, ↓ in bile salts → precipitation of cholesterol and calcium
   B. Black pigment stones: ↑ hemolysis → ↑ in serum unconjugated bilirubin → ↑ uptake and conjugation → precipitation of bilirubin
   C. Brown stones: infection leading to increased β-glucuronidase → increased hydrolysis of conjugated bilirubin → precipitation of cholesterol, calcium carbonate and calcium bilirubinate

III. Cholelithiasis: Risk Factors
   A. Cholesterol stones
      1. Four "Fs": Fat, Female, Forty, Fertile
      2. Represents obesity, female sex, age, pregnancy or multiparity
      3. Rapid weight loss, total parenteral nutrition
   B. Black pigment stones: chronic hemolysis, total parenteral nutrition
   C. Brown pigment stones: bacterial or parasitic infection of biliary tract, cholangitis

IV. Cholelithiasis: Clinical Features
   A. Most gallstones are asymptomatic
   B. Biliary colic
      1. Right upper quadrant pain (dull and aching) < 6 hours
      2. Postprandial pain due to cholecystokinin → gallbladder contraction of stone against cystic duct
      3. Radiation to epigastrium, right shoulder (Kehr's sign), and back
   C. Nausea, vomiting, dyspepsia, bloating

V. Cholelithiasis: Diagnosis
   A. Asymptomatic cholelithiasis: no workup required
   B. Symptomatic cholethiasis
      1. Initial diagnostic study: right upper quadrant ultrasound
      2. If high clinical suspicion and U/S nondiagnostic: endoscopic ultrasound
   C. Ultrasound
      1. Echogenic foci in gallbladder
      2. Posterior acoustic shadow
      3. Biliary sludge: no acoustic shadow, moves with changing patient position
   D. Lab studies: normal in uncomplicated cholelithiasis

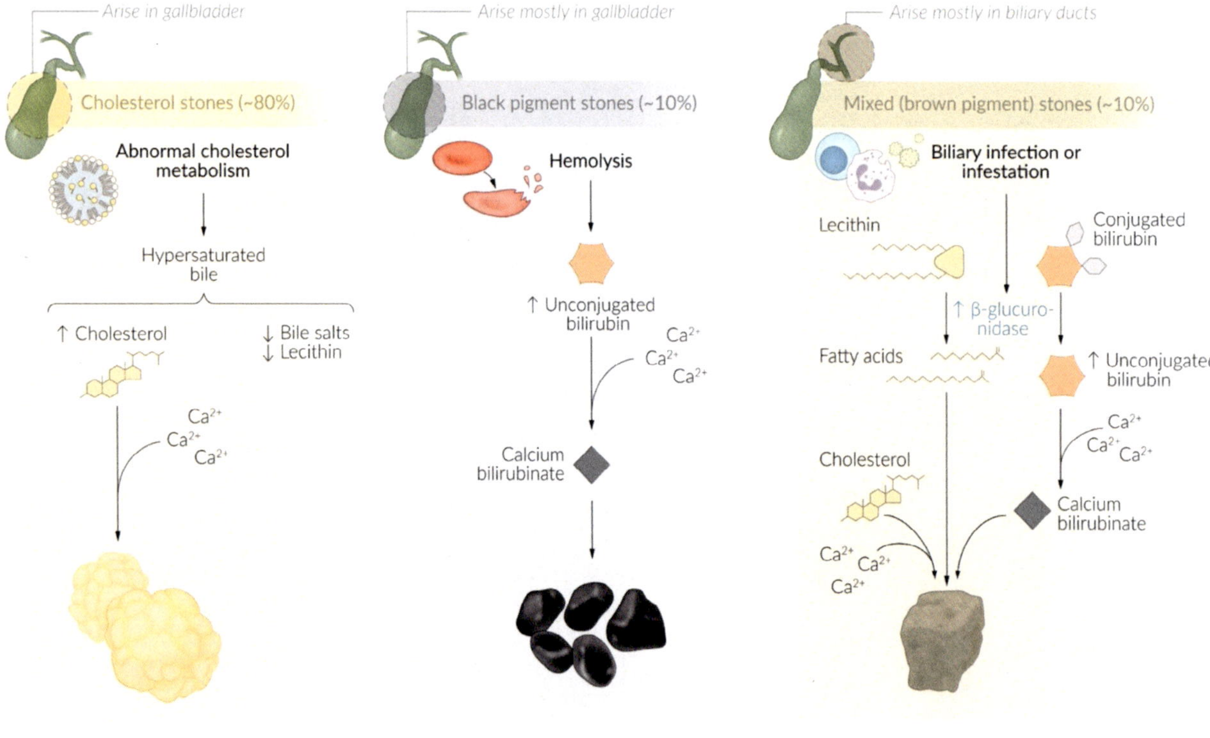

FIGURE 21.5.23 - Pathophysiology of Different Types of Gallstones

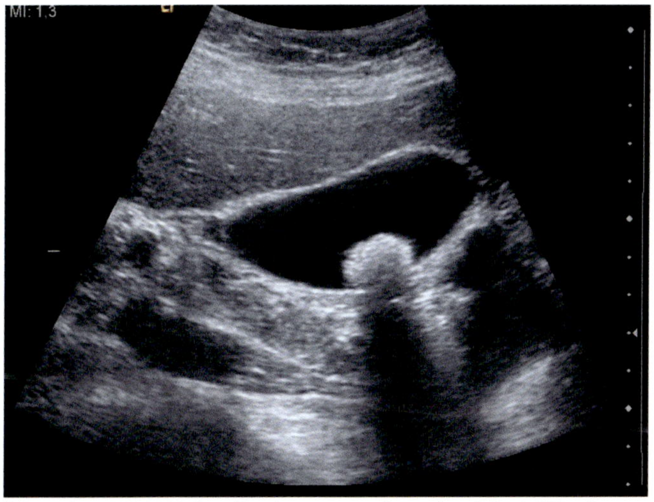

FIGURE 21.5.24 - Gallstones on Ultrasound

VI. Cholelithiasis: Management
  A. Asymptomatic: expectant management
  B. Symptomatic uncomplicated cholelithiasis
    1. NPO, analgesics (NSAIDs or opioids), antiemetics
    2. Elective cholecystectomy as soon as possible after episode

VII. Acute Cholecystitis: Definition
  A. Inflammation of the gallbladder
    1. Calculous cholecystitis: blockage by stone in the cystic duct
    2. Emphysematous cholecystitis: infection with gas-forming bacteria

VIII. Acute Cholecystitis: Pathophysiology
  A. Calculous cholecystitis
    1. Cholelithiasis → obstruction of cystic duct → gallbladder distension → gallbladder inflammation ± secondary bacterial infection
  B. Acalculous cholecystitis
    1. Bile stasis and gallbladder hypoperfusion → gallbladder inflammation
  C. Infection of gallbladder with gas-forming bacteria (e.g. *Clostridium* species or *E. coli*) → gallbladder inflammation and air within gallbladder wall

IX. Acute Cholecystitis: Risk Factors
  A. Acute calculous cholecystitis: similar risk factors to cholelithiasis
  B. Risk factors for emphysematous cholecystitis
    1. Immunocompromised (e.g. diabetes)
    2. Infection with gas-forming bacteria (e.g. *Clostridium* spp., *E. coli*, *Klebsiella* spp., anaerobic streptococci)

X. Acute Cholecystitis: Clinical Features
  A. Prolonged and severe RUQ pain
    1. Radiation to right scapula
  B. Fever, malaise and anorexia
  C. Nausea/vomiting
  D. Guarding
  E. Positive Murphy's sign
    1. Inspiratory arrest on deep palpation of RUQ

XI. Acute Cholecystitis: Diagnosis
  A. Laboratory studies
    1. CBC: leukocytosis with increased neutrophils
    2. Elevated CRP/ESR
    3. Blood cultures for patients with suspicion for biliary sepsis
  B. Best initial test: RUQ abdominal ultrasound
      i. Gallbladder wall thickening
    1. Gallbladder wall edema and pericholecystic fluid
    2. Presence of gallstones in gallbladder
    3. Gallbladder distention
    4. Air in gallbladder wall in emphysematous cholecystitis

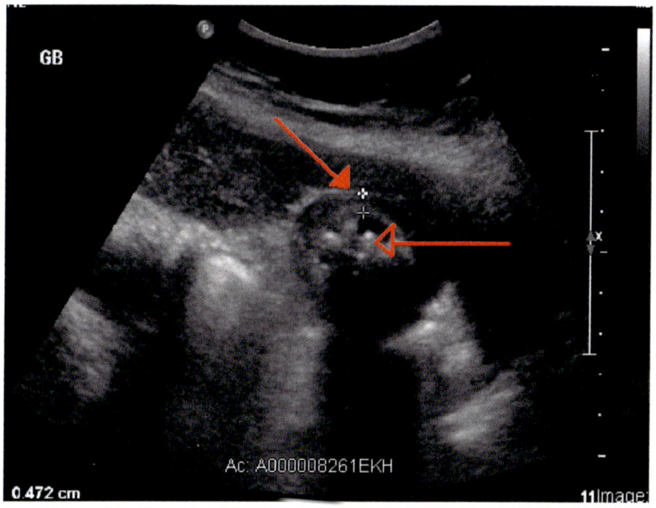

FIGURE 21.5.25 Gallbladder Wall Thickening on Ultrasound in Cholecystitis

XII. Acute Cholecystitis: Diagnosis
  A. Hepatobiliary iminodiacetic acid (HIDA scan)
    1. Radioactive tracer is injected, taken up by hepatocytes and excreted into bile
    2. Gallbladder takes up the tracer if cystic duct is patent
    3. No visualization of gallbladder > 4 hours from administration of tracer: cholecystitis
    4. Best confirmatory test if U/S inconclusive

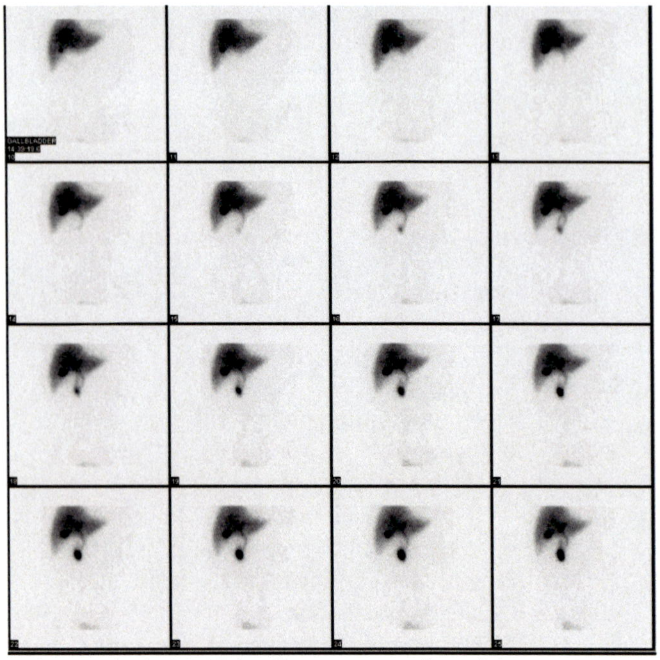

FIGURE 21.5.26 - Normal HIDA Scan Showing Tracer Entering Gallbladder

XIII. Acute Cholecystitis: Management
- A. NPO, IV fluids, electrolyte repletion, analgesics
- B. Empiric antibiotic therapy
  1. Metronidazole and ciprofloxacin
  2. Piperacillin-tazobactam
- C. Cholecystectomy
- D. Early laparoscopic cholecystectomy (if < 10 days from symptom onset)
- E. Delayed laparoscopic cholecystectomy

XIV. Acute Cholecystitis: Complications
- A. Gangrenous cholecystitis or suppurative cholecystitis
- B. Gallbladder perforation
- C. Chronic cholecystitis
- D. Cholecystoenteric fistula
  1. May lead to gallstone ileus with bowel obstruction or bile acid diarrhea

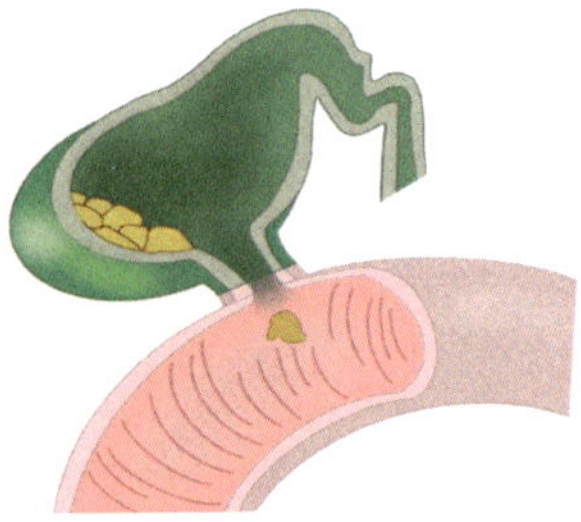

FIGURE 21.5.27 - Cholecystoenteric Fistula

XV. Acute Acalculous Cholecystitis: Definition
- A. Inflammation of the gallbladder not caused by gallstones
  1. Can be secondary to biliary sludge, gallbladder hypoperfusion

XVI. Acute Acalculous Cholecystitis: Pathophysiology
- A. Bile stasis and gallbladder hypoperfusion → inflammation of gallbladder
- B. Inflammation and distension can eventually lead to necrosis

XVII. Acute Acalculous Cholecystitis: Risk Factors
- A. Total parenteral nutrition
- B. Critically ill patients (ICU, multiorgan failure, sepsis)
- C. Severe trauma or burns
- D. CMV infection
- E. Immunodeficiency
- F. Prolonged fasting/malnutrition

XVIII. Acute Acalculous Cholecystitis: Clinical Features
- A. Similar clinical presentation to acute calculous cholecystitis
- B. Patients usually severely ill and symptoms may not be as obvious as in acute calculous cholecystitis

XIX. Acute Acalculous Cholecystitis: Diagnosis
- A. Lab studies: leukocytosis and elevated CRP
- B. Imaging
  1. Initial test: RUQ ultrasound
     - a) Gallbladder inflammation, distention, pericholecystic fluid
     - b) Absence of cholelithiasis
     - c) Biliary sludge may be present

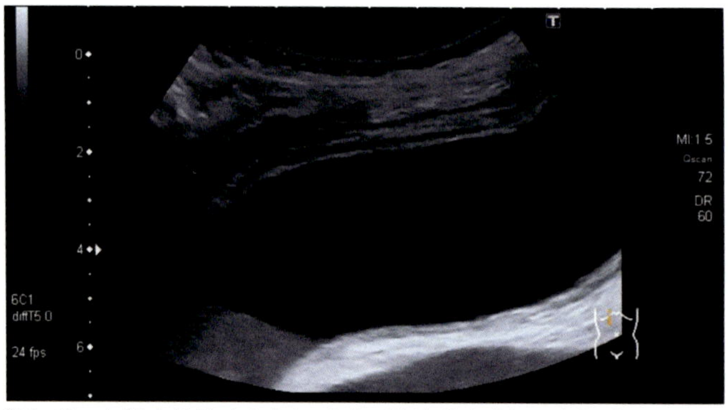

FIGURE 21.5.28 - Gallbladder Wall Thickening and Biliary Sludge on Ultrasound in Acalculous Cholecystitis

XX. Acute Acalculous Cholecystitis: Management
- A. NPO, IV fluids, analgesics, empiric antibiotics
- B. Surgery
  1. Low risk: emergent cholecystectomy
  2. High risk: percutaneous cholecystostomy (gallbladder drainage)
  3. Necrosis, perforation, emphysematous cholecystitis, lack of improvement after drainage requires cholecystectomy

REVIEW QUESTIONS

1. A 42-year-old woman comes to the emergency department because of a dull, achy pain in her right upper quadrant for the last 3-4 hours. She also mentions that the pain radiates to her back and right shoulder. Physical examination shows an overweight woman with right upper quadrant tenderness. What is the best next step in management?

   - **The initial step in diagnosing cholelithiasis is a right upper quadrant ultrasound. If the ultrasound were to be non-diagnostic, then the second step would be an MRCP.**
   - A 42-year-old female who is overweight presents with dull, achy right upper quadrant pain.
   - The pain radiates to her back and right shoulder and there is tenderness in her right upper quadrant.
   - These symptoms are highly indicative of biliary colic.
   - Additionally, the patient is in her forties, overweight, and female, all of which are risk factors for cholelithiasis.

2. A 78-year-old woman is evaluated in an intensive care unit for right upper quadrant abdominal pain for the past day. She was admitted to the ICU 3 weeks ago due to acute decompensated heart failure with left ventricular ejection fraction of 10% (55-70%). Her past medical history includes two myocardial infarctions and GOLD 3 chronic obstructive pulmonary disease. Her vital signs include a temperature of 39 °C (102.2 °F), a blood pressure of 125/75 mmHg, a heart rate of 115 beats/min, and a respiratory rate of 15 breaths/min. Physical examination shows inspiratory arrest on deep right upper quadrant palpation. There is no rebound tenderness or abdominal rigidity. Right upper quadrant ultrasound shows a thickened gallbladder wall with pericholecystic fluid but no gallstones. The common bile duct is of normal diameter. Which of the following is the best next step in the management of this patient?

   A. Emergent cholecystectomy
   B. Percutaneous cholecystostomy
   C. ERCP
   D. HIDA scan

- **The correct answer is option B.**
- This elderly woman complains of right upper abdominal pain for the past day.
- She was admitted to the ICU 3 weeks ago due to acute decompensated heart failure with a very low left ventricular ejection fraction of 10%.
- Additionally, she has a past medical history of two myocardial infarctions and GOLD 3 chronic obstructive pulmonary disease.
- Prolonged ICU stay and all these comorbidities increase her risk of acute acalculous cholecystitis.
- The physical examination reveals inspiratory arrest on deep right upper quadrant palpation. This is known as Murphy's sign and is indeed suggestive of acute cholecystitis.
- Right upper quadrant ultrasound reveals a thickened gallbladder wall with pericholecystic fluid but no gallstones.
- Absence of gallstones along with classic radiographic signs of cholecystitis confirms the diagnosis of acute acalculous cholecystitis.
- This patient is at high risk for surgery due to her comorbidities.
- Therefore, the best next step in the management of this patient's acalculous cholecystitis is percutaneous cholecystostomy.
- Option A is incorrect because this patient is at high risk for surgery. Therefore, cholecystectomy could compromise her clinical status even further.
- Option C is incorrect because endoscopic retrograde cholangiopancreatography, also known as ERCP, is used for choledocholithiasis and acute cholangitis. This patient's common bile duct is of normal diameter, making both choledocholithiasis and acute cholangitis less likely.
- Finally, option D is incorrect because HIDA scan is used when right upper quadrant ultrasound is equivocal or indeterminate. This patient's ultrasound clearly shows signs of gallbladder inflammation along with no gallstones. Therefore, there is no need to perform a HIDA scan.

Gastroenterology | Section 6: Pancreatic Cancer

I. Pancreatic Cancer: Definition
  A. Highly lethal malignancy of the exocrine pancreas
  B. Typically refers to a ductal adenocarcinoma of the pancreas

II. Pancreatic Cancer: Pathophysiology
  A. Can occur in the head, body, or tail of the pancreas
  B. Obstructive jaundice
    1. Due to impaired excretion of bilirubin from liver to intestines
  C. Clay-colored stool
    1. Biliary obstruction decreases bilirubin in intestines
    2. Decreases stercobilin which creates the brown color of stool

III. Pancreatic Cancer: Risk Factors
  A. Chronic pancreatitis
  B. Smoking
  C. High-fat diets
  D. Family history
  E. Primary sclerosing cholangitis

IV. Pancreatic Cancer: Clinical Presentation
  A. Painless jaundice
  B. Weight loss, weakness, loss of energy, anorexia
  C. May be associated with abdominal or epigastric pain
  D. Tea-colored urine and clay-colored stools
  E. Trousseau's syndrome
    1. Unexplained superficial thrombophlebitis due to hypercoagulable state
  F. Courvoisier sign
    1. Painless palpable RUQ mass
    2. Nontender enlarged gallbladder due to obstruction
  G. Sister Mary Joseph nodule
    1. Periumbilical mass that can be seen with GI malignancies

V. Pancreatic Cancer: Diagnosis
  A. Laboratory evaluation
    1. Comprehensive metabolic panel
    2. Lipase to evaluate for pancreatitis
    3. Urine urobilinogen
    4. GGT
    5. CA 19-9 may be elevated but has low specificity
  B. Imaging
    1. Transabdominal ultrasound: biliary dilatation and level of obstruction
    2. CT scan: can confirm diagnosis if a mass is seen on transabdominal ultrasound
  C. Biopsy

VI. Pancreatic Cancer: Management
  A. Whipple procedure
    1. Also known as a pancreaticoduodenectomy
    2. Removes pancreas, duodenum, proximal jejunum, distal stomach, gallbladder, and common bile duct
    3. Distant metastases or tumor invasion into superior mesenteric, celiac, or hepatic arteries prevents surgical intervention
  B. Chemotherapy

REVIEW QUESTIONS ?

1. A 74-year-old woman comes to the physician because of a rash on her left forearm. She first noticed similar lesions on her right foot which have now resolved. The patient states she has lost 20 kg over the last 4 months, and her stools are now clay-colored. She has a 80pack/year smoking history. Physical examination shows jaundice and erythematous, indurated cords on her left forearms. What is the most likely cause of this patient's skin findings?
   - **The most likely cause of this patient's skin findings is pancreatic cancer.**
   - This patient with significant smoking history presents with erythematous, indurated cords on her left forearm.
   - She noticed similar lesions on her right foot which have since resolved..
   - Trousseau's syndrome, which is a superficial migratory thrombophlebitis and is often associated with malignancy.

Gastroenterology | Section 7: Diseases of the Esophagus: Esophageal Cancer & Achalasia

I. Esophageal Cancer: Definition
   A. Adenocarcinoma
      1. More common in the United States
      2. Lower ⅓ of esophagus
   B. Squamous cell carcinoma
      1. More common worldwide
      2. Upper ⅔ of esophagus

II. Esophageal Cancer: Risk Factors
   A. Adenocarcinoma
      1. Gastroesophageal reflux disease (GERD)
      2. Barrett esophagus
      3. Obesity, smoking
   B. Squamous cell carcinoma
      1. Smoking, alcohol, Plummer-Vinson syndrome
      2. Hot liquids, caustic ingestion, achalasia

III. Esophageal Cancer: Pathophysiology
   A. Irritant stimulus → metaplasia or dysplasia of esophageal epithelium → irreversible malignant transformation of esophageal epithelium

IV. Esophageal Cancer: Clinical Presentation
   A. Weight loss, fatigue, low-grade fever
   B. Progressive dysphagia (first solids, then liquids) due to enlarging mass
   C. Odynophagia
   D. Chest pain
   E. Hoarseness (recurrent laryngeal nerve involvement)
   F. Rapid spread due to lack of serosa in esophageal wall
   G. Poor prognosis due to advanced stage at presentation

V. Esophageal Cancer: Diagnosis
   A. Endoscopy with biopsy
      1. Exophytic (protruding) or endophytic (ulcerating) mass
      2. Adenocarcinoma
         a) Mucin-positive cells arranged in tubules
      3. Squamous cell carcinoma
         a) Keratin pearls
         b) Intercellular bridges (desmosomes)
   B. Full metastatic work-up
      1. Transesophageal ultrasound (local metastasis)
      2. CT of the abdomen and pelvis
      3. Bone scan

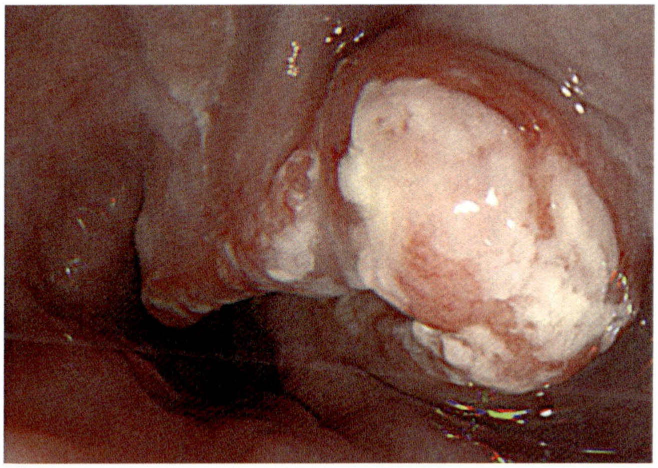

FIGURE 21.5.29 - Esophagogastroduodenoscopy: Exophytic Mass in Esophageal Adenocarcinoma

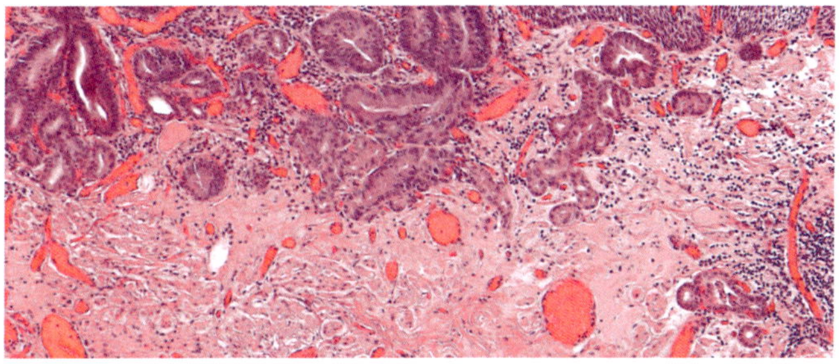

FIGURE 21.5.30 - Metaplastic Tubules in Esophageal Adenocarcinoma

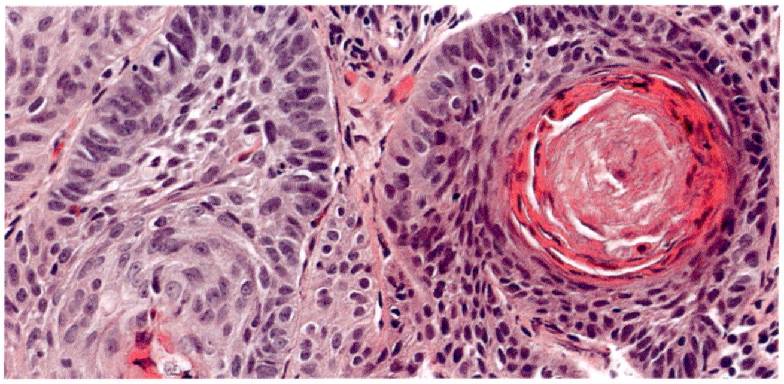

FIGURE 21.5.31 - Keratin Pearl in Esophageal Squamous Cell Carcinoma

VI. Esophageal Cancer: Management
   A. Chemotherapy (e.g. cisplatin, 5-fluorouracil, paclitaxel)
   B. Radiation therapy
   C. Esophagectomy
   D. Hospice care for patients with advanced-stage disease

VII. Achalasia: Definition
   A. Failure of lower esophageal sphincter to relax
   B. Mostly idiopathic

VIII. Achalasia: Causes
- A. Primary achalasia: idiopathic
- B. Secondary achalasia
  - 1. Chagas disease due to *Trypanosoma cruzi*
  - 2. Esophageal cancer
  - 3. Extraesophageal malignancies
    - a) Mediastinal cancer exerting mass effect

IX. Achalasia: Pathophysiology
- A. Destruction of inhibitory neurons in myenteric (Auerbach) plexus → ↓ NO and VIP → ↓ relaxation of lower esophageal sphincter → achalasia

X. Achalasia: Clinical Presentation
- A. Dysphagia to both solids and liquids due to impaired esophageal peristalsis
- B. Regurgitation of food
- C. Halitosis (unpleasant smell in oral cavity)
- D. ↑ risk for esophageal cancer

XI. Achalasia: Diagnosis
- A. Barium swallow
  - 1. "Bird's beak" appearance
- B. Esophageal manometry
  - 1. Weak peristalsis throughout the esophagus
  - 2. Increased lower esophageal sphincter pressure
- C. Chest X-ray
  - 1. Widened mediastinum
  - 2. Absent gastric air bubble
- D. Endoscopy with biopsy
  - 1. Rules out esophageal cancer as the cause of achalasia

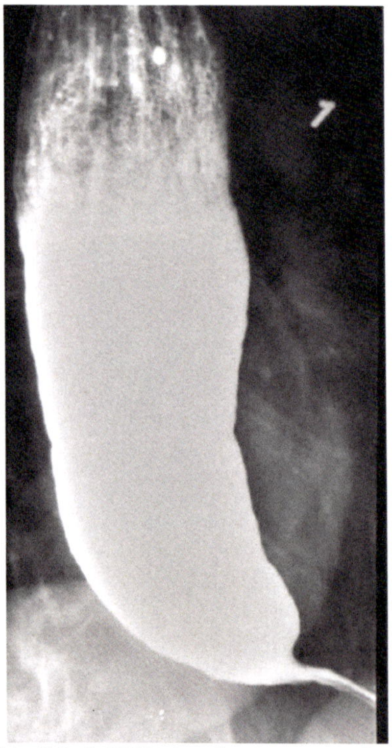

FIGURE 21.5.32 - Barium Swallow: "Bird's Beak" Sign in Achalasia

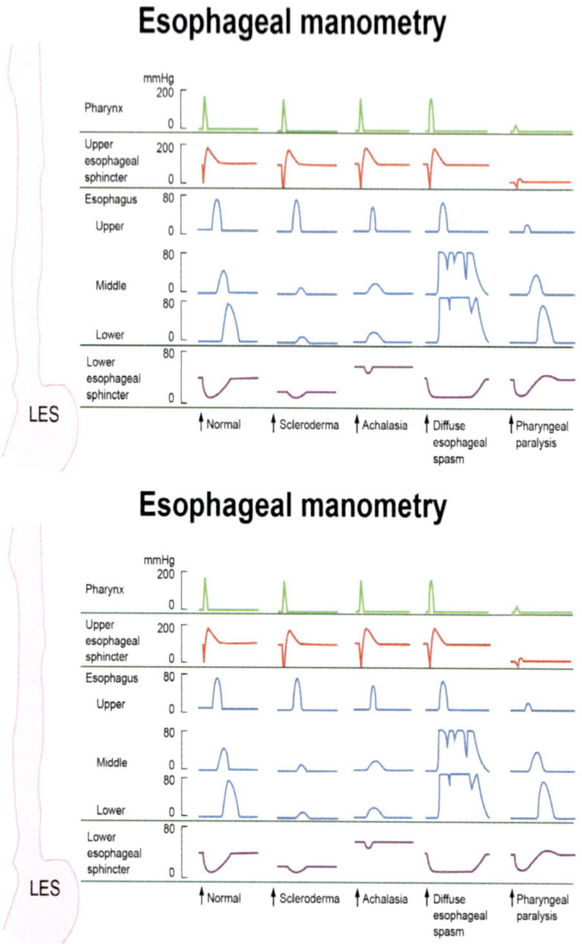

FIGURE 21.5.33 - Manometry Findings in Achalasia

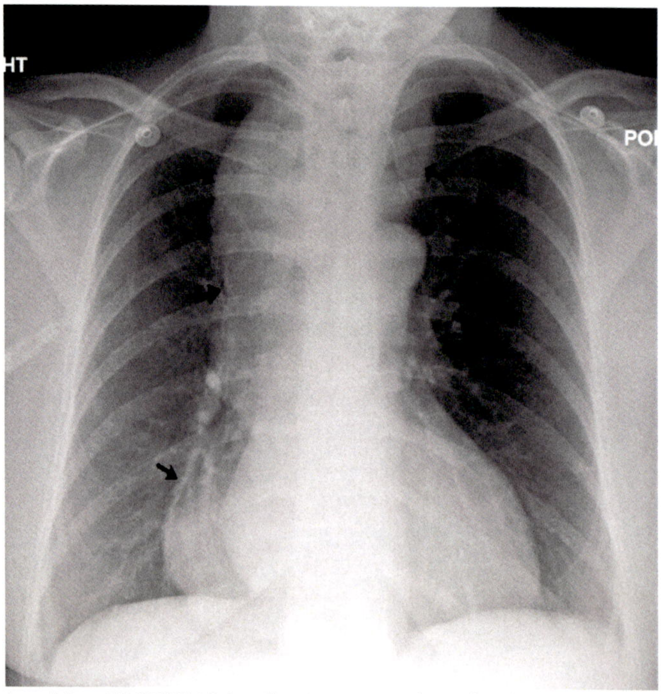

FIGURE 21.5.34 - Chest X-Ray: Widened Mediastinum and Absent Gastric Air Bubble in Achalasia

XII. Achalasia: Management
  A. Pneumatic dilation
    1. Temporary measure
    2. Risk for esophageal perforation
  B. Botulinum toxin (botox) injection
    1. Temporary measure
    2. Relaxes lower esophageal sphincter
  C. Heller myotomy: incision of LES muscle (↑ risk for GERD)

REVIEW QUESTIONS

1. A 67-year-old man comes to the physician due to a 20-kg unintentional weight loss over the past 4 months, low-grade fever, and progressive dysphagia. He has been smoking 2 packs of cigarettes per day for 40 years, and he has been drinking one bottle of wine daily for the last 10 years. Recently, he has also noticed hoarseness of his voice. He is diagnosed with esophageal squamous cell carcinoma. What is the most likely underlying cause of this patient's hoarseness?
   - **This patient's hoarseness is caused by invasion of the recurrent laryngeal nerve by malignancy.**
   - This patient with a long-term smoking and drinking history has a 20-kg unintentional weight loss over the past 4 months, low-grade fever, and progressive dysphagia.
   - Recently, he has noticed hoarseness of his voice.
   - He is diagnosed with esophageal squamous cell carcinoma.
   - Hoarseness in the context of esophageal cancer is best explained by recurrent laryngeal nerve invasion by malignancy.

2. A 78-year-old woman with a 20-year history of gastroesophageal reflux disease comes to the emergency department because of unintentional weight loss, low-grade fever, and progressive dysphagia for the past 2 months. Endoscopy shows an exophytic esophageal mass. Biopsy confirms esophageal adenocarcinoma. What is most likely to be seen on the biopsy of this patient's lesion?
   - **Biopsy will show mucin-positive, light-colored cells arranged in tubules.**
   - This patient with a long-term history of gastroesophageal reflux disease presents with unintentional weight loss, low-grade fever, and progressive dysphagia.
   - Biopsy of an exophytic esophageal mass confirms esophageal adenocarcinoma.
   - Biopsy of esophageal adenocarcinoma typically shows mucin-positive, light-colored cells arranged in tubules.

3. A 45-year-old man comes to the office because of an unpleasant taste in the mouth and difficulty swallowing solids and liquids. He has occasional regurgitation of undigested food at night. Barium studies show proximal widening and distal narrowing of the esophagus. Esophageal manometry is performed. What are expected findings on esophageal manometry?
   - **Esophageal manometry will show weak peristalsis throughout the esophagus and increased baseline LES pressure.**
   - This patient presents with an unpleasant taste in the mouth, dysphagia to solids and liquids, and occasional regurgitation of undigested food at night.
   - Barium studies show proximal widening and distal narrowing of the esophagus.
   - All of these findings are consistent with the diagnosis of achalasia.
   - Esophageal manometry in the case of achalasia shows weak peristalsis throughout the esophagus and an increased baseline pressure of the lower esophageal sphincter.

Gastroenterology | Section 8: Plummer-Vinson Syndrome, Schatzki Ring & Zenker Diverticulum

I. Plummer-Vinson Syndrome: Definition and Risk Factors
   A. Definition
      1. Esophageal webs causing dysphagia
   B. Risk factor
      1. Iron deficiency anemia

II. Plummer-Vinson Syndrome: Pathophysiology
   A. Iron deficiency → abnormal maturation of esophageal mucosa → reactive mucosal hyperplasia → esophageal webs

III. Plummer-Vinson Syndrome: Clinical Presentation
   A. Esophageal webs
      1. Dysphagia to solids but not liquids
      2. ↑ risk of esophageal squamous cell carcinoma
   B. Iron deficiency anemia
      1. Fatigue
      2. Koilonychia (spoon nails)
      3. Glossitis (inflammation of the tongue), angular cheilitis

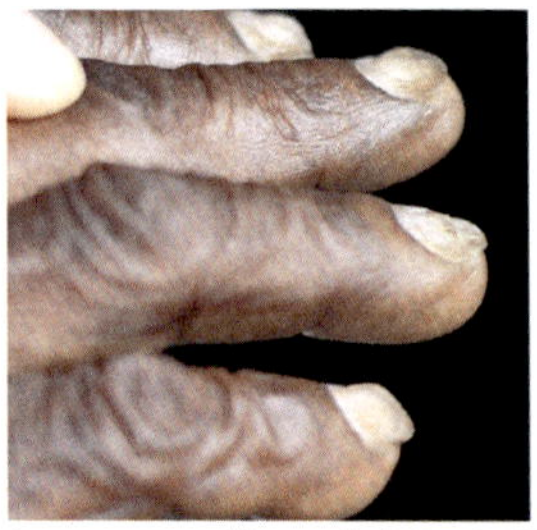

FIGURE 21.5.35 - Koilonychia

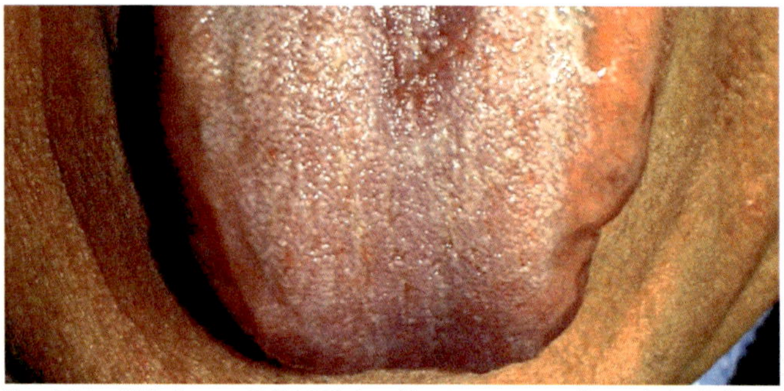

FIGURE 21.5.36 - Glossitis

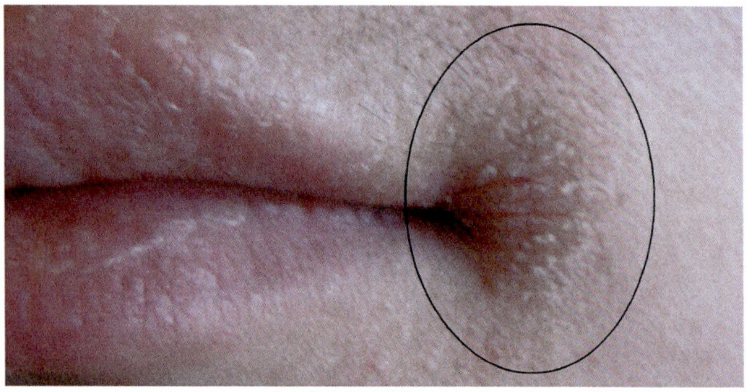

FIGURE 21.5.37 - Angular Cheilitis

IV. Plummer-Vinson Syndrome: Diagnosis
   A. Endoscopy
      1. Esophageal webs
   B. Complete blood count
      1. Microcytic hypochromic anemia (↓ Hgb, ↓ Hct, ↓ MCV)
   C. Iron panel
      1. ↓ serum iron, ferritin, and transferrin saturation
      2. ↑ total iron binding capacity (TIBC)

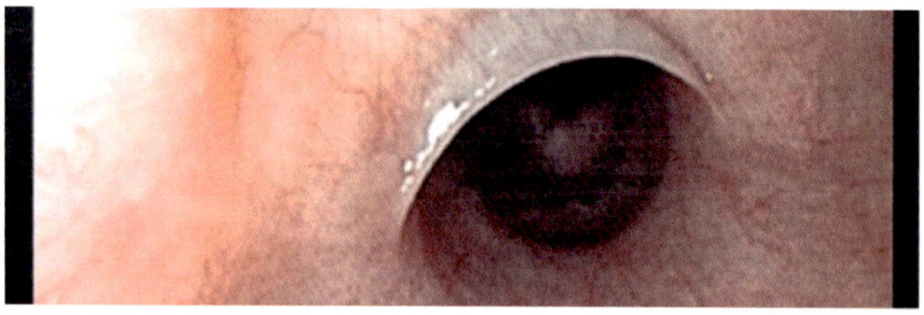

FIGURE 21.5.38 - Esophagogastroduodenoscopy Showing Esophageal Webs

V. Plummer-Vinson Syndrome: Management
   A. Surgical excision of esophageal webs
      1. Improves dysphagia
      2. Reduces risk of esophageal squamous cell carcinoma
   B. Iron supplementation

VI. Schatzki Ring: Definition
   A. Circular band of mucosal tissue (stricture) at the gastroesophageal junction

VII. Schatzki Ring: Risk Factors
   A. Gastroesophageal reflux disease (GERD)
   B. Caustic ingestion
   C. Esophagitis

VIII. Schatzki Ring: Pathophysiology
   A. Irritant stimulus (e.g. gastric acid, caustic material, infection) → esophageal wall fibrosis and reactive epithelial hyperplasia → circular mucosal band at the gastroesophageal junction

IX. Schatzki Ring: Clinical Presentation
   A. Asymptomatic (minor obstruction)
   B. Dysphagia to solids but not liquids
   C. Heartburn
   D. Chest pain
   E. Food impaction in the distal esophagus

X. Schatzki Ring: Diagnosis
   A. Barium swallow
      1. Narrowed gastroesophageal junction
      2. Not highly sensitive for Schatzki ring
   B. Endoscopy (gold standard)
      1. Circular mucosal band at the gastroesophageal junction

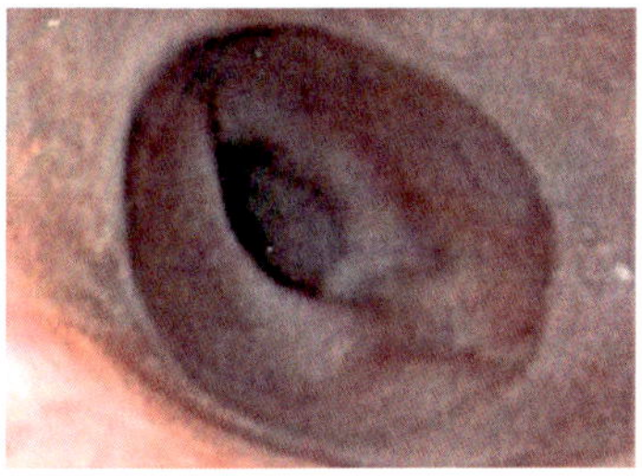

FIGURE 21.5.39 - Esophagogastroduodenoscopy of a Schatzki Ring

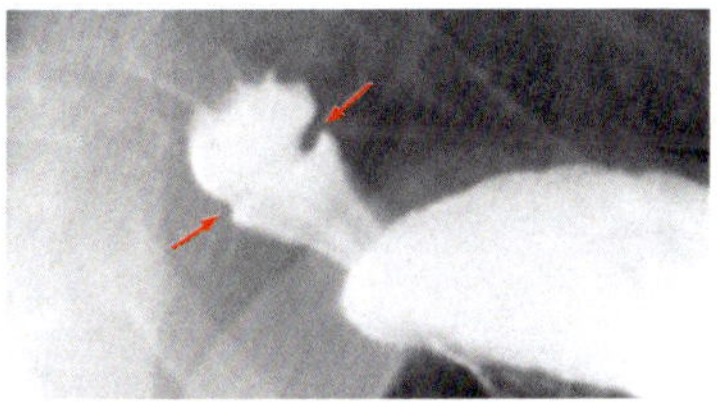

FIGURE 21.5.40 - Barium Swallow: Schatzki Ring

XI. Schatzki Ring: Management
  A. Esophageal dilation
    1. Not curative
    2. Risk for esophageal perforation
  B. Surgical excision in refractory cases

XII. Zenker Diverticulum: Definition
  A. False diverticulum (mucosa and submucosa) at the pharyngoesophageal junction
  B. Common in elderly men

XIII. Zenker Diverticulum: Risk Factors
  A. Esophageal dysmotility
    1. Prior stroke
    2. Diabetes mellitus
    3. Scleroderma
    4. Amyotrophic lateral sclerosis
    5. Myasthenia gravis

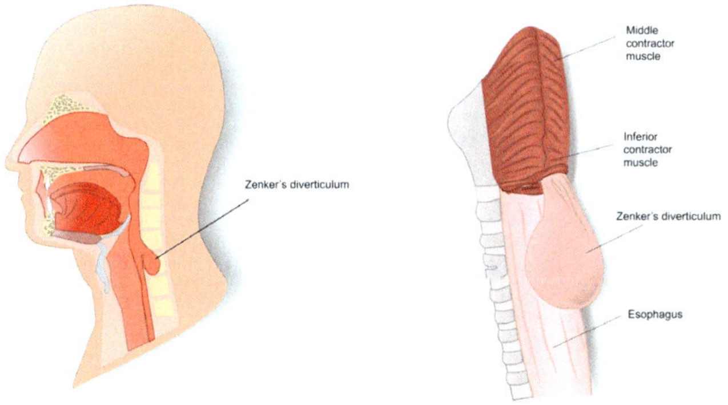

FIGURE 21.5.41 - Zenker DIverticulum

XIV. Zenker Diverticulum: Clinical Presentation
  A. Dysphagia to solids and liquids
  B. Gurgling
  C. Regurgitation of food in supine position
  D. Halitosis
  E. Sensation of neck mass

XV. Zenker Diverticulum: Diagnosis and Management
  A. Diagnosis
  B. Barium swallow
  C. Endoscopy
    1. Mucosal pouch at pharyngoesophageal junction
  D. Management
    1. Surgical incision of inferior pharyngeal constrictor muscle (diverticulotomy) or excision or pouch (diverticulectomy)

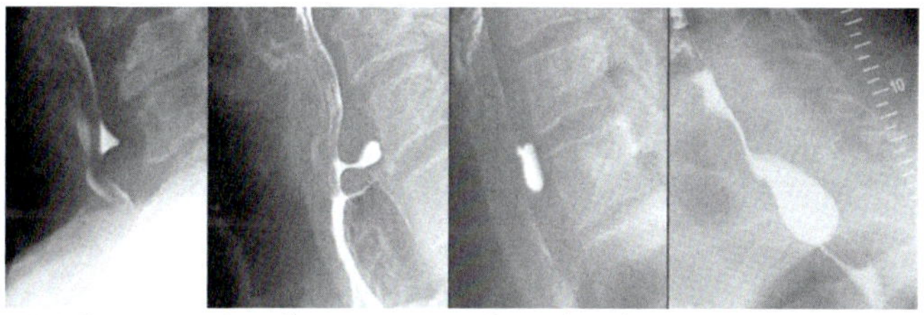

FIGURE 21.5.42 - Barium Swallow: Zenker Diverticulum

REVIEW QUESTIONS

1. A 38-year-old man comes to the physician because of difficulty swallowing the past 6 months. Physical examination shows pale conjunctiva and shiny, erythematous tongue. Vital signs are within normal limits. Endoscopy is performed and shows multiple mucosal protrusions in the esophageal lumen. Which nutrient should be supplemented in this patient's diet?
   - **Iron should be supplemented in this patient's diet.**
   - This patient presents with dysphagia food.
   - Pale conjunctiva suggests anemia while shiny, erythematous tongue suggests glossitis.
   - Multiple mucosal protrusions in the esophageal lumen are consistent with esophageal webs.
   - Esophageal webs, dysphagia, anemia, and glossitis suggest the diagnosis of Plummer-Vinson syndrome.
   - Anemia in Plummer-Vinson syndrome is due to iron deficiency. Therefore, iron should be supplemented in this patient's diet.

2. An 88-year-old man comes to the physician because of difficulty swallowing both solids and liquids. He states there is an unpleasant taste in mouth, and he occasionally regurgitates undigested food. He mentions a sensation of a deep neck mass. What is the best initial diagnostic test for this patient's condition?
   - **The best initial diagnostic test for this patient's condition is barium studies.**
   - This patient presents with dysphagia to solids and liquids, unpleasant taste in mouth, and occasional regurgitation of undigested food.
   - He also has a sensation of a deep neck mass.
   - All of these findings are consistent with the diagnosis of Zenker diverticulum.

Gastroenterology | Section 9: Gastric Malignancies

I. Gastric Adenocarcinoma: Definition
   A. Two histological types
      1. Intestinal: ulcerative
      2. Diffuse: thickened (linitis plastica), poorer prognosis

II. Gastric Adenocarcinoma: Risk Factors
   A. Consuming nitrosamines in smoked foods
   B. Cigarette smoking
   C. *H. pylori*, chronic gastritis → intestinal metaplasia
   D. Other risk factors include gastric ulcers, gastric polyps, and partial gastrectomy

III. Gastric Adenocarcinoma: Clinical Features
   A. History of present illness
      1. Involuntary weight loss, abdominal pain, early satiety
      2. Leser-Trelat sign: multiple seborrhoeic keratoses suddenly appear
      3. Acanthosis nigricans: dark, velvety discoloration in body folds and creases
      4. Signs of upper GI bleeding: hematemesis, melena
   B. Signs of metastasis
      1. Virchow node: left supraclavicular lymphadenopathy
      2. Krukenberg tumor: signet cells, bilateral ovaries
      3. Sister Mary Joseph nodule: periumbilical metastasis
      4. Blumer shelf: mass on digital rectal exam, metastasis to pouch of Douglas

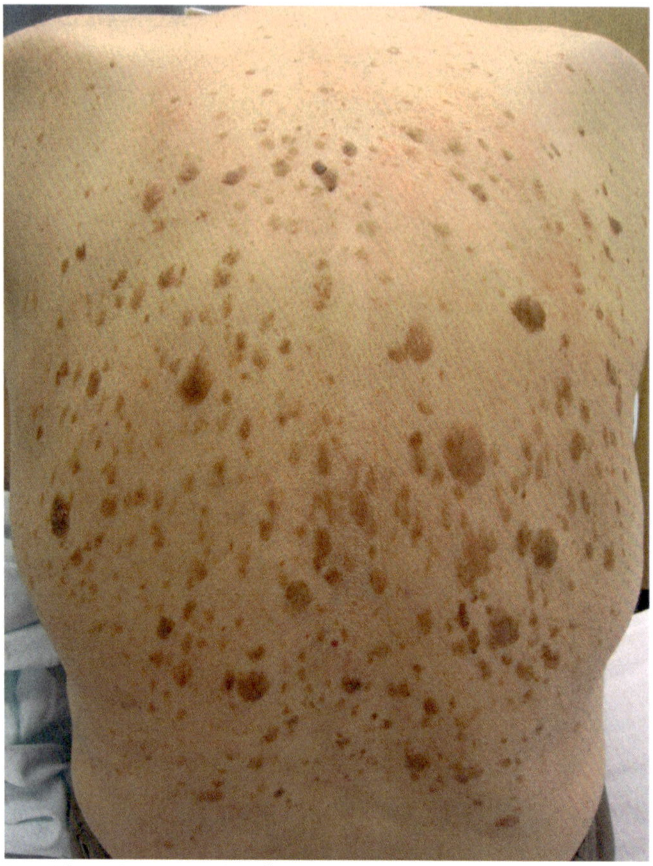

FIGURE 21.5.44 - Seborrheic Keratosis

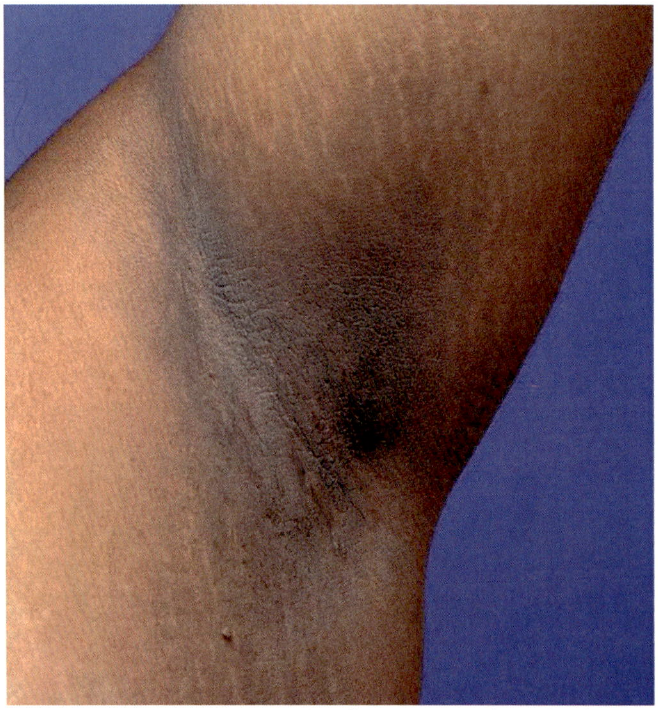

FIGURE 21.5.43 - Acanthosis Nigricans

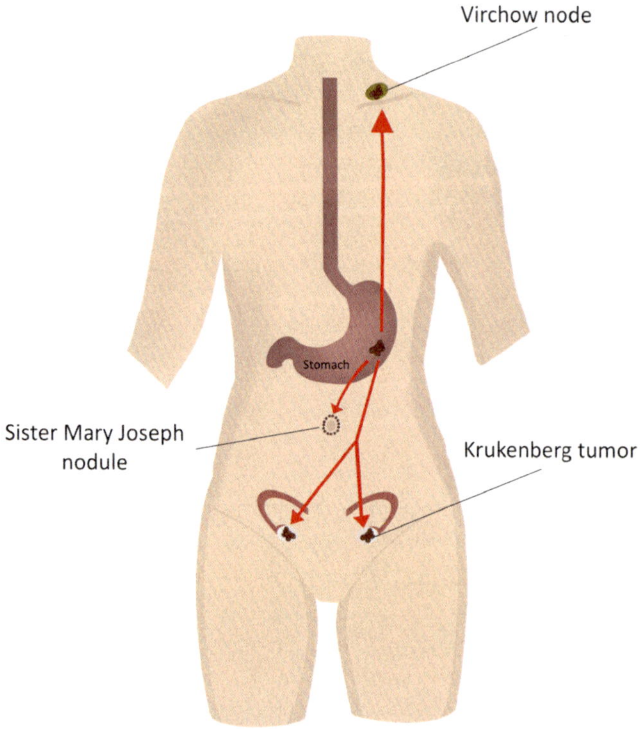

FIGURE 21.5.45 - Location of Metastasis in Gastric Cancer

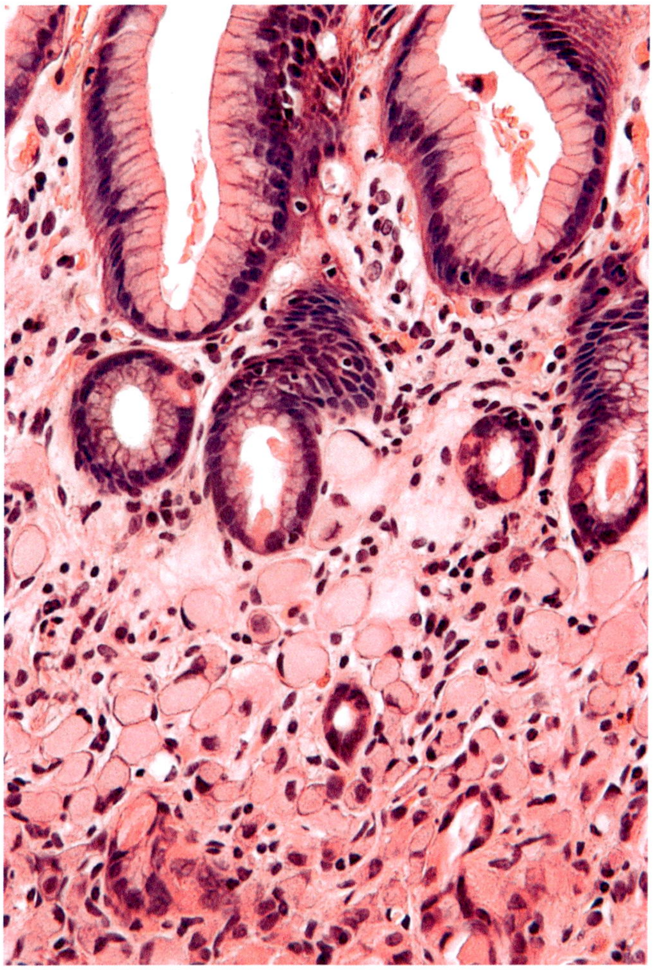

FIGURE 21.5.46 - Signet Cells on Histology

IV. Gastric Adenocarcinoma: Diagnosis
  A. Upper GI endoscopy with multiple biopsies
    1. Intestinal: lesser curvature, ulcer with raised margins
    2. Diffuse: thickened and leathery
  B. Abdominal CT scan for metastasis and stage

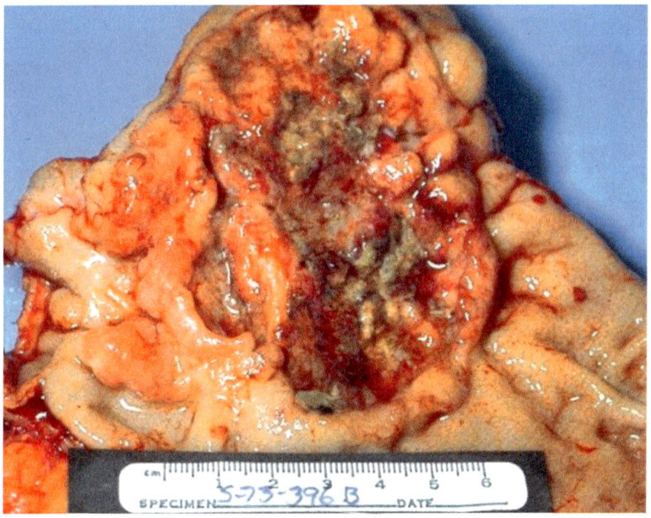

FIGURE 21.5.47 - Gross Image of Intestinal Adenocarcinoma of the Stomach

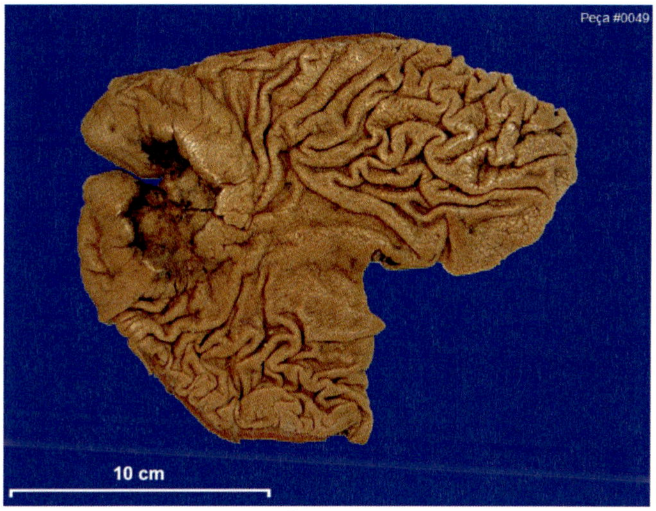

FIGURE 21.5.48 - Gross Image of Diffuse Adenocarcinoma of Stomach

V. Gastric Adenocarcinoma: Treatment
  A. Management
    1. Endoscopic resection
    2. Gastrectomy and lymphadenectomy
    3. Roux-en-Y procedure
    4. Chemotherapy

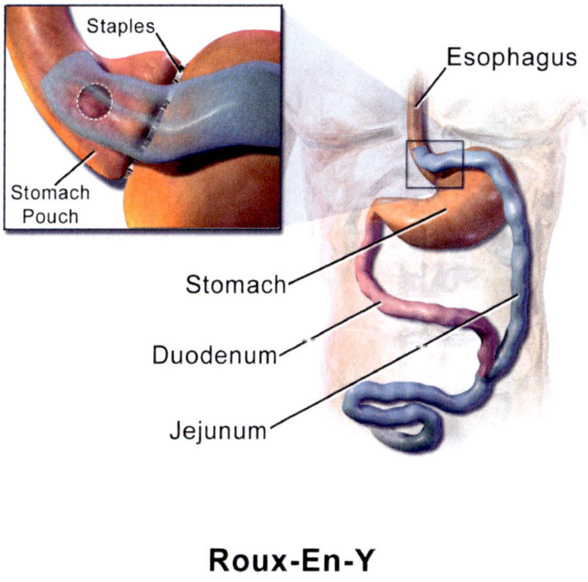

FIGURE 21.5.49 - Roux-En-Y Surgery

VI. Gastric Lymphoma: Definition
  A. Diffuse large B-cell lymphoma
  B. MALT lymphoma (mucosa associated lymphoid tissue)

VII. Gastric Lymphoma: Etiology
  A. Chronic *H. pylori* infection is associated with MALT lymphoma

VIII. Gastric Lymphoma: Clinical Features
  A. History of present illness
    1. Involuntary weight loss, abdominal pain, early satiety, melena
    2. Unremarkable physical exam

IX. Gastric Lymphoma: Diagnosis
  A. Endoscopy with biopsy
    1. Identify *H. pylori* infection or malignancy
  B. Histopathology and immunochemistry
    1. Histopathology findings: thick infiltrates of lymphoid cells
    2. Immunochemistry findings: immunologic markers of B-cell such as *CD20*
  C. CT or MRI for tumor staging

X. Gastric Lymphoma: Treatment
  A. Triple therapy or quadruple therapy (*H. pylori*)
    1. Triple: Amoxicillin, clarithromycin, proton pump inhibitors (PPI)
    2. Quadruple: Macrolides, tetracyclines, bismuth, PPI
  B. If *H. pylori* negative or unresponsive to *H. pylori* treatment
    1. Local radiotherapy; chemotherapy for refractory cases
      a) Rituximab: inhibits CD20, downregulating B cells that cause tumor burden

XI. GI Stromal Tumors: Definition
  A. Stromal tumor found anywhere in the GI tract
    1. Most common in the stomach
  B. Arises from the interstitial cells of Cajal in the stomach; pacemaker cells for peristalsis

XII. GI Stromal Tumors: Pathophysiology
  A. Activating mutation in c-*Kit* proto-oncogenes

XIII. GI Stromal Tumors: Clinical Features
  A. History of present illness
    1. Bloating and early satiety
    2. Abdominal pain, melena

XIV. GI Stromal Tumors: Diagnosis
  A. Contrast CT scan: solid, smoothly contoured mass
  B. MRI: necrosis and hemorrhage with larger tumors
  C. Immunochemistry and histopathology
  D. *c-Kit* receptor analysis

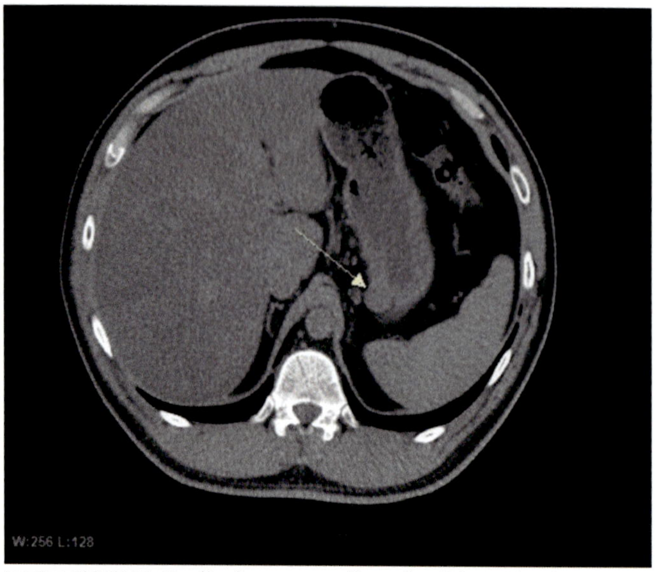

FIGURE 21.5.50 - Abdominal CT Scan of GIST

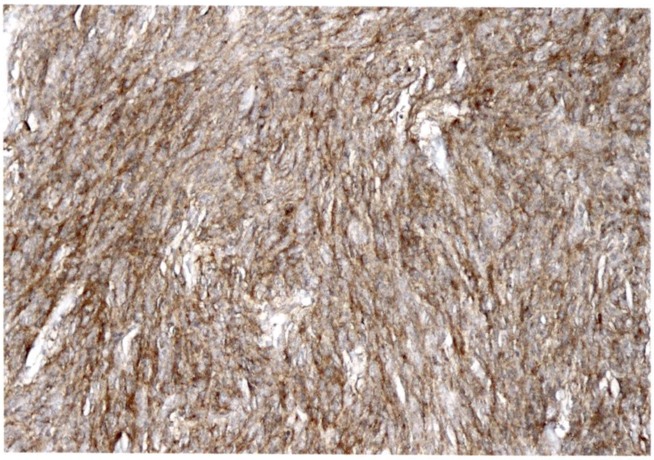

FIGURE 21.5.51 - GIST Under Immunohistochemistry for *c-Kit*

XV. GI Stromal Tumors: Treatment
  A. Resection for localized tumors
  B. *C-kit* tyrosine kinase inhibitors
    1. Imatinib
    2. Sunitinib

REVIEW QUESTIONS

1. A 54-year-old man comes to the clinic because of abdominal pain and dyspepsia for 3-months. He is an immigrant from China. Physical examination shows epigastric pain, mild hepatomegaly, and a palpable nodule just above the left clavicle. Initial laboratory studies show Hgb 8.2 g/dL and MCV 74 μm^3. What is the next best step in the diagnosis?

   - **The next best step in the diagnosis would be to refer this patient for upper endoscopy as there's a high likelihood that this patient may have gastric cancer.**
   - Gastric cancer is particularly prevalent in Eastern Asia, Eastern Europe, and certain parts of South America as a result of diets rich in carcinogenic nitrosamine compounds.
   - Findings of epigastric pain in conjunction with mild hepatomegaly and the Virchow node should always prompt suspicion of gastric cancer.
   - Findings of a microcytic anemia on initial laboratory evaluation is also highly suspicious of and consistent with a diagnosis of gastric cancer.
   - Hence, this patient needs to undergo endoscopy and all suspicious lesions must be biopsied and sent for analysis.

2. A 55-year-old woman comes to her primary care provider to follow-up on results of biopsy. Recently a biopsy was taken from a 3-cm mass that was found in her stomach. Histological report shows lymphoma arising from the mucosa-associated lymphoid tissue. What is the next best step in management?

   - **The next best step in management is to test for *H. pylori.***
   - A lymphoma arising from the mucosa-associated lymphoid tissue is the description of MALT lymphoma.
   - All patients diagnosed with MALT lymphoma must be tested for *H. pylori* infection as it is present in about 90% of patients with MALT lymphomas.
   - Interestingly, early-stage MALT lymphomas can be treated solely by eradicating the *H. pylori* infection.

3. A 67-year-old man with a history of osteoarthritis presents to his primary care provider because of intermittent abdominal pain and heartburn for the last 4-months. He describes the pain as "burning" and localizing just above his belly button. He says the pain often gets worse soon after he eats. He has never had anything similar before. The only medication he takes is daily ibuprofen "for a bad knee." Vital signs include a blood pressure of 139/75 mmHg, pulse of 75 bpm, and temperature of 37.0° C (98.6° F). BMI is 26 kg/m^2, down from 29 kg/m^2 during his prior clinic visit four months ago. Abdominal examination shows mild tenderness to palpation in the epigastric region. Rectal examination is unremarkable. In addition to laboratory work-up, which of the following options is the next best step in management of this patient?

   A. Order a urea breath test
   B. Initiate omeprazole, amoxicillin, and clarithromycin
   C. Refer for upper endoscopy
   D. Order a stool guaiac test

   - **The correct answer is option C.**
   - This is a case of a patient presenting with burning epigastric pain that worsens after he eats, which is suggestive of peptic ulcer disease.
   - However, this 67-year-old patient also lost a significant amount of weight since his prior visit given that his BMI has decreased from 29 to 26.
   - His old age and unintentional weight loss are concerning for underlying malignancy, which would be best evaluated with upper endoscopy.
   - A urease breath test can be ordered to test for presence of *H. pylori* infection.
   - Unfortunately, this patient's high-risk features of old age and weight loss warrant an assessment for cancer, not just *H. pylori* infection.
   - Since endoscopic biopsy of a presumed gastric ulcer can be diagnostic of both cancer and *H. pylori* infection, it is preferred over the urea breath test, so option A is incorrect.
   - Option B describes the triple therapy that can be employed in eradication of *H. pylori* infection. This option is incorrect because we must first evaluate this patient for the presence of cancer.
   - Option D would determine whether this patient is experiencing occult gastrointestinal blood loss. Though somewhat useful, the diagnostic yield of a stool guaiac test pales in comparison to the diagnostic yield of an upper endoscopy in a patient with presumed gastric cancer, which is why option D is incorrect.

Gastroenterology | Section 10: Small Bowel Obstruction

I. Small Bowel Obstruction: Definition
   A. Mechanical small bowel obstruction is due to either intraluminal obstruction or extraluminal compression
   B. Partial obstruction vs. complete obstruction
      1. Partial: some intestinal content can pass through the blocked segment
      2. Complete: total blockage with no passage of intestinal content
   C. Closed-loop: a segment of bowel is obstructed at two points
   D. Simple vs. strangulated
      1. Simple: no evidence of ischemia
      2. Strangulated: compromised blood flow leading to ischemia and necrosis, associated with severe abdominal pain and localized tenderness
      3. Fever, tachycardia, leukocytosis are associated with strangulation

II. Small Bowel Obstruction: Pathophysiology
   A. Proximal to the blockage: progressive dilation and increased pressure
      1. Increased peristalsis to overcome the obstruction
   B. Distal to the obstruction: decompression of bowel
   C. Bowel becomes edematous and loses absorptive function → fluid accumulates in the lumen
   D. Ischemic necrosis
      1. Bowel or mesentery twists around adhesive band or attachment
      2. Excessive bowel dilation compromises vasculature
      3. Increased bowel wall permeability → translocation of intestinal microbes → sepsis
      4. Perforation of bowel → peritonitis
      5. Anaerobic metabolism creates lactic acid

III. Small Bowel Obstruction: Etiologies
   A. Extraluminal compression
      1. Adhesions due to prior surgeries or inflammatory processes are the most common cause of SBO
      2. Volvulus
      3. Incarcerated hernias
      4. Intussusception
      5. Superior mesenteric artery syndrome
   B. Incarcerated hernia
      1. Intestines herniate through abdominal wall and cannot be reduced
      2. Causes obstruction of that portion of the intestine
   C. Intussusception
      1. Proximal portion of small bowel telescopes into distal portion
      2. Usually due to a lead point that becomes stuck during peristalsis, dragging the bowel forward; Meckel diverticulum is most common
   D. Superior mesenteric artery syndrome
      1. Portion of the duodenum becomes trapped underneath the superior mesenteric artery
      2. Usually protected by abdominal fat pad
      3. Significant weight loss → loss of abdominal fat pad that surrounds the duodenum → compression and obstruction of the duodenum
   E. Intraluminal obstruction
      1. Tumors
      2. Strictures, associated with Crohn's disease
      3. Gallstones
      4. Foreign bodies

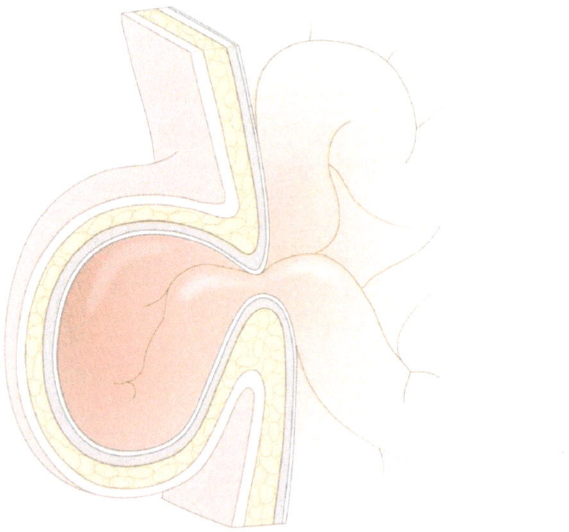

FIGURE 21.5.52 - Illustration of a Hernia

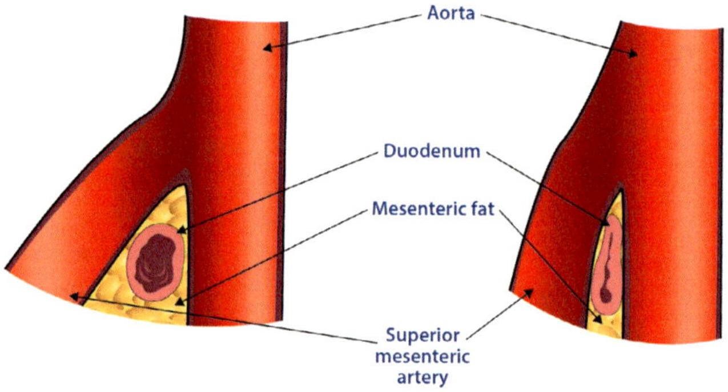

FIGURE 21.5.53 - Superior Mesenteric Artery Syndrome

IV. Small Bowel Obstruction: Clinical Features
   A. Nausea and vomiting
   B. Colicky abdominal pain and distension
   C. Constipation or obstipation
   D. Signs of dehydration: tachycardia, orthostatic hypotension
   E. Change in bowel sounds
      1. Early: increased high-pitched tinkling bowel sounds
      2. Late: absent bowel sounds

F. Metabolic derangements
   1. Loss of fluid through vomiting and third-space volume loss into the lumen
   2. Lose sodium, potassium, hydrogen ions, and chloride when vomiting
   3. Results in hypovolemia with a hypokalemic, hypochloremic metabolic alkalosis

V. Small Bowel Obstruction: Diagnosis
   A. Laboratory evaluation
      1. Complete blood count: leukocytosis may indicate complications
      2. Basic metabolic panel: establish the severity of hypovolemia and electrolyte abnormalities
      3. Serum lactate: detect the presence of ischemia or necrosis
      4. Arterial blood gas: evaluate for acid-base changes (alkalosis, acidosis)
   B. Imaging
      1. Abdominal series: chest film, upright and supine abdominal films
      2. Chest radiograph: investigate for free air
      3. Upright abdominal radiograph: air-fluid levels and the presence of air in the colon
      4. Supine abdominal radiograph: estimate distention
   C. CT scan can confirm the presence of a small bowel obstruction
      1. Reveals transition point between the area proximal to the obstruction and distal to the obstruction
      2. Target sign: concentric circles; intussusception
      3. Whirl sign: twisting of bowel around mesentery; volvulus
      4. Pneumatosis: gas in wall of intestine; ischemia and necrosis
      5. Pneumoperitoneum: free air under the diaphragm, spleen, or liver

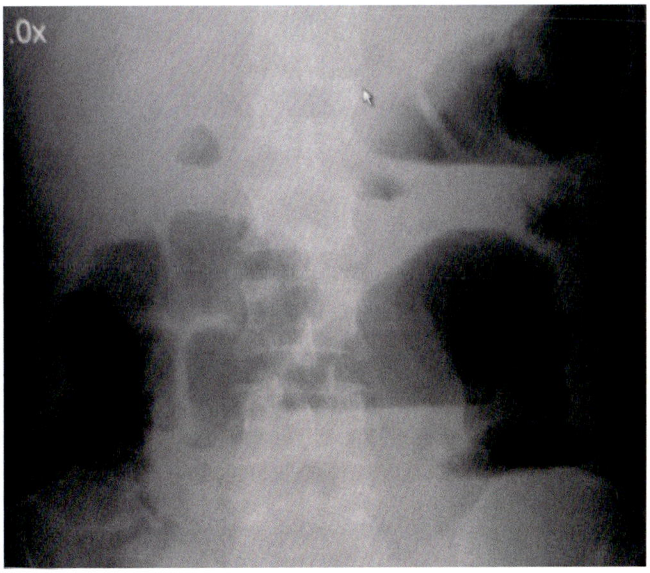

FIGURE 21.5.54 - Plain Upright Abdominal X-Ray of Small Bowel Obstruction

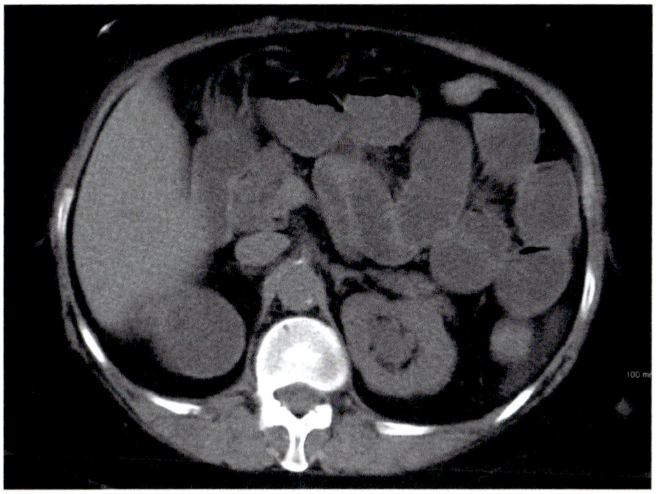

FIGURE 21.5.55 - Abdominal CT Showing Dilated Loops of Bowel with Air Fluid Levels

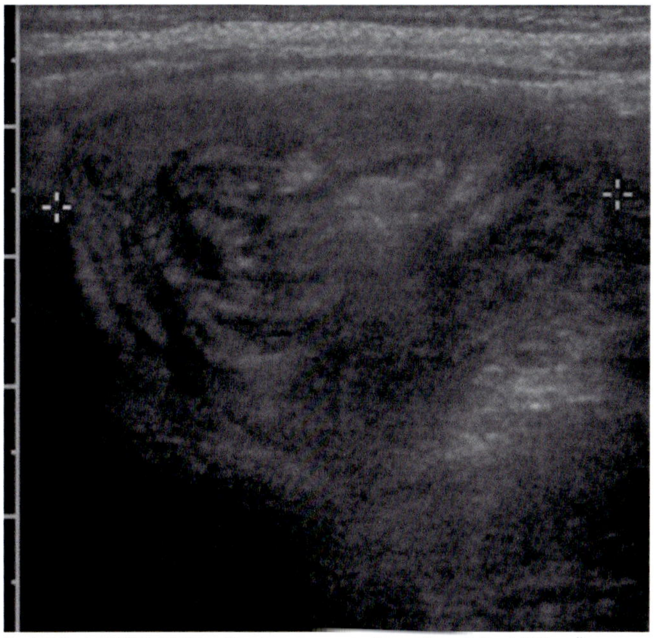

FIGURE 21.5.56 - Ultrasound Study of a Patient with Intussusception

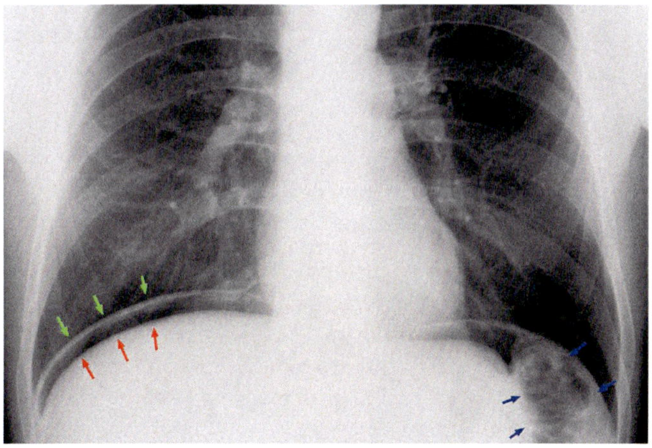

FIGURE 21.5.57 - Upright Chest X-Ray Showing Pneumoperitoneum

VI. Small Bowel Obstruction: Management
   A. Conservative
      1. Partial obstruction or no signs of ischemia
      2. IV fluids and correction of electrolytes
      3. Decompression with NG tube
      4. NPO for bowel rest
      5. Analgesics and antiemetics; avoid metoclopramide
      6. Serial abdominal assessments (to detect changes)
   B. Surgical management required if
      1. Complete obstruction with hemodynamic instability or sepsis
      2. Signs of ischemia or necrosis
      3. Closed-loop obstructions
      4. Persistent obstructions
   C. Exploratory laparotomy
      1. Resection of nonviable bowel if present
      2. Examine for abnormal color, the absence of peristalsis, and the absence of arterial pulsations in the mesentery

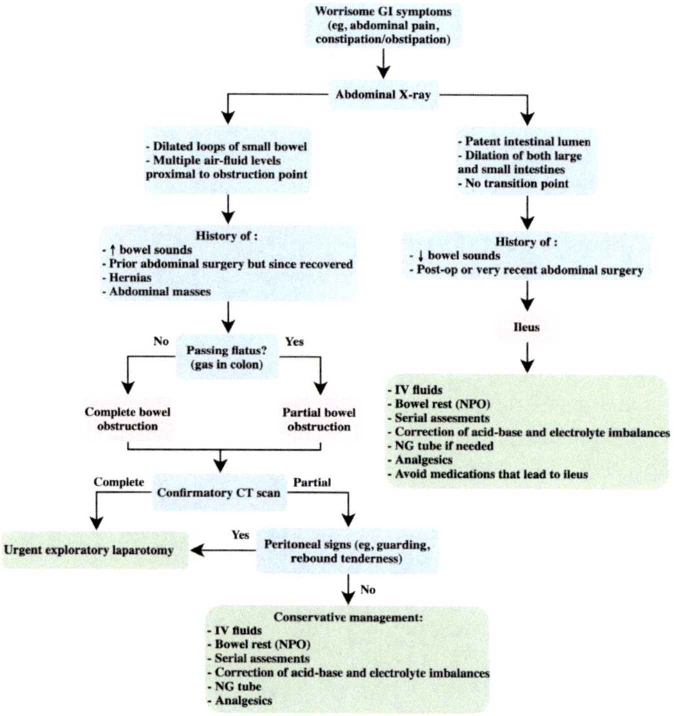

FIGURE 21.5.58 - Small Bowel Obstruction Algorithm

REVIEW QUESTIONS

1. A 57-year-old woman is brought to the emergency department due to intractable vomiting and abdominal pain for the past day. Past medical history is significant for cholecystectomy for acute cholecystitis. She has not had a bowel movement for the last 3 days. Vital signs include a blood pressure of 85/70 mmHg, heart rate of 130 beats/min, and respiratory rate of 13 breaths/min. Abdominal X-ray shows dilated duodenal and jejunal loops with air-fluid levels, and a gasless ileum. Which acid-base disturbance is most likely present in this patient?
   - **The acid-base disturbance most likely present in this patient is hypokalemic hypochloremic metabolic alkalosis.**
   - This patient presents with vomiting, abdominal pain, and absent bowel movements for the last 3 days.
   - Her abdominal X-ray reveals dilated duodenal and jejunal loops with air-fluid levels, and a gasless ileum.
   - Considering that she has a history of cholecystectomy, she likely developed intraperitoneal adhesions.
   - Her vital signs reveal hypotension and tachycardia, likely due to intractable vomiting.
   - Severe volume depletion activates renin-angiotensin-aldosterone system, and causes contraction alkalosis with hypokalemia.
   - This patient is losing chloride by vomiting the gastric acid, so she likely has hypochloremia as well.
   - If bowel obstruction is so severe that it compromises blood flow, it can lead to ischemic necrosis of the bowel wall.
   - Prolonged tissue ischemia and anaerobic metabolism can result in lactic acidosis.

REVIEW QUESTIONS

2. A 75-year-old man is brought to the emergency department due to severe abdominal pain and vomiting for the past 2 days. His last bowel movement was 4 days ago. Past medical history is significant for sigmoidectomy due to recurrent diverticulitis. Vital signs include blood pressure of 70/60 mmHg, heart rate of 130 beats/min, and respiratory rate of 20 breaths/min. Arterial blood gasses show metabolic acidosis with anion gap of 20 mEq/L (10-14 mEq/L). Abdominal X-ray shows dilated jejunal loops with air-fluid levels and a gasless colon. IV fluids have been administered. What is the best next step in the management of this patient?

    - **Since IV fluids have been administered, the best next step in the management of a hemodynamically unstable patient with bowel obstruction or infarction is exploratory laparotomy.**
    - This patient presents with severe abdominal pain, vomiting, and absent bowel movements for the last 4 days.
    - Considering that he has a past medical history of sigmoidectomy possibly leading to adhesions, this patient likely has bowel obstruction.
    - Abdominal X-ray findings of dilated jejunal loops with air-fluid levels and a gasless colon indicate a complete bowel obstruction.
    - This patient is hemodynamically unstable with hypotension, tachycardia, and anion gap metabolic acidosis, suggesting a possible bowel infarction.

3. A 60-year-old man is brought to the emergency department because of multiple episodes of bilious vomiting, diffuse abdominal pain, and bloating for 1 day. He denies alcohol, or illicit drug use. Physical examination shows a tender mass in his abdomen that can't be reduced by pressing. Guarding and rebound tenderness is also noted. Vital signs include, temperature of 38° C (100.4° F), heart rate of 110 beats/min, respiratory rate of 23 breaths/min, and blood pressure of 139/85 mmHg. Which of the following laboratory values is most likely to be elevated in this patient?

    A. AST > ALT
    B. Serum lipase
    C. Serum urate
    D. Serum lactate
    E. Serum potassium

- **The correct answer is option D.**
- This patient's symptoms are typical for bowel obstruction, which include bilious vomiting, diffuse abdominal pain, and bloating.
- He likely developed bowel obstruction secondary to incarcerated hernia, suggested here by the tender mass in his abdomen that can't be pushed back by pressing
- The strangulated hernia likely also resulted in ischemia, necrosis of the intestinal tissue, and peritonitis, manifesting here as rigid abdomen, guarding, rebound tenderness, and signs of distress like fever, tachycardia, tachypnea, and an elevated blood pressure.
- The ischemia and necrosis of the intestine can lead to an increase in lactic acid as this portion of the bowel undergoes anaerobic metabolism.
- The tissue within the hernia can become strangulated if the blood supply is compromised, leading to ischemia and necrosis of the intestines.
- Elevated AST > ALT is seen in the case of alcoholic hepatitis. The patient doesn't drink alcohol, which makes this answer option A less likely.
- Option B is incorrect because elevated serum lipase is evident in the case of acute pancreatitis, which is less likely since it typically presents with epigastric pain radiating to the back and it wouldn't explain the non-reducible abdominal mass.
- Option C is incorrect because elevated serum urate can be seen in tumor lysis syndrome and some other metabolic disorders like gout. However, uric acid levels are not necessarily increased in bowel obstruction or incarcerated hernia.
- Option E is incorrect because elevated serum potassium vomiting typically leads to dehydration and hypovolemia, which activates the renin-angiotensin-aldosterone system and results in potassium wasting.

Gastroenterology | Section 11: Hernias

I. General Overview
   A. A hernia is a protrusion of tissue through the abdominal wall
   B. Can result from loss of mechanical integrity of the abdominal wall
   C. Usually present in areas of discontinuity of the abdominal wall (e.g. groin, umbilicus, or incisional sites)

II. Inguinal Hernias: Introduction
   A. Indirect
      1. The most common type of abdominal hernia
      2. The majority of inguinal hernias in children are indirect hernias
      3. Herniates lateral to the inferior epigastric vessels
   B. Direct
      1. Herniates medial to the inferior epigastric vessels

III. Inguinal Hernias: Etiology
   A. Indirect hernia
      1. Congenital: persistent processus vaginalis
   B. Direct hernia
      1. Acquired: focal weakening of the transversalis fascia

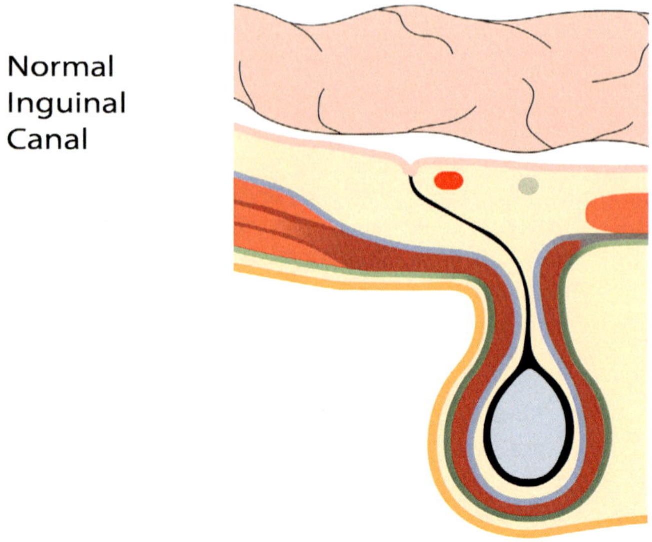

FIGURE 21.5.60 - Normal Inguinal Canal

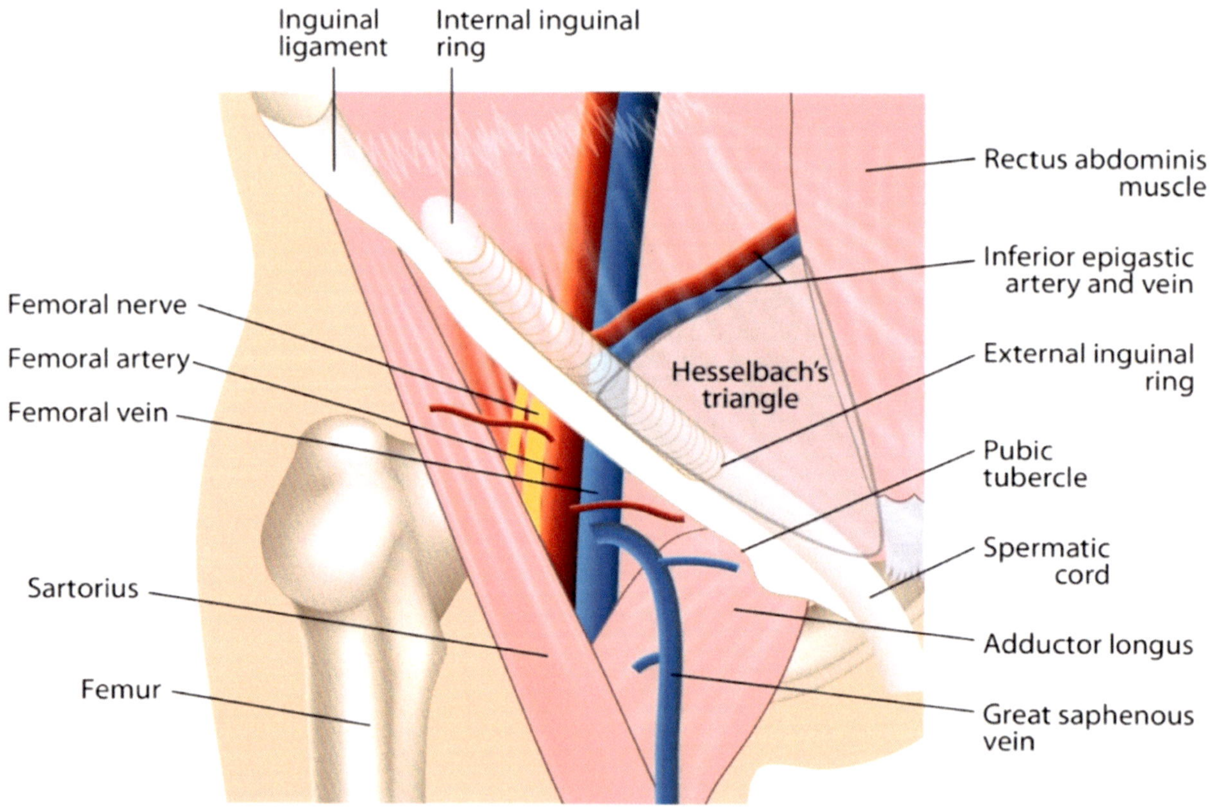

FIGURE 21.5.59 - Anatomy of Inguinal Canal

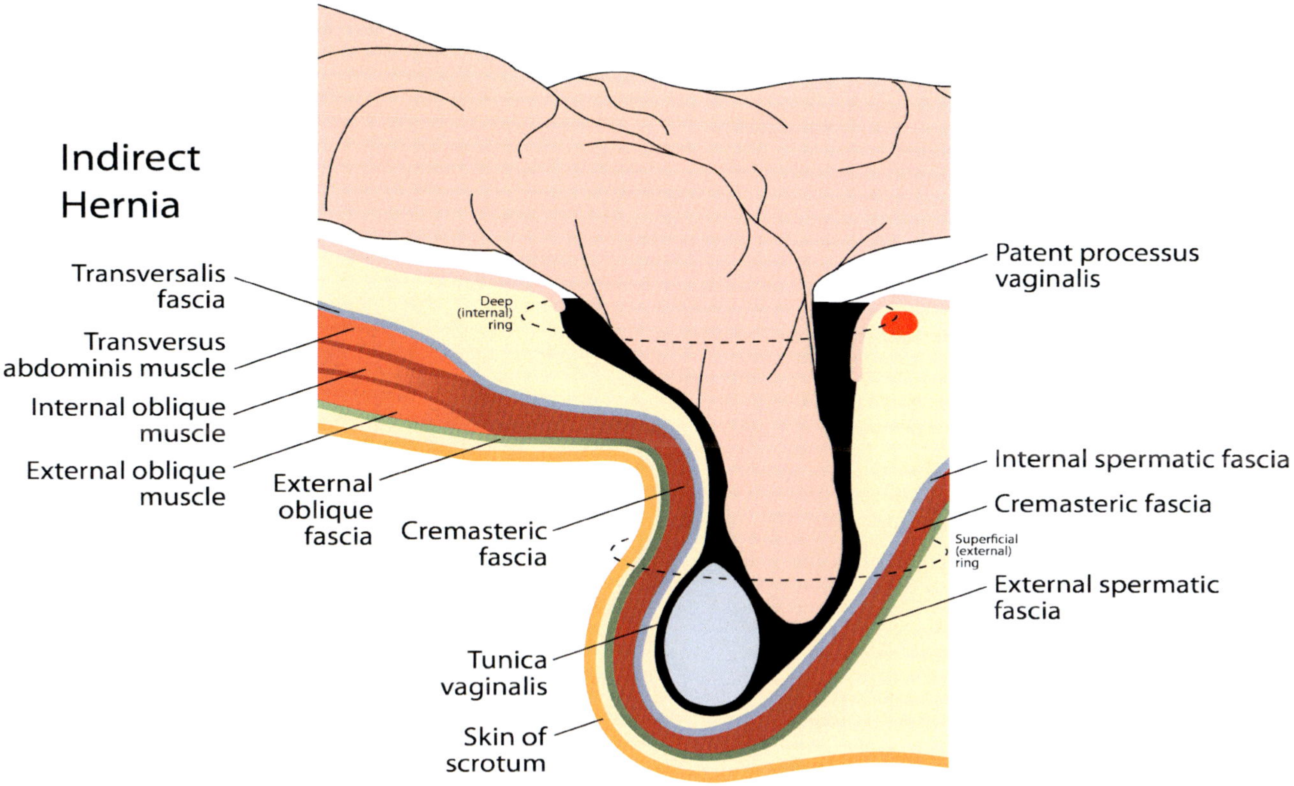

FIGURE 21.5.61 - Indirect Hernia

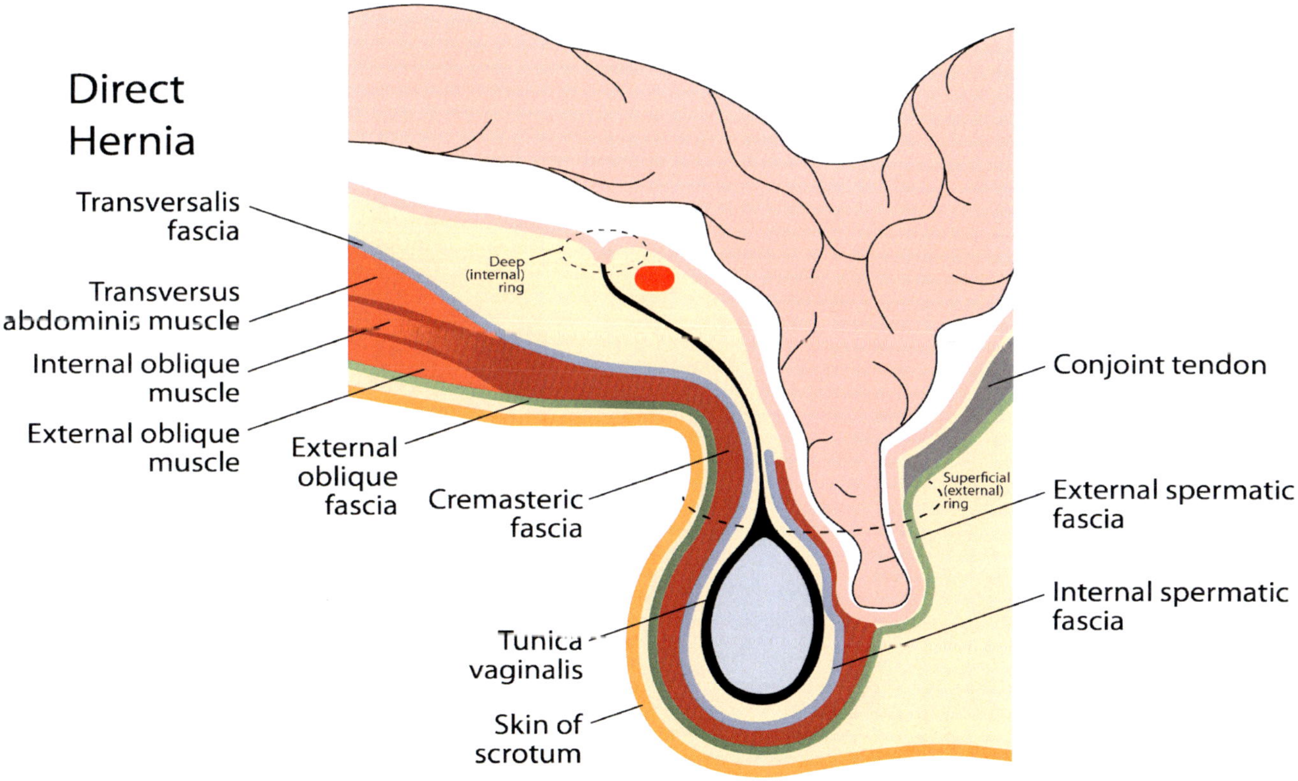

FIGURE 21.5.62 - Direct Inguinal Hernia

IV. Inguinal Hernias: Risk Factors
   A. Direct hernia
      1. Older men
      2. Family history of hernias
      3. Smoking
      4. Chronic cough
      5. Heavy lifting
      6. Collagen vascular disease

V. Inguinal Hernias: Clinical Presentation
   A. Indirect hernia
      1. Asymptomatic
      2. Intermittent mass noted with the increase of abdominal pressure
   B. Direct hernia
      1. Asymptomatic
      2. Bulge in the groin
      3. Discomfort
   C. Incarceration
      1. The hernia cannot be reduced back into the abdomen or pelvis
      2. The bowel gets trapped the hernia sac
      3. Symptoms of mechanical obstruction (e.g. pain, nausea, vomiting)
   D. Strangulation
      1. Cutoff of the bowel blood supply in the hernia sac
      2. Painful, red, swollen mass in the groin
   E. Physical examination
      1. Asymptomatic: not present on physical examination
      2. Reducible: mass reducible with pressure, not tender to palpation
      3. Incarcerated: signs of intestinal obstruction (e.g. abdominal distention), intact skin
      4. Strangulated: sepsis signs, redness of the skin

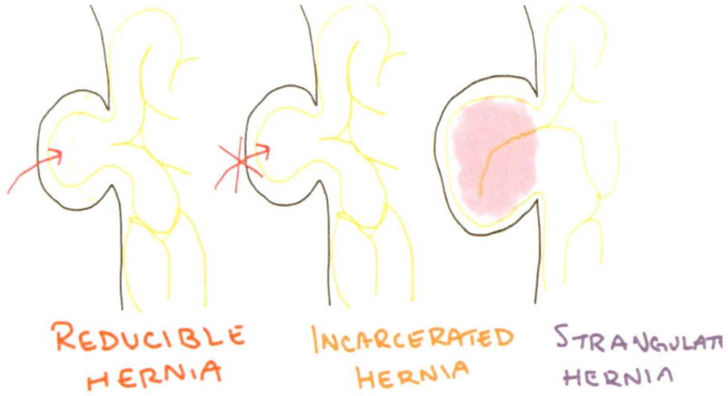

FIGURE 21.5.63 - Complications of Inguinal Hernia

VI. Inguinal Hernias: Diagnosis
   A. Mainly a clinical diagnosis
   B. Patient history
   C. Physical examination
      1. Indirect hernia: mass comes from superolateral to inferomedial, directly touching the distal fingertip
      2. Direct hernia: mass comes from deep to superficial, touching the finger pad
   D. Role of imaging
      1. Useful if the diagnosis is unclear, presence of occult or recurrent inguinal hernia, or in the preoperative setting
      2. Best initial imaging test: ultrasound
      3. CT with IV contrast if the ultrasound is normal with a high suspicion
      4. Known hernia + strangulation/incarceration: no imaging needed

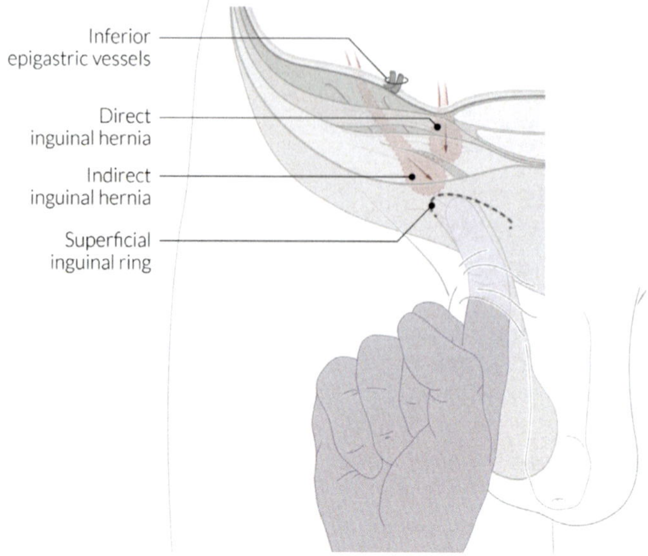

FIGURE 21.5.64 - Physical Examination of Inguinal Hernia

VII. Inguinal Hernias: Management
   A. Uncomplicated hernias (asymptomatic or reducible mass)
      1. Elective surgical repair
      2. Surgery is always recommended to avoid complications
      3. Inform about signs and symptoms of incarceration and strangulation
   B. Complicated hernias
      1. Surgical repair always indicated
      2. Incarcerated: manual reduction then surgical repair to avoid complications
      3. Strangulated: urgent surgical repair
   C. Hernioplasty: mesh placement
      1. Gold standard
      2. Open surgery: presence of complications, patients with contraindications to laparoscopic surgery
      3. Laparoscopic surgery: bilateral hernia, recurrent hernia after an open repair
   D. Herniorrhaphy: repair of hernial defect using autologous tissue

VIII. Femoral Hernia: Definition
   A. A protrusion of tissue through the femoral ring
   B. Located inferior to the inguinal ligament and medial to the femoral vessels
   C. More common in women
   D. More susceptible to strangulation due to narrow neck

Injury	Presentation
Genital branch of the genitofemoral nerve	- Loss of the cremasteric reflex in men, and loss of sensation in the scrotum or labia majora
Ilioinguinal nerve	- Loss of sensation of the skin along the inguinal ligament, medial groin, labia majora, scrotum, and inner thigh
Iliohypogastric nerve	- Hypoesthesia of the suprapubic region
Lateral femoral cutaneous nerve (meralgia paresthetica)	- Loss of sensation in the lateral side of the thigh

TABLE 21.5.2 - Common Nerve Injuries During Surgical Repair of Inguinal Hernia

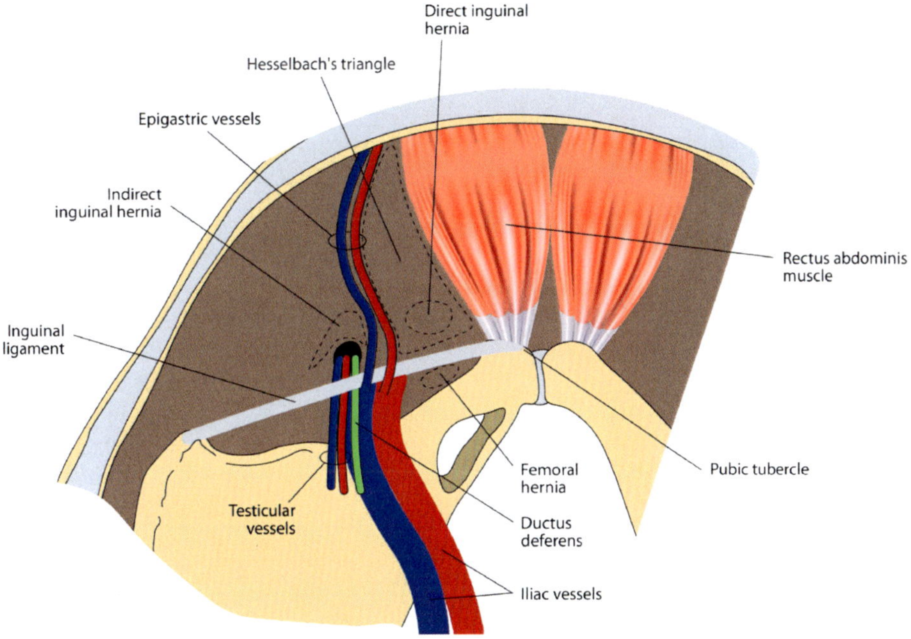

FIGURE 21.5.65 - Protrusion Sites of Different Hernia Types

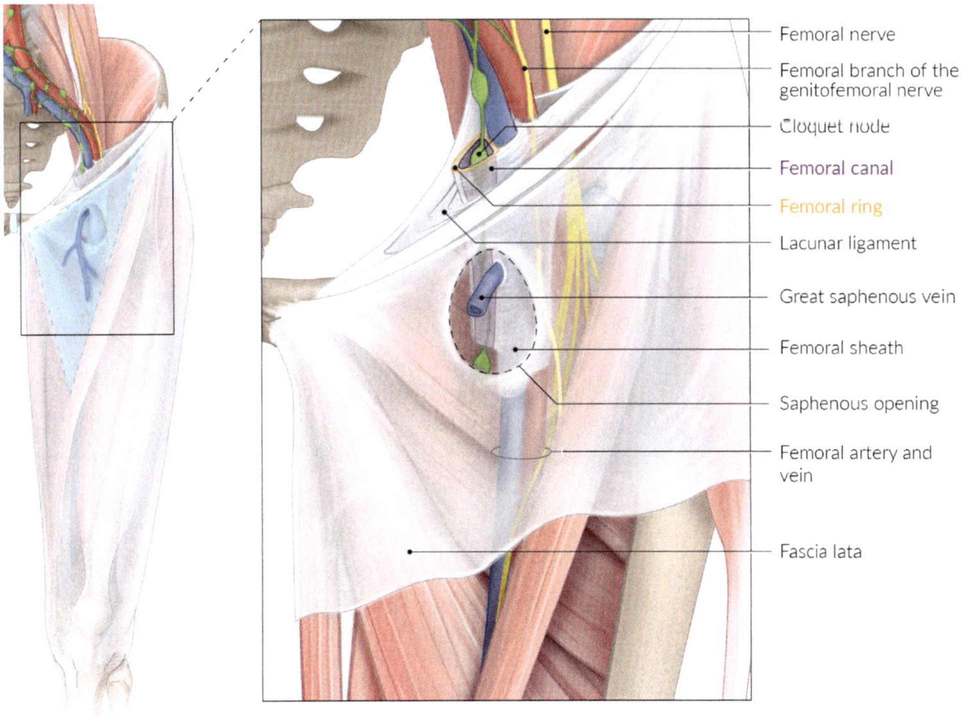

FIGURE 21.5.66 - Anatomy of Femoral Ring

IX. Femoral Hernia: Risk Factors
   A. Female
   B. Multiple pregnancies
   C. Increased intra-abdominal pressure (e.g. constipation, obesity, chronic cough)

X. Femoral Hernia: Clinical Presentation
   A. Uncomplicated
      1. Occult hernia (difficult to diagnose clinically)
      2. Swelling in the groin that enlarges with Valsalva maneuver
   B. Complicated
      1. Incarceration: irreducible mass without skin changes
      2. Strangulation: tenderness and discoloration over the mass, signs of sepsis, abdominal distention, high-pitched bowel sounds

XI. Femoral Hernia: Diagnosis
   A. Mainly a clinical diagnosis
   B. Physical examination
      1. Bulge below the inguinal ligament that enlarges with coughing or Valsalva maneuver
   C. If the physical examination is inconclusive, ultrasound is indicated

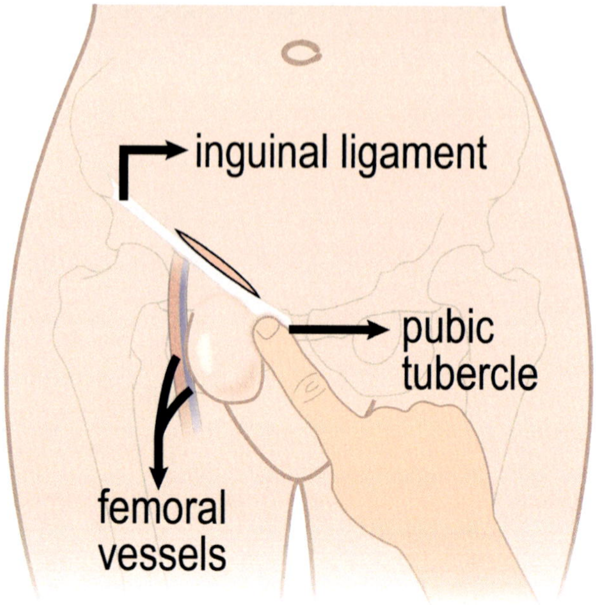

FIGURE 21.5.67 - Location of Femoral Hernia

XII. Femoral Hernia: Management
   A. Asymptomatic/uncomplicated
      1. Elective surgical repair
      2. Laparoscopic approach is preferred (unless any contraindications)
   B. Complicated: incarcerated or strangulated
      1. Urgent, open surgical repair

Condition	Pathophysiology	Risk Factors
Direct	- Leaves the abdomen through a weakness in the transversalis fascia, through the floor of Hesselbach triangle, medial to the inferior epigastric vessels	- Old age, family history of hernias, smoking, chronic cough, collagen vascular disease, heavy weight lifting
Indirect	- Goes through the deep inguinal ring, lateral to the inferior epigastric vessels	- Congenital defect caused by persistence of processus vaginalis
Femoral	- Protrudes below the inguinal ligament and lateral to the pubic tubercle through the femoral ring	- Female, multiple pregnancies

TABLE 21.5.3 - Overview of Abdominal Hernias

REVIEW QUESTIONS

1. A 4-year-old boy is brought to the emergency department because of a protruding mass in his left groin noticed by his mother today. The bulge is displaced downward when the boy cries. The physician inverts the scrotal sac with his index finger and asks the patient to cough. The bulge is felt at the tip of the physician's finger during the cough. What is the most likely pathophysiology of this patient's condition?

   - **This patient has an indirect inguinal hernia due to failure of the processus vaginalis to obliterate.**
   - This patient presents with a protruding mass in his left groin covered with skin. The bulge is displaced downward when he cries. These findings are consistent with the diagnosis of a non-incarcerated inguinal hernia.
   - The physician inverts the scrotal sac with his index finger and asks the patient to cough. The bulge is felt at the tip of the physician's finger.
   - This finding is consistent with an indirect inguinal hernia because this type of hernia travels through both the internal and external inguinal rings.
   - Therefore, part of the intestine can go through the patent processus vaginalis all the way with the spermatic cord.
   - This is why the bulge is felt at the tip of an examiner's finger rather than on the side.

2. A 63-year-old man comes to the emergency department because of worsening abdominal pain that started 2 hours ago. Physical examination shows a tender, erythematous, and edematous inguinal mass. He first noticed this protrusion after lifting heavy boxes at work last week. It has never been painful until today. What is the best next step in the management of this patient?

   - **This patient requires urgent surgical repair.**
   - This patient with abdominal pain has a tender, erythematous, and edematous inguinal mass.
   - This presentation is consistent with an incarcerated inguinal hernia.
   - Considering his age and the appearance of a hernia after lifting heavy boxes, he likely has a direct inguinal hernia.
   - The best next step in the management of an incarcerated hernia is an urgent surgical repair to avoid necrosis and subsequent peritonitis and sepsis.

3. A 57-year-old woman comes to the physician because of a protruding mass in her right groin. BMI is 34 kg/m^2. Physical examination shows a protruding mass below the right inguinal ligament. The mass is displaced downward when the patient coughs, and it disappears when the patient lies down. What are the modifiable risk factors for this patient's condition?

   - **The modifiable risk factors for femoral hernia include obesity, constipation, and smoking-related lung diseases that cause cough.**
   - This woman presents with a protruding mass in her right groin.
   - The physical exam reveals a protruding mass below the right inguinal ligament.
   - The mass is displaced downward when the patient coughs, and it disappears when she lies down.
   - All these clues point to the diagnosis of non-incarcerated femoral hernia.

REVIEW QUESTIONS

4. A 75-year-old man comes to the physician because of a protruding mass in his left groin. He first noticed the mass after he was moving furniture in his new home last week. He has smoked 2-packs of cigarettes per day for the last 50 years. Vital signs include temperature of 36 °C (96.8 °F), blood pressure of 145/80 mmHg, heart rate of 75 beats/min, and respiratory rate of 15 breaths/min. Physical examination shows a bulge that is displaced downward when the patient coughs and disappears when the patient lies down. The physician inverts the scrotal sac with his index finger and asks the patient to cough. The bulge is felt at the side of the physician's finger during the cough. Which of the following is the most likely underlying cause of this patient's physical exam findings?

    A. Weakness of transversalis fascia
    B. Persistence of processus vaginalis
    C. Pleuroperitoneal membrane defect
    D. Phrenoesophageal membrane laxity

- **The correct answer is option A.**
- This patient presents with a protruding mass in his left groin. He first noticed the mass after he was moving heavy furniture. The physical examination shows a bulge that is displaced downward when the patient coughs and disappears when he lies down.
- All of these findings suggest the diagnosis of an inguinal hernia.
- The physician inverts the scrotal sac with his index finger and asks the patient to cough. The bulge is felt at the side of the physician's finger during coughing.
- This clue indicates that the patient most likely has a direct inguinal hernia, because this type of hernia travels from the Hesselbach triangle to the external inguinal ring.
- This is why the bulge is felt at the side of the examiner's finger.
- The underlying cause of a direct inguinal hernia is weakness of the transversalis fascia.
- Option B is incorrect because persistence of the processus vaginalis causes an indirect, rather than direct, inguinal hernia.
- Option C is incorrect because pleuroperitoneal membrane defect causes congenital diaphragmatic hernia.
- Finally, option D is incorrect because phrenoesophageal membrane laxity is the cause of sliding hiatal hernia.

Gastroenterology | Section 12: Abdominal Compartment Syndrome

I. Abdominal Compartment Syndrome: Definition
   A. Increased pressure in an anatomic compartment resulting in decreased perfusion of those tissues and eventually resulting in end organ dysfunction without intervention

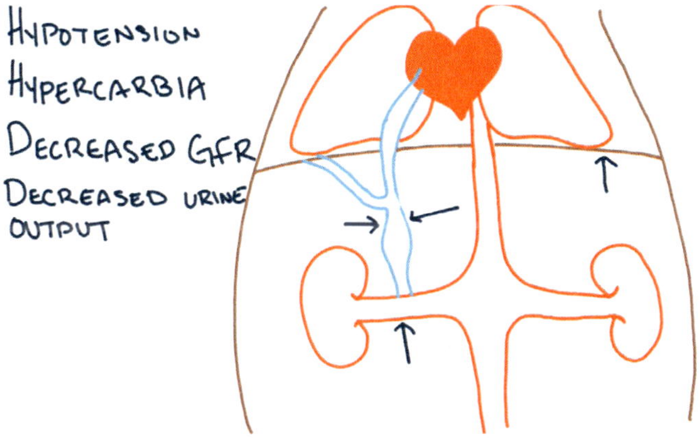

FIGURE 21.5.68 - Pathophysiology of Organ Failure due to Compartment Syndrome

II. Abdominal Compartment Syndrome: Pathophysiology
   A. Increased central venous pressure and systemic vascular resistance
   B. Decreased cardiac output and hypotension
   C. Increased central venous pressure leads to increased intracranial pressure
   D. Decreased thoracic volumes and elevated peak pressures
   E. Decreased GFR and urine output

III. Abdominal Compartment Syndrome: Risk Factors
   A. Multiple traumatic injuries with large volume fluid resuscitation
      1. Intra-abdominal
      2. Retroperitoneal
   B. Circumferential burns around the abdomen
   C. Intra-abdominal edema
   D. Inflammatory processes such as pancreatitis and sepsis

IV. Abdominal Compartment Syndrome: Clinical Features
   A. Shortness of breath
   B. Abdominal pain
   C. Increased jugular venous distension
   D. Lower extremity edema
   E. Acute kidney injury

V. Abdominal Compartment Syndrome: Diagnosis
   A. Bladder pressures
   B. > 25-30 mmHg

VI. Abdominal Compartment Syndrome: Treatment
   A. Airway, breathing, circulation (ABCs)
   B. Decompressive laparotomy
   C. Maintenance of open abdomen with vacuum-assisted suction
   D. Delayed closure of abdomen once swelling has decreased
   E. Treat the underlying cause (e.g. evacuate hematoma)

REVIEW QUESTIONS

1. What supportive measures can be taken to decrease the risk of developing abdominal compartment syndrome?
    - **There are three main things to consider that can help prevent the development of abdominal compartment syndrome: positioning of the patient, adequate draining, and adequate pain control.**
    - Positioning of the patient: having the patient supine without elevation of the head decreases the amount of pressure on the abdomen. This, of course, has to be balanced with the risk of ventilator-associated pneumonia or aspiration.
    - Adequate draining: this includes nasogastric tubes, rectal tubes, paracentesis, and hematoma drainage.
    - Adequate pain control: pain medication and paralytics decrease the risk due to increased abdominal wall compliance.

2. A retrospective study is investigating mortality associated with abdominal compartment syndrome. The researcher is hoping to establish the leading cause of mortality in these patients and then develop a protocol addressing the leading cause. Which of the following patients would most likely be excluded from this study?

    A. A 57-year-old male with caput medusae
    B. A 45-year-old female alcoholic with pain in the epigastric area that radiates around the right side of the abdomen to the back
    C. A 45-year-old male with unilateral 2+ pitting lower extremity edema and shortness of breath
    D. A 52-year-old male who is the victim of an auto-pedestrian accident who is severely hypotensive in the emergency department
    E. A 75-year-old women with vaginal bleeding for 3 years

- **The correct answer is option C.**
- One of the reasons abdominal compartment syndrome has such a high mortality rate is because it can lead to multisystem organ failure. It can also be caused by many pathologies that lead to increased inflammation and edema of the abdomen.
- The 45-year-old with unilateral 2+ pitting edema and shortness of breath likely has a pulmonary embolism, which is unlikely to lead to abdominal compartment syndrome.
- Caput medusae is dilatation and distension of the superficial epigastric veins associated with liver cirrhosis, which is a classic volume overload state. Blood gets congested passing through the damaged liver, which causes the blood to back up into the veins that feed into the liver. This can lead to increased abdominal pressure and compartment syndrome, so answer choice A is wrong.
- RUQ pain that radiates to the back in an alcoholic patient is likely pancreatitis, which is a massive inflammatory state causing significant abdominal swelling and increased pressure with potential for compartment syndrome, so answer choice B is wrong.
- Answer choice D is wrong because this patient with major trauma and hypotension is going to receive a massive amount of fluid, which places him at very high risk for abdominal compartment syndrome.
- The 75-year-old woman who has vaginal bleeding has endometrial cancer until proven otherwise. Since it has been going on for 3 years, it is likely the cancer has grown to a significant size. This places the patient at a doubly increased risk for compartment syndrome: she has both inflammation associated with malignancy and an intra-abdominal mass. This makes answer choice E wrong.

ENDOCRINOLOGY

Endocrine | Section 1: Obesity, Metabolic Syndrome, and Pancreatic Neuroendocrine Tumors

I. Obesity
  A. BMI ≥ 30 kg/m^2
  B. Caused by genetic and environmental factors (overeating, sedentary lifestyle)
  C. Obesity is the greatest modifiable risk factor for hypertension
  D. Increases the risk of coronary heart disease, diabetes mellitus, dyslipidemia

II. Obesity: Treatment
  A. Lifestyle modification: diet, exercise
  B. If this fails, pharmacotherapy
    1. Orlistat (pancreatic lipase inhibitor), combination phentermine and topiramate
  C. Bariatric surgery is the most effective treatment
    1. Indicated in patients with severe obesity (BMI ≥ 40 kg/m^2) who have failed medical therapy and have complications

III. Metabolic Syndrome
  A. ≥ 3 of the following
    1. Central obesity (waist circumference ≥ 40 inches in men, ≥ 35 inches in women)
    2. Hypertension (> 130/80 mmHg)
    3. Hypertriglyceridemia (> 150 mg/dl)
    4. HDL (< 40 mg/dl in men, < 50 mg/dl in women)
    5. Hyperglycemia (FBS ≥ 100 mg/dl)
  B. Associated with increased cardiovascular mortality
  C. Insulin resistance is the central abnormality
  D. Other abnormalities associated with insulin resistance
    1. Polycystic ovarian syndrome, non-alcoholic fatty liver disease, acanthosis nigricans, hyperuricemia and uric acid stones
  E. Treatment: lifestyle modification, metformin, antihypertensive agents, statins

IV. Insulinoma
  A. Beta-cell tumor producing insulin
  B. Benign, associated with multiple endocrine neoplasia type 1
  C. Whipple's triad
    1. Symptoms of hypoglycemia
    2. Documented low blood glucose during symptoms
    3. Rapid resolution of symptoms with administration of glucose

V. Insulinoma: Diagnosis
  A. 72-hour fast test is the most accurate test
    1. Whipple's triad fulfilled
    2. ↑ insulin, ↑ C-peptide, negative sulfonylurea screen
  B. CT/MRI of the abdomen to locate the tumor

VI. Insulinoma: Management
  A. Surgical resection
  B. Regular carbohydrate consumption
  C. Octreotide
    1. Somatostatin analog
    2. Inhibits insulin secretion

VII. Gastrinoma
  A. Pancreatic or duodenal tumor producing gastrin
    1. ↑ gastrin → ↑ H^+ by parietal cells → peptic ulcers, mucosal damage
  B. Zollinger-Ellison syndrome
    1. Recurrent peptic ulcer disease, refractory to over-the-counter antacids and H_2 blockers
  C. Associated with multiple endocrine neoplasia type 1

VIII. Gastrinoma: Diagnosis
  A. Clinical features: abdominal pain, epigastric tenderness, occult GI bleed, nausea, vomiting, diarrhea, weight loss
  B. ↑ fasting serum gastrin
  C. Secretin stimulation test
    1. Diagnostic test of choice
    2. Increase in gastrin level with secretin administration
  D. CT abdomen to localize the tumor

IX. Gastrinoma: Treatment
  A. Surgical resection
  B. High dose proton pump inhibitors
  C. Chemotherapy for metastatic cancer

X. Glucagonoma
  A. Glucagon-producing tumor in the pancreas
  B. Clinical features
    1. Necrolytic migratory erythema (erythematous, painful rash affecting lower limbs, perineum)
    2. New onset diabetes mellitus (often mild)
    3. Weight loss, diarrhea, venous thromboembolism, depression, psychosis
  C. Diagnosis
    1. Markedly elevated glucagon level
    2. Hyperglycemia, normocytic normochromic anemia
    3. CT to localize the tumor
  D. Treatment
    1. Surgical resection

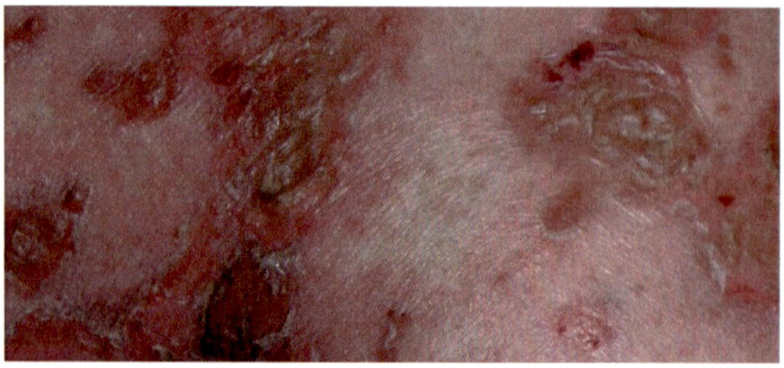

FIGURE 21.6.1 - Necrolytic Migratory Erythema

XI. VIPoma
- A. Tumor producing vasoactive intestinal peptide
  1. VIP increases intestinal fluid secretion
  2. VIP inhibits gastrin secretion
- B. WDHA syndrome
  1. Watery diarrhea
  2. Hypokalemia
  3. Achlorhydria
- C. Diagnosis
  1. Low stool osmotic gap (secretory diarrhea)
  2. High VIP level
  3. CT to localize the tumor
- D. Treatment
  1. Surgical resection
  2. Fluid and electrolyte replacement, octreotide to reduce diarrhea

XII. Somatostatinoma
- A. Somatostatin producing tumor
- B. Somatostatin inhibits secretion of various hormones
  1. ↓ Cholecystokinin (gallstones)
  2. ↓ Pancreatic secretion (steatorrhea)
  3. ↓ Insulin (hyperglycemia)
- C. Majority malignant
- D. Treatment: surgical resection, chemotherapy, octreotide

REVIEW QUESTIONS ?

1. A 40-year-old female with metabolic syndrome comes to her primary care physician asking for a referral to a bariatric surgeon. What kind of discussion should the physician have with her?

- **The discussion should establish what the patient has already tried.**
- First line treatment should include lifestyle changes such as dietary modifications and physical activity.
- Graded exercise is important to prevent injury, and dietary modifications should be lasting.
- Second line would be the use of pharmacologic agents such as orlistat, phentermine, and topiramate.
- If these interventions fail and there is morbid obesity, surgical intervention may be considered.

REVIEW QUESTIONS ?

2. A 58-year-old male comes to the emergency department with three weeks of abdominal pain. His stools have become dark colored for the past day, though the consistency is the same. He also reports associated nausea without vomiting. The blood work is pending, but a mass is seen on his CT scan. What lab values are most consistent with this patient's likely pathophysiology?

   A. Increased insulin and C-peptide
   B. Increased insulin, normal C-peptide
   C. Increased gastrin
   D. Hyperglycemia, normocytic normochromic anemia
   E. Hypokalemia, low stool osmotic gap
   F. Hyperglycemia, and decreased cholecystokinin

- **The correct answer is option C.**
- This patient has abdominal pain, discoloration of the stool, nausea, and a mass found on imaging.
- The stool color change is likely the result of blood in the gastrointestinal tract and the abdominal pain suggest peptic ulcers.
- Increased acid production by parietal cells and the mass suggests a potential source.
- A gastrin producing tumor, gastrinoma, would account for this patient's symptoms, which would have increased gastrin on laboratory evaluation.
- Option A is incorrect, because increased insulin and C-peptide is consistent with an insulinoma which would present with symptoms of hypoglycemia such as weakness, blurry vision, and irritability.
- Option B is incorrect, because increased insulin without changes in C-peptide is found in sulfonylurea use. This is abused in people who are trying to lose weight, and is usually surreptitious use of a family member's medication.
- Option D is incorrect because hyperglycemia with a normocytic normochromic anemia would be the laboratory findings with glucagonoma. Glucagon in excess leads to tissue necrosis presenting as necrotising migratory erythema. It may also present with new-onset diabetes, weight-loss, diarrhea, depression, and psychosis.
- Option E is incorrect because This patient does not have changes in stool consistency. A VIPoma presents with watery diarrhea, low stool osmotic gap, and hypokalemia.
- Option F is incorrect because hyperglycemia with decreased cholecystokinin would be found with somatostatinoma, which is more likely to present with symptoms of cholecystitis such as RUQ pain that is worse with meals, and no changes in stool color.

Endocrine | Section 10: Diseases of Thyroid Gland: Thyroiditis, Thyroid Nodules & Neoplasms

I. Thyroiditis: Definition
   A. Inflammation of the thyroid tissue
   B. Release of preformed hormones from the colloid space, causing hyperthyroidism, followed by recovery or hypothyroidism

II. Thyroiditis: Causes
   A. Painful thyroiditis
      1. Subacute granulomatous thyroiditis (De Quervain)
         a) Typically preceded by flu-like illness
   B. Painless thyroiditis
      1. Postpartum thyroiditis
      2. Drug-induced thyroiditis (e.g. amiodarone, IL-2, lithium)
      3. Riedel's thyroiditis

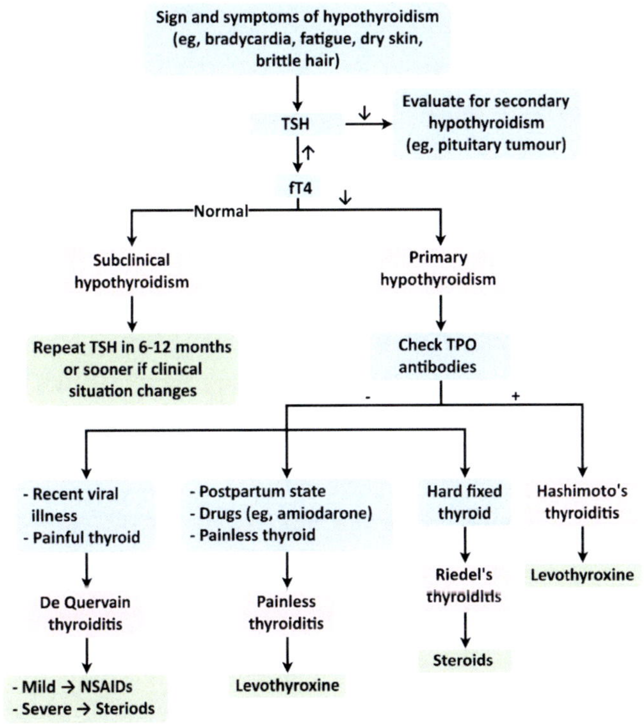

FIGURE 21.6.2 - Algorithm for Thyroiditis

III. Thyroid Nodules: Definition
   A. Abnormal mass within the thyroid gland
   B. Found during physical examination or ultrasound
   C. Can be benign (most common) or malignant

IV. Thyroid Nodules: Clinical Presentation
   A. Malignant characteristics
      1. Solitary nodule
      2. Fixed nodule
      3. Firm or irregular consistency
      4. Vocal cord paralysis (e.g. hoarseness)
      5. History of rapid development

V. Thyroid Nodules: Diagnosis
   A. Suspicious sonographic criteria
      1. Hypoechoic
      2. Taller-than-wide shape
      3. Microcalcifications
      4. Central vascularity
      5. Irregular margins

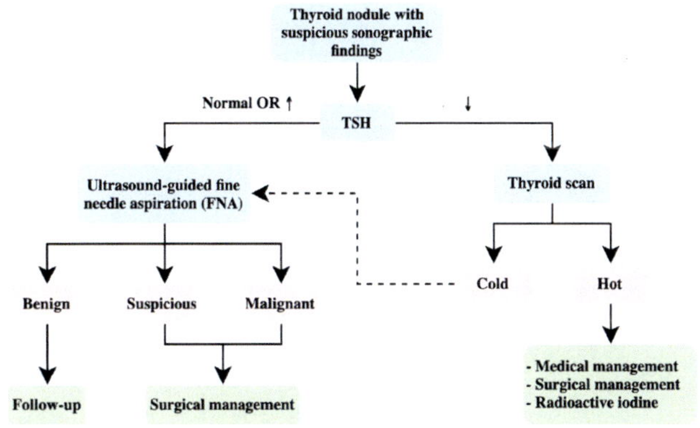

FIGURE 21.6.3 - Algorithm for Thyroid Nodule

VI. Thyroid Nodules: Complications
   A. Surgery complications
      1. Injury of the recurrent laryngeal nerve (e.g. hoarseness)
      2. Injury of the external branch of the superior laryngeal nerve
      3. Parathyroid glands injury → hypoparathyroidism

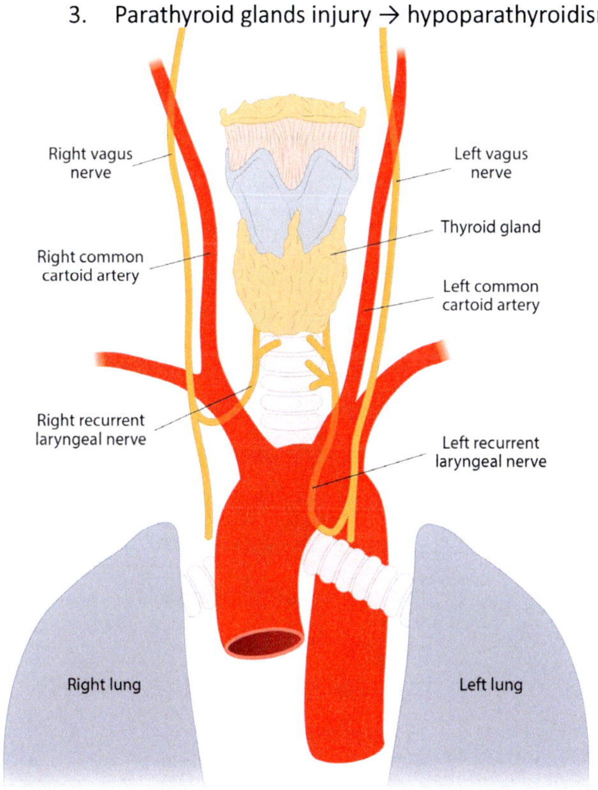

FIGURE 21.6.4 - Thyroid and Its Relation to Major Nerves and Vessels

Condition	Key Features
Follicular adenoma	- Benign, solitary growth - Non-functional (most common) - No vascular invasion
Papillary carcinoma	- Radiation of the head/neck is a risk factor - Classical finding: psammoma bodies - Lymphatic spread
Follicular carcinoma	- Invades the capsule and vessels - Hematogenous spread
Medullary carcinoma	- Arises from parafollicular cells - Produces calcitonin - Histologic features: polygonal cells in amyloid stroma - May be associated with MEN II
Anaplastic carcinoma	- Rapidly growing mass and metastasizes - Undifferentiated and disorganized architecture on histologic exam - Typically arises in elderly patients

TABLE 21.6.1 - Summary of Thyroid Neoplasms

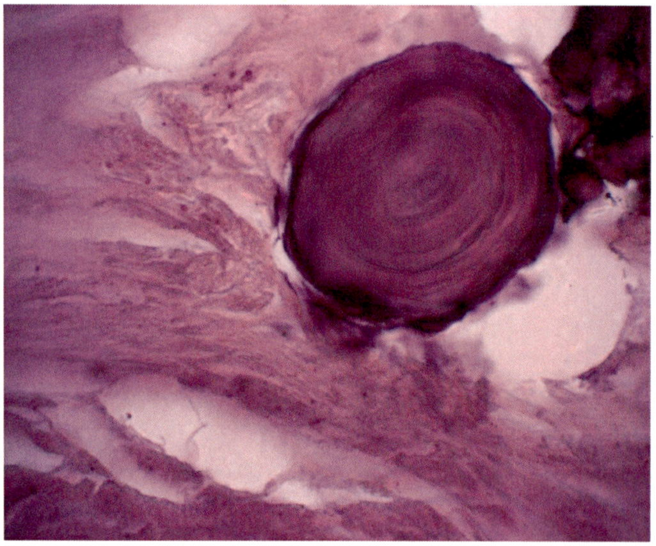

FIGURE 21.6.5 - Psammoma Body

REVIEW QUESTIONS

1. A 37-year-old female patient presents to the office with complaints of weight gain and fatigue. She has a history of bipolar disorder, for which she takes medications. What abnormalities in laboratory values would be expected in this patient?

    - **Free T3 and T4 are low with high TSH and creatinine kinase would be expected in this patient.**
    - The patient is likely on lithium because it is the most common drug used to treat bipolar, and it is a known cause of thyroiditis.
    - She is now experiencing symptoms of hypothyroidism due to the destruction of the cells containing thyroid hormone.
    - The lithium levels do not need to be elevated for this side effect to occur, so they are expected to be normal.

2. A 25-year-old man comes to the physician reporting anterior neck pain for the past 3 days. He has recently recovered from viral upper respiratory infection. The physical examination reveals a tender mass in the anterior neck. Laboratory findings are significant for ESR of 50 mm/hr (0 mm/hr - 15 mm/hr). What is the best initial treatment option for this patient's condition?

    - **The best initial treatment option for subacute thyroiditis is NSAIDs that will decrease the inflammation. However, if the condition is severe, steroids may need to be considered.**
    - This young man presents with anterior neck pain and a tender neck mass after recovering from viral upper respiratory infection.
    - His ESR is high at 50 mm/hr indicating underlying inflammation.
    - This is a classic scenario for subacute granulomatous thyroiditis, also known as De Quervain thyroiditis, that follows the viral infection.

3. What are the histologic findings that would be expected on a fine needle aspiration of a patient's thyroid nodule if they have been diagnosed with MEN IIB?

    - **For medullary thyroid cancer, histologic examination reveals sheets of polygonal cells in amyloid stroma.**
    - MEN IIB places patients at risk for pheochromocytoma, mucosal neuromas, and medullary thyroid carcinoma.

4. A 35-year-old woman is evaluated for a thyroid nodule discovered on thyroid ultrasound 1 week ago. She has no health concerns. Her vital signs include a temperature of 36° C (96.8° F), a blood pressure of 115/75 mmHg, a heart rate of 84 beats/min, and a respiratory rate of 15 breaths/min. The physical examination reveals a well-circumscribed rubbery mass in the right thyroid lobe. Serum TSH is 6 mIU/L (0.5 mIU/L - 5 mIU/L). Which of the following is the best next step in the management of this patient?

    A. Radioactive iodine uptake scan
    B. Fine needle aspiration
    C. Surgical referral
    D. Regular follow-up

    - **The correct answer is option B.**
    - This 35-year-old woman has a thyroid nodule.
    - She has no health concerns and her vital signs are unremarkable.
    - However, her serum TSH is slightly high with the value of 6 mIU/L.
    - High TSH may indicate a cold, or hypofunctioning, nodule.
    - Hypofunctioning thyroid nodules have a considerably high risk of malignancy.
    - Therefore, in order to rule out malignancy, fine needle aspiration should be performed which will allow for the evaluation of nodular histology.
    - Option A is incorrect because radioactive iodine uptake scan is typically performed when the thyroid nodule is accompanied by low TSH.
    - This is because low TSH may indicate hot, also known as toxic, nodule.
    - Option C is incorrect because surgical referral is premature for now.
    - If malignancy were confirmed or highly suspected on histological examination, then surgical referral would be appropriate.
    - Option D is incorrect because the thyroid nodule should be extensively investigated for malignancy before regular follow-up is arranged.

Endocrine | Section 2: Acromegaly & Craniopharyngioma

I. Acromegaly: Definition
   A. Excessive secretion of growth hormone in adults
   B. Most commonly due to pituitary somatotroph adenoma

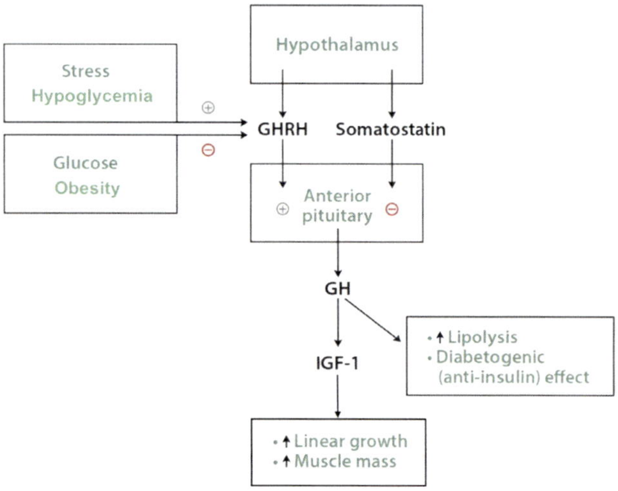

FIGURE 21.6.6 - Regulation of Growth Hormone Secretion

II. Acromegaly: Clinical Features
   A. Overgrowth of tissues (e.g. bones, cartilages, soft tissues, viscera)
      1. Coarse facial features, enlarged hands and feet
      2. Macrognathia, arthralgia
      3. Macroglossia, deepening of the voice
      4. Enlargement of visceral organs (e.g. heart, thyroid)
   B. Metabolic effects
      1. Insulin resistance
   C. Mass-effects of adenoma
      1. Headache
      2. Visual disturbances

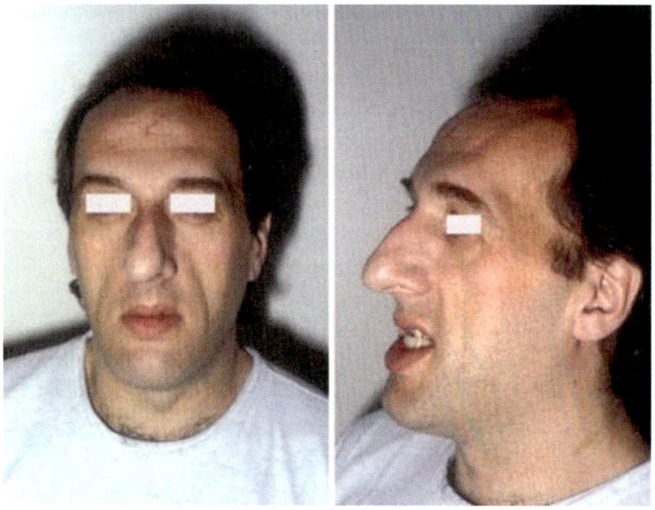

FIGURE 21.6.7 - Patient with Acromegaly with Prognathism

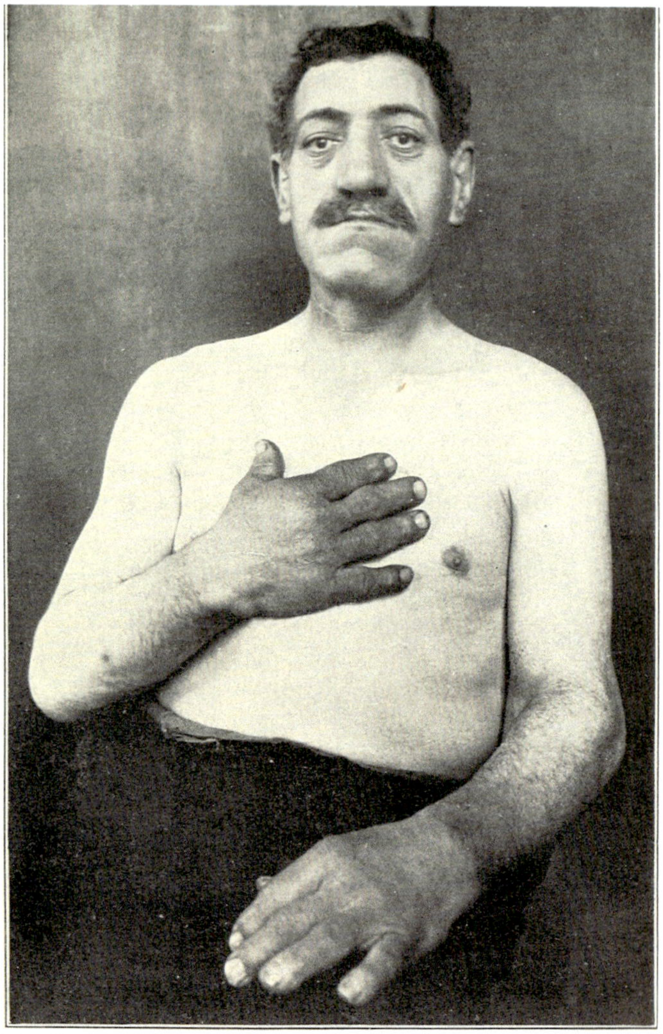

FIGURE 21.6.8 - Patient with Acromegaly

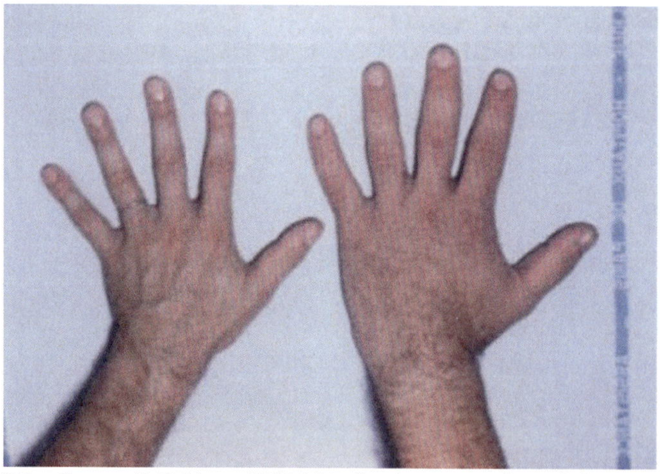

FIGURE 21.6.9 - Normal Hand (Left) Compared to Hand of a Patient with Acromegaly (Right)

III. Acromegaly: Complications
  A. Carpal tunnel syndrome
  B. Pulmonary (e.g. obstructive sleep apnea)
  C. Cardiovascular (e.g. hypertension, left ventricular hypertrophy, heart failure, mitral regurgitation)
  D. Gastrointestinal (e.g. colon polyps, colonic diverticula)
  E. Metabolic (e.g. secondary diabetes mellitus)

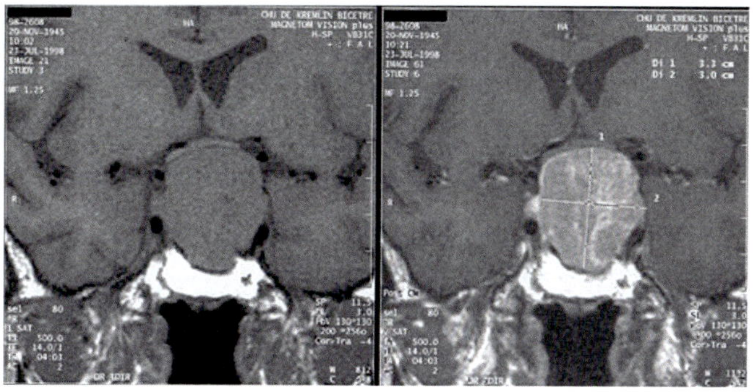

FIGURE 21.6.10 - MRI of a Patient Brain with Acromegaly

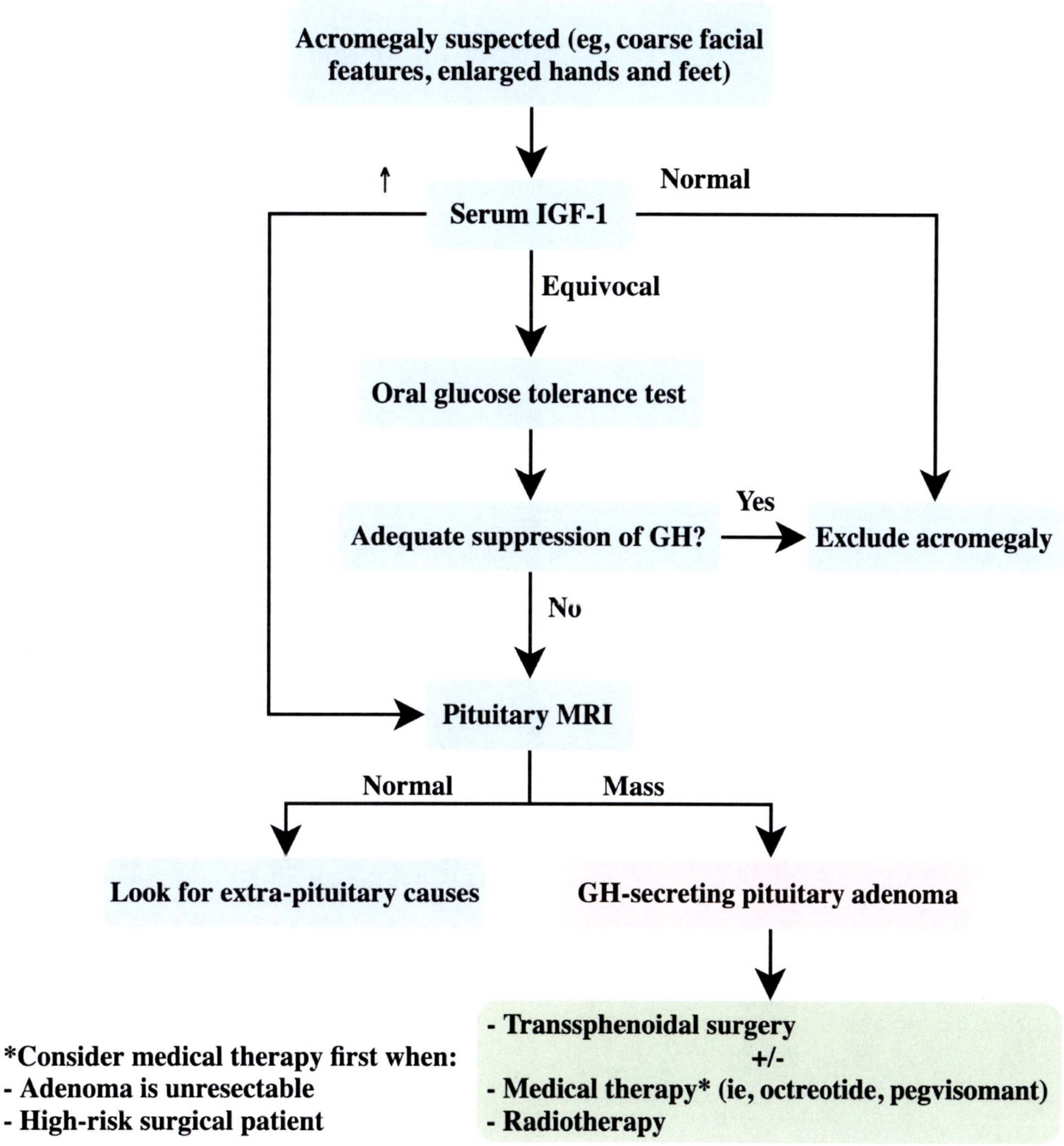

FIGURE 21.6.11 - Algorithm of Acromegaly

IV. Craniopharyngioma: Definition
   A. Benign tumor arising from embryological remnants of Rathke's pouch, forming a sellar mass
   B. Commonly mixed solid and cystic components
   C. Grows gradually and slowly over time
   D. Two incidence peaks
      1. In children 5-14 years
      2. In adults 50-75 years

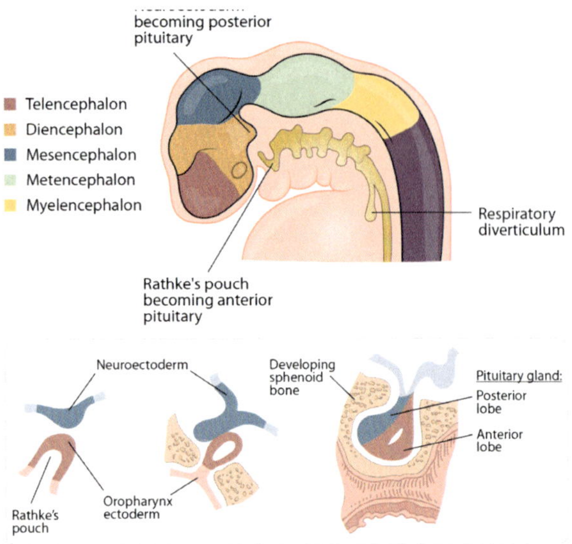

FIGURE 21.6.12 - Embryology of Pituitary Gland

V. Craniopharyngioma: Clinical Features
   A. Mass-effect symptoms
      1. Headache
      2. Visual disturbances
   B. Features of hypopituitarism (e.g. growth failure in children, sexual dysfunction in adults)

VI. Craniopharyngioma: Diagnosis & Management
   A. Diagnosis: neuroimaging (MRI, CT)
      1. Most commonly cystic calcified lesion in parasellar area
   B. Management
      1. Surgical resection (preferred)
      2. Radiation therapy

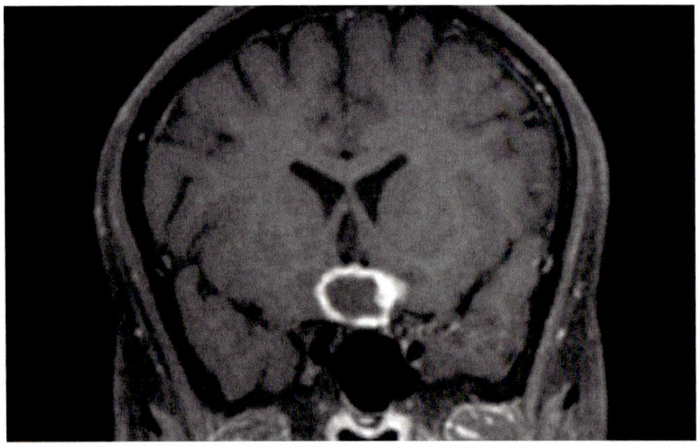

FIGURE 21.6.13 - MRI of a Patient Brain with Craniopharyngioma

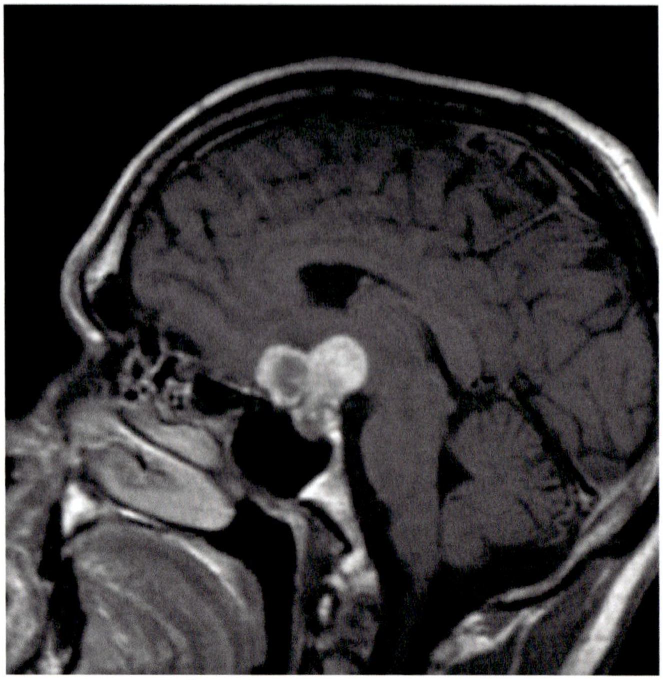

FIGURE 21.6.14 - MRI of a Patient Brain with Craniopharyngioma

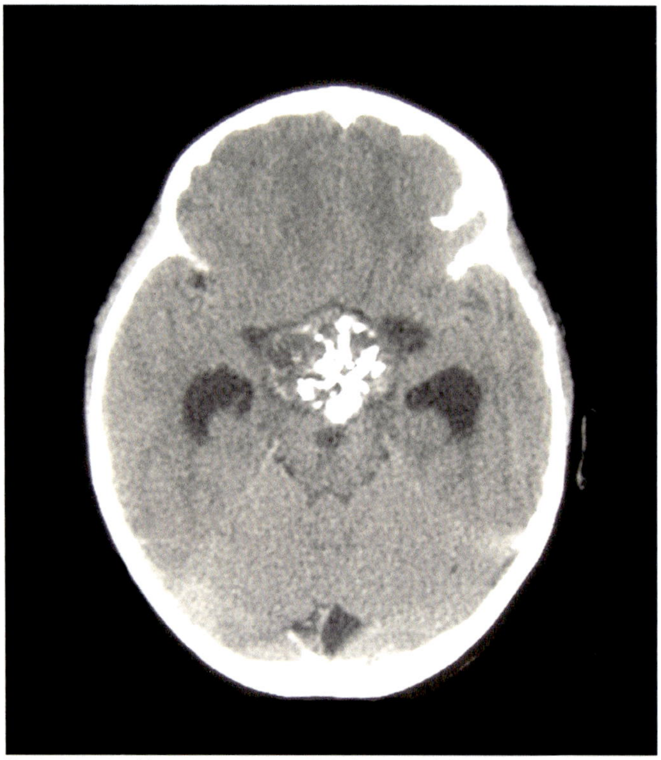

FIGURE 21.6.15 - CT Scan of a Patient with Craniopharyngioma

REVIEW QUESTIONS

1. A patient that is previously diagnosed with acromegaly presents to the office complaining of shortness of breath on exertion. It started three weeks ago and got worse over time. His history of cardiopulmonary diseases is insignificant. What is the most likely finding on echocardiogram?

- **The most likely finding on echocardiogram of this patient is concentric left ventricular hypertrophy.**
- This patient was diagnosed with acromegaly.
- He complains of worsening shortness of breath on exertion.
- Acromegaly can lead to left ventricular hypertrophy, which is exacerbated further by hypertension that is likely to be found in acromegaly as well.
- Diastolic dysfunction can ensue.
- And a patient can present with fatigue and worsening dyspnea on exertion.
- This can be complicated later by heart failure and arrhythmias.

2. A 10-year-old boy is brought to the physician by his mother due to severe headaches for the last 6 months. Headache commonly wakes him up from sleep and is more severe in the mornings. He also complains of decreased vision. The ophthalmological exam reveals bitemporal hemianopsia. His vital signs include a temperature of 36° C (96.8° F), a blood pressure of 110/70 mmHg, a heart rate of 91 beats/min, and a respiratory rate of 14 breaths/min. Brain MRI shows a calcified parasellar mass with solid and cystic components. Which of the following is the preferred management option for this patient's condition?

   A. Chemotherapy
   B. Radiotherapy
   C. Surgical excision
   D. Observation

- **The correct answer is option C.**
- This patient presents with headaches for the last 6 months.
- Headache commonly wakes him up from sleep and is more severe in the mornings. This pattern of headache suggests an increased intracranial pressure due to space occupying lesions.
- This is because the supine posture decreases the cerebral venous drainage raising the intracranial pressure.
- If the patient also has a space-occupying lesion, then the intracranial pressure increases to the point that the headache wakes the patient up from sleep.
- Bitemporal hemianopsia on the ophthalmological exam indicates that the intracranial mass compresses the optic chiasm.
- Brain MRI shows a calcified parasellar mass with solid and cystic components.
- This is the classic description for craniopharyngioma.
- The preferred management option for craniopharyngioma is surgical excision.
- Option A is incorrect because chemotherapy is not typically used in the treatment of craniopharyngioma.
- Option B is incorrect because although radiotherapy is used to treat craniopharyngioma, it's not the preferred management option and is considered for residual tumors or recurrent cases.
- Option D is incorrect because this patient is symptomatic and needs prompt intervention.

MUSCULOSKELETAL SYSTEM

MSK | Section 1: Common Adult Orthopedic Injuries of the Upper Extremities

I. Anterior Shoulder Dislocation
   A. Most common type of shoulder dislocation
   B. Mechanism of injury: direct blow to externally rotated, abducted arm or a fall on an outstretched arm
   C. Physical exam: abducted and externally rotated upper extremity, flattening of the anterior shoulder or deltoid prominence
   D. Associated with injury of the axillary artery and the axillary nerve

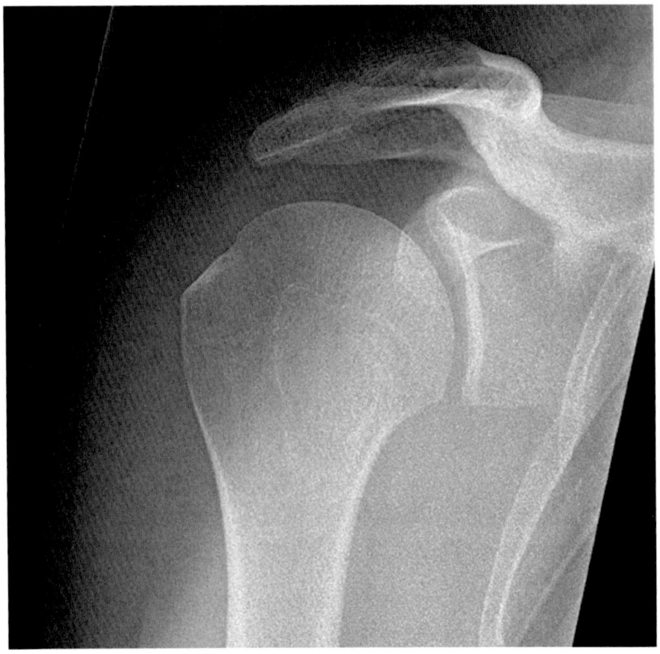

FIGURE 21.7.1 - X-Ray of a Healthy Shoulder Joint

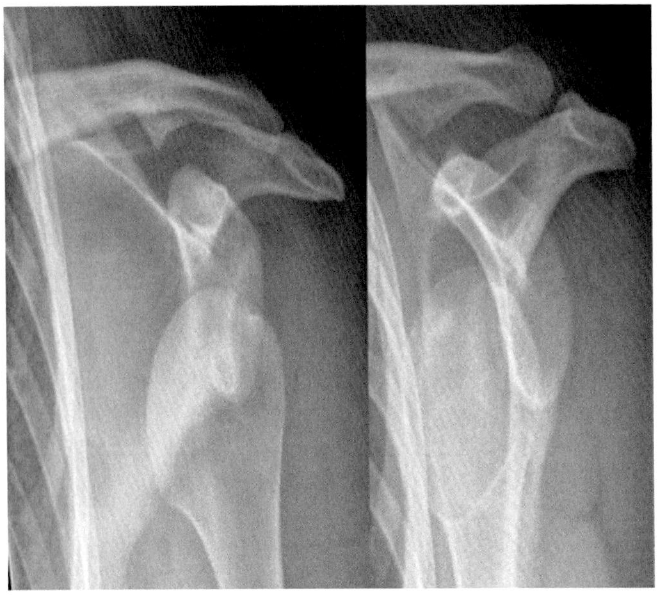

FIGURE 21.7.2 - X-ray of Displaced Humerus Head

II. Posterior Shoulder Dislocation
   A. Uncommon
   B. Mechanism of injury
      1. Seizure
      2. Electrocution
   C. Physical exam
      1. Adducted and internally rotated upper extremity
      2. Flattening of the anterior shoulder or deltoid prominence

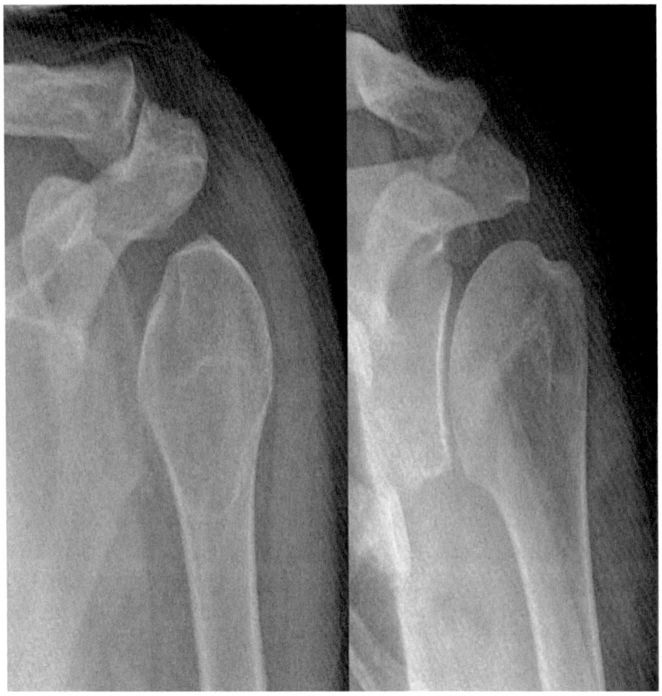

FIGURE 21.7.3 - X-Ray Showing an Overlapping Between the Head of the Humerus and the Glenoid Cavity of the Scapula

III. Shoulder Dislocation
   A. Diagnosis confirmed with X-ray of the affected shoulder
   B. Treatment steps
      1. Closed reduction of the dislocated shoulder
      2. Immobilization with a collar and cuff or a sling and swathe
      3. Physical therapy
      4. Surgery
   C. Recurrence rate remains high despite optimal treatment

IV. Rotator Cuff Injury
   A. Rotator cuff muscles: supraspinatus, infraspinatus, teres minor, and subscapularis
      1. Supraspinatus is the most commonly injured rotator cuff muscle
   B. Rotator cuff tendinopathy
   C. Rotator cuff tear

V. Rotator Cuff Tendinopathy
   A. Mechanism of injury: overuse, impingement, inflammation (tendinitis)
   B. Physical exam
      1. Pain
      2. No weakness
      3. Positive impingement tests: Hawkins Kennedy test and Neer test
   C. Diagnosis: ultrasound
   D. Treatment: conservative (e.g. rest, ice, pain meds, physical therapy)

VI. Rotator Cuff Tear
   A. Risk factor: age > 40
   B. Mechanism of injury: trauma, fall on an outstretched arm
   C. Physical exam: pain, weakness, positive drop arm test or positive empty can test
   D. Diagnosis: MRI
   E. Treatment: surgical repair for acute tears
      1. Chronic tears: conservative management, surgical repair

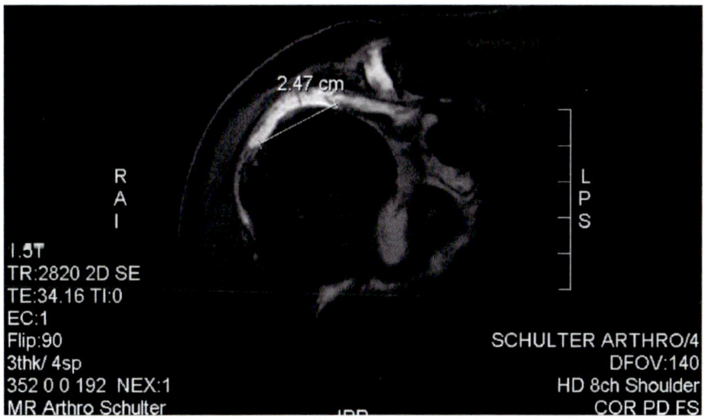

FIGURE 21.7.4 - MRI of a Shoulder Depicting a Complete Supraspinatus Tear

VII. Adhesive Capsulitis
   A. Stiffness and limited range of motion of the affected shoulder
   B. Associated with type 2 diabetes, thyroid disease, shoulder injuries
   C. Physical exam
      1. Stiffness, dull pain, decreased passive and active range of motion, no weakness
   D. Diagnosis: ultrasound, X-ray, or MRI to rule out rotator cuff injury
   E. Self-limited disorder, treated conservatively

VIII. Humerus Shaft Fracture
   A. Mechanism of injury: trauma
   B. Associated with radial nerve injury
   C. Diagnosis: X-ray
   D. Treatment
      1. Nonsurgical: closed reduction, arm immobilization
      2. Surgery for open fractures, significantly displaced fractures, or if there's evidence of neurovascular compromise

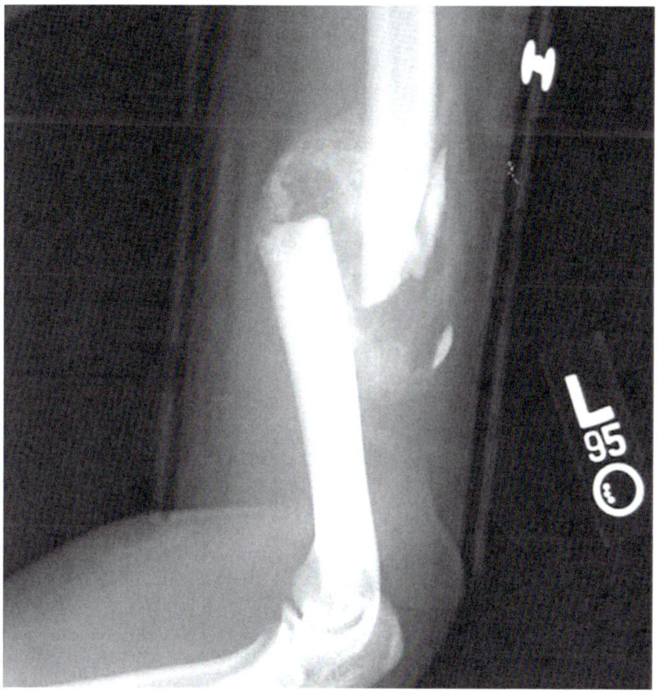

FIGURE 21.7.5 - X-Ray Depicting a Displaced Humerus Shaft Fracture

IX. Colles Fracture
   A. Fracture of the distal radius with dorsal angulation and impaction
   B. Mechanism of injury: fall on an outstretched hand
   C. Physical examination: "dinner fork deformity" of the wrist and median nerve palsy
   D. Diagnosis: X-ray
   E. Treatment: closed reduction and cast immobilization
      1. Surgery is reserved for unstable fractures

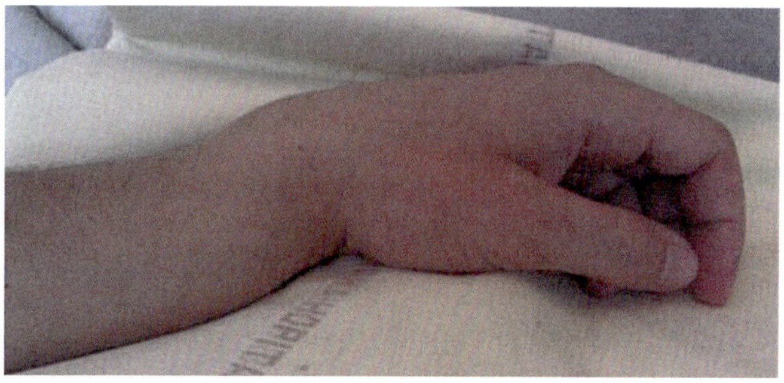

FIGURE 21.7.6 - "Dinner-Fork" Deformity in a Colles Fracture

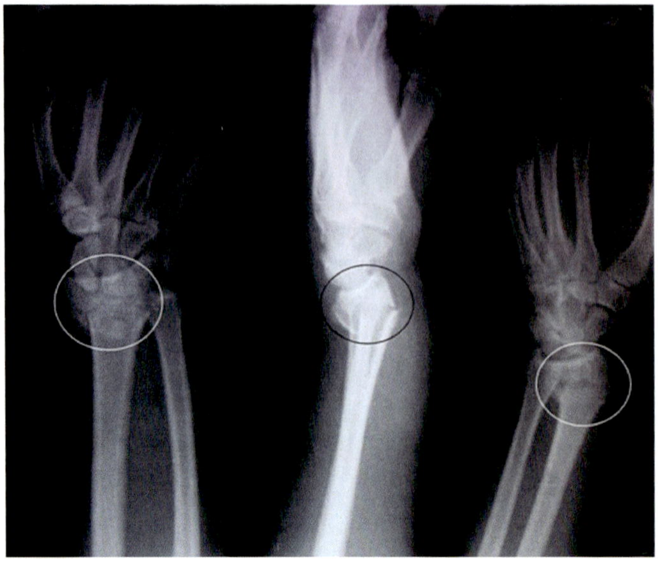

Ashish j29, CC BY 3.0 <https://creativecommons.org/licenses/by/3.0>, via Wikimedia Commons

FIGURE 21.7.7 - X-Ray Showing a Colles Fracture

X. Scaphoid Fracture
   A. Scaphoid bone is the most commonly fractured carpal bone
   B. Mechanism of injury: fall on an outstretched hand
   C. Physical exam: pain in the anatomical snuffbox and pain on pinching
   D. Diagnosis: X-ray (often falsely negative), CT scan or MRI
   E. Treatment: thumb spica splint, repeat imaging in 7-10 days
      1. Surgery for displaced fractures or if there is high risk for nonunion
   F. Complications: nonunion or avascular necrosis

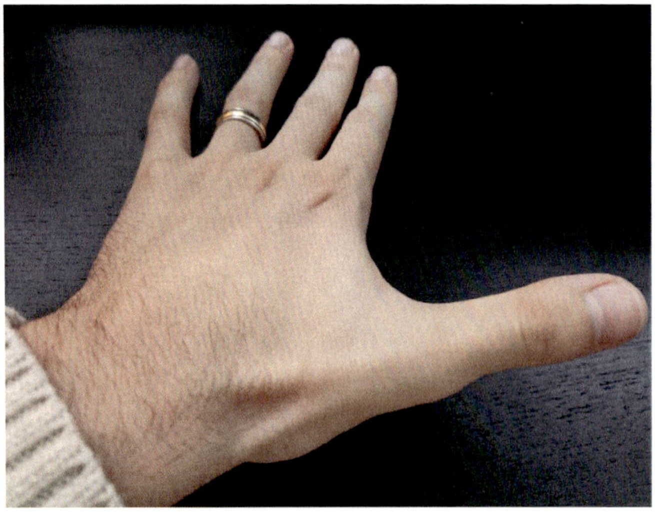

FIGURE 21.7.8 - Snuffbox

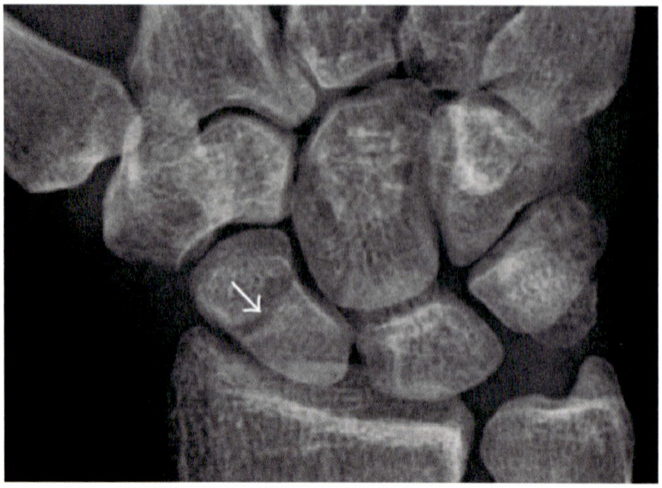

Mohamed Jarraya, Daichi Hayashi, Frank W. Roemer, Michel D. Crema, Luis Diaz, Jane Conlin, Monica D. Marra, Nabil Jomaah, and Ali Guermazi, CC BY 3.0 <https://creativecommons.org/licenses/by/3.0>, via Wikimedia Commons

FIGURE 21.7.9 - X-Ray Showing a Scaphoid Fracture

XI. Boxer's Fracture
   A. Fracture of the neck of the 5th metacarpal bone
   B. Mechanism of injury: direct trauma to a clenched fist
   C. Physical exam: pain and swelling at the fracture site
   D. Diagnosis: X-ray
   E. Treatment
      1. Nonsurgical: closed reduction, ulnar gutter splint
      2. Surgery reserved for complex fractures

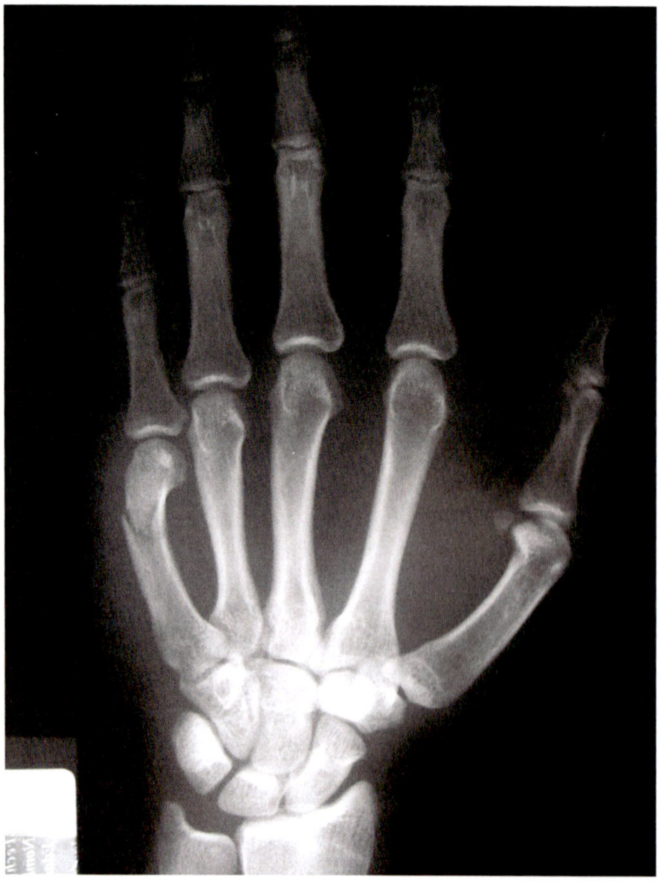

Roberto J. Galindo, CC BY-SA 4.0 <https://creativecommons.org/licenses/by-sa/4.0>, via Wikimedia Commons

FIGURE 21.7.10 - Fracture in the Neck of the Fifth Metacarpal Bone

XII. Monteggia Fracture
A. Diaphyseal fracture of the proximal third of the ulnar shaft with dislocation of the radial head
B. Mechanism of injury: fall on pronated, outstretched arm
C. Physical exam: pain and swelling at the elbow joint
D. Diagnosis: X-ray
E. Treatment: surgical

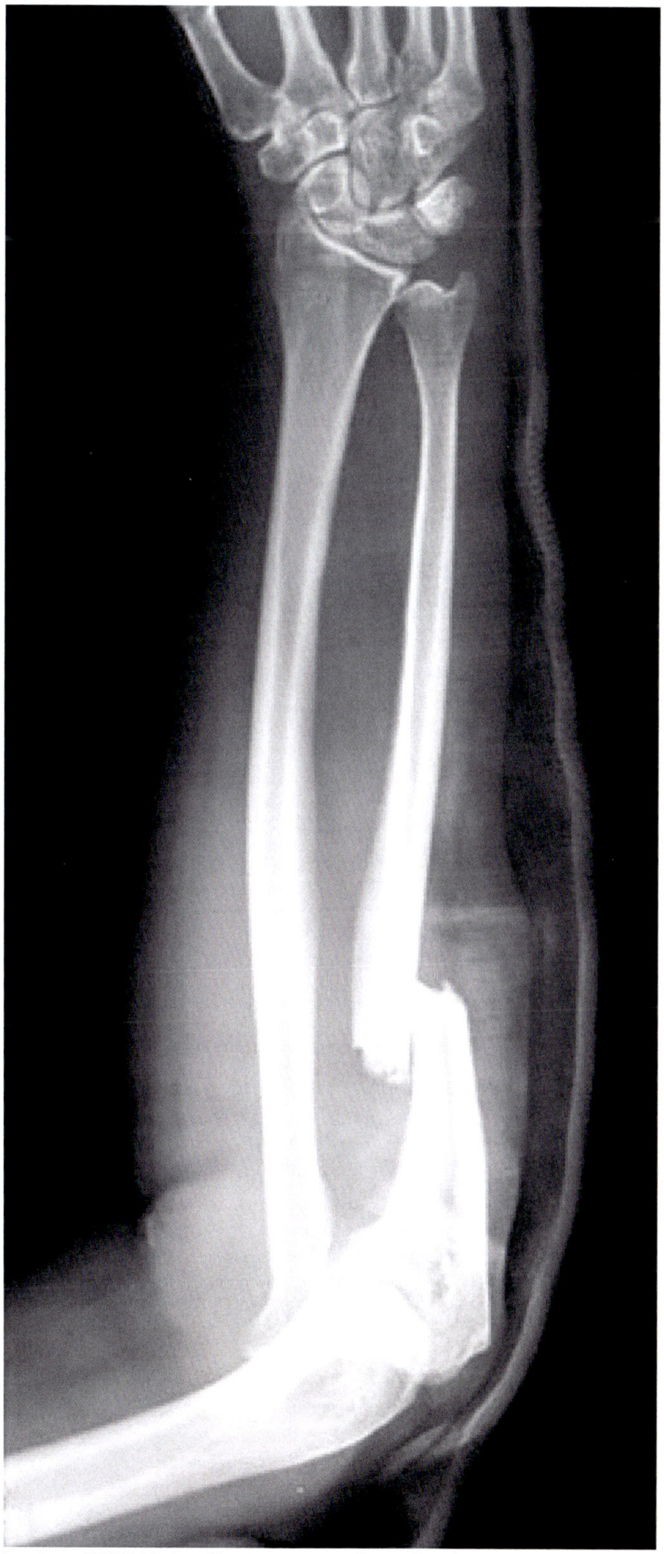

FIGURE 21.7.11 - X-Ray Depicting a Monteggia Fracture

XIII. Galeazzi Fracture
A. Fracture of the distal third of the radius shaft with dislocation of the distal radioulnar joint
B. Mechanism of injury: direct wrist trauma or fall onto outstretched hand with forearm in pronation
C. Physical exam: pain over fracture site, swelling, deformity
D. Diagnosis: X-ray
E. Treatment: surgical

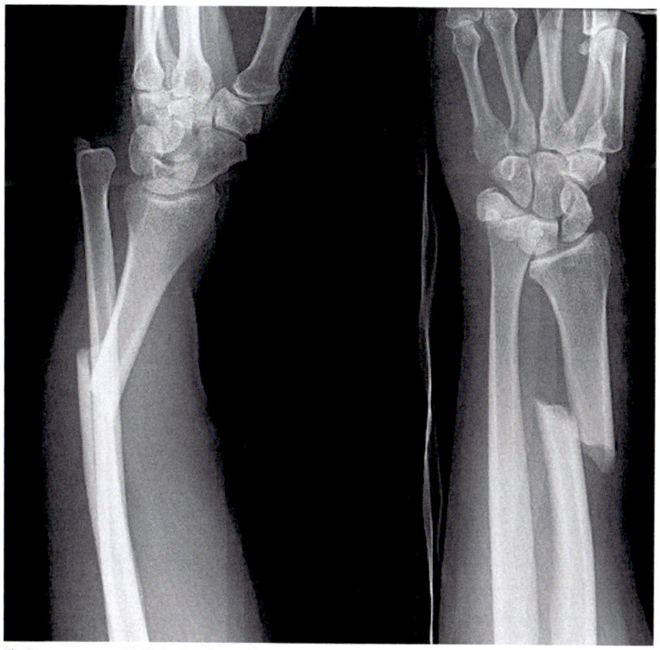

FIGURE 21.7.12 - X-Ray Depicting a Galeazzi Fracture

XIV. De Quervain Tenosynovitis
A. Pain at the radial side of the wrist
B. Mechanism of injury: overuse of abductor pollicis longus and extensor pollicis brevis
C. Women > men; classic patient is a first-time mom
D. Clinical diagnosis: positive Finkelstein test
E. Treatment: thumb spica splint, pain medications

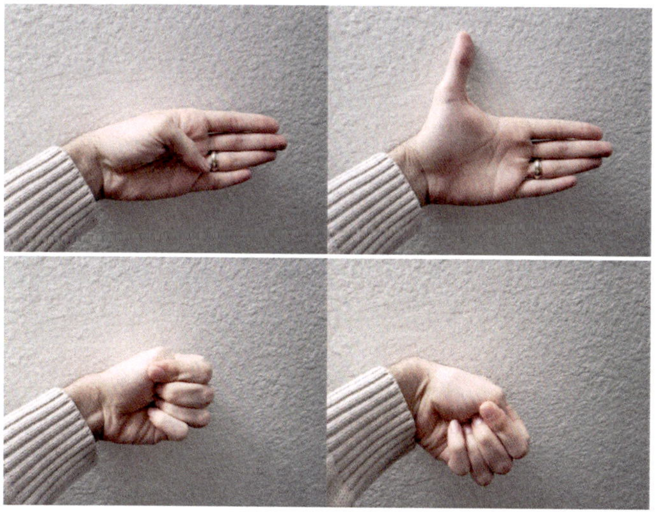

FIGURE 21.7.13 - Series of Images Demonstrating the Finkelstein Test

XV. Dupuytren's Contracture
   A. Disorder characterized by painless fascial nodules and contractures on the palmar side of the hand
   B. Pathophysiology: abnormal connective tissue formation
   C. Classic presentation: contracture of the ring finger in an older male
   D. Diagnosis: clinical
   E. Treatment: physical therapy, steroid injections, clostridial collagenase injections, fasciotomy

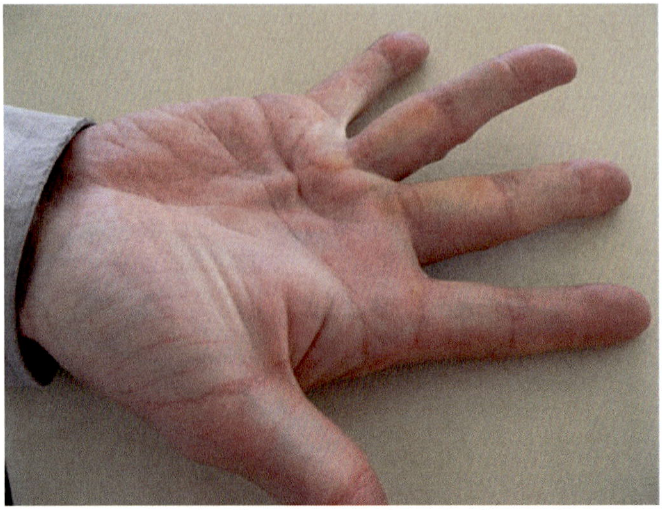

FIGURE 21.7.14 - Dupuytren's Contracture

Injury	Key Feature(s)	Key Management
Shoulder dislocation	- Anterior: abducted, externally rotated extremity; axillary nerve injury - Posterior: adducted, internally rotated extremity; seizures; light bulb sign	- Diagnosis with X-ray - Treatment with closed reduction and immobilization - Recurrence rate is high, especially in younger patients
Rotator cuff injury	- Tendinopathy: pain, no weakness, + Hawkins-Kennedy, Neer tests - Tear: pain and weakness, + drop arm test, + empty can test	- Tendinopathy: conservative treatment - Tear: surgery for acute tear, conservative treatment for chronic tear
Adhesive capsulitis	- "Frozen shoulder:" stiffness, limited active and passive range of motion	- Conservative treatment (self-limited disorder)
Humerus shaft fracture	- Associated with radial nerve palsy	- Closed reduction, immobilization - Surgery for open/displaced fractures or neurovascular compromise
Colles fracture	- Fracture in distal radius with dorsal angulation - "Dinner fork" deformity, median nerve palsy	- Closed reduction, cast immobilization - Surgery for unstable fractures
Scaphoid fracture	- Pain in anatomical snuffbox - High risk for avascular necrosis and nonunion	- Initial X-rays may be negative - Treat with thumb spica splint, repeat imaging in 7-10 days
Boxer's fracture	- Fracture in neck of 5th metacarpal bone	- Closed reduction, ulnar gutter splint
Monteggia fracture	- Fracture in proximal ulnar shaft, dislocated radial head	- Treat surgically
Galeazzi fracture	- Fracture in distal radius shaft, dislocated radioulnar joint	- Treat surgically
De Quervain Tenosynovitis	- Overuse of abductor pollicis longus and extensor pollicis brevis, + Finkelstein test	- Thumb spica splint, pain medications
Dupuytren contracture	- Painless fascial nodules and contractures in palmar fascia - Ring finger most commonly affected	- Physical therapy, steroid injections, clostridial collagenase injections, and surgery if refractory

TABLE 21.7.1 - Common Orthopedic Injuries of the Upper Extremities

REVIEW QUESTIONS

1. A 19-year-old woman with a history of epilepsy is brought into the emergency department following a tonic-clonic seizure 30 minutes ago. Physical examination shows an adducted and internally rotated right arm with flattening of the deltoid prominence. What is the most likely diagnosis?

   - **The most likely diagnosis for this patient is a posterior shoulder dislocation.**
   - This patient has had a recent seizure episode.
   - The physical examination reveals an adducted and internally rotated upper extremity.
   - Posterior shoulder dislocations are rare and typically follow either a seizure or an electrocution episode.
   - Patients with posterior shoulder dislocations typically hold the affected arm in adduction and internal rotation, which is in contrast to patients with anterior shoulder dislocations who typically hold the affected arm in abduction and external rotation.

2. An 18-year-old woman comes to urgent care because of left shoulder pain for 2 weeks. She is the pitcher on her school's softball team. Physical examination shows full active and passive range of motion. Strength is 5/5 in bilateral upper extremities. However, when the clinician brings the patient's left glenohumeral joint into full flexion, she reports pain. What is the most likely diagnosis?

   - **The most likely diagnosis is rotator cuff tendinopathy secondary to shoulder overuse.**
   - This patient is a pitcher on a softball team, which puts her at risk of overuse injury to her shoulder.
   - When the clinician performs the Neer test by bringing the patient's left shoulder into full flexion, she reports pain.
   - Adhesive capsulitis and rotator cuff tear are unlikely for two reasons.
   - First, the patient in question is young, and both adhesive capsulitis and rotator cuff tears are more common in patients over 40.
   - Second, on physical examination, she had full active and passive range of motion, which makes adhesive capsulitis unlikely, and full strength, which makes a rotator cuff tear unlikely as well.

3. A 24-year-old man is brought to the trauma bay by EMS following a high-speed motor vehicle collision 15 minutes ago. The patient's right upper extremity is visibly shortened when compared to the left upper extremity. Portable X-ray of the right arm shows a right humerus shaft fracture. What is the next best step in management of the fracture?

   - **Visible shortening of an extremity indicates a significantly displaced fracture, which warrants prompt operative repair with open reduction and internal exploration.**

4. A 44-year-old man comes to his primary care provider because of worsening left shoulder pain for 3 month. He works in construction and has had to take days off of work due to the pain. Past medical history is notable for type 2 diabetes and hypothyroidism for which he takes metformin and levothyroxine, respectively. There is no record of prior shoulder injuries or surgeries. Vital signs are within normal limits. Examination of the left shoulder shows decreased passive and active range of motion, but no weakness. Passive flexion of the left glenohumeral joint does not elicit pain. There are no sensory deficits of the left upper extremity. The remainder of the musculoskeletal examination is normal. Which of the following is the most likely diagnosis?

   A. Rotator cuff tendinopathy
   B. Rotator cuff tear
   C. Adhesive capsulitis
   D. Glenohumeral osteoarthritis

   - **The correct answer is option C.**
   - This patient endorses insidious shoulder pain over the course of three months.
   - He has a history of type 2 diabetes and hypothyroidism, which are considered to be risk factors for adhesive capsulitis.
   - His physical examination is notable for decreased passive and active range of motion, which is strongly suggestive of adhesive capsulitis.
   - Option A is incorrect. Rotator cuff tendinopathy is less likely in this patient because passive flexion of his left glenohumeral joint, i.e. the Neer test, did not elicit any pain.
   - Option B is incorrect. Rotator cuff tear is unlikely in this patient because he had no weakness on examination of his left shoulder, and rotator cuff tears are almost always present with weakness.
   - Option D is incorrect because shoulder arthritis is typically caused by repeated trauma to the joint. Since this patient does not have a record of prior shoulder injuries or surgeries, glenohumeral osteoarthritis is less likely than adhesive capsulitis.

MSK | Section 2: Common Adult Orthopedic Injuries of the Hip

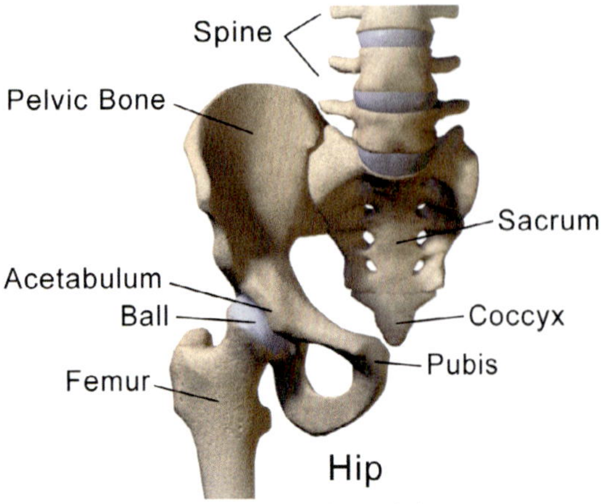

FIGURE 21.7.15 - Anatomy of the Hip

I. Hip Fracture
   A. Femoral neck fractures and intertrochanteric fractures are the most common types of hip fracture
   B. Osteoporosis is the primary risk factor
   C. Presentation: acute pain in the groin, inability to bear weight, externally rotated and shortened leg
   D. Complications: avascular necrosis, nonunion, sciatic nerve injury, VTE
   E. Treatment: open reduction, internal fixation; VTE prophylaxis

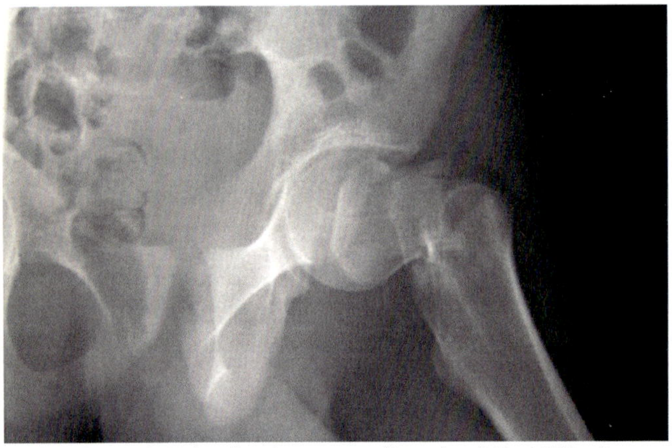

FIGURE 21.7.16 - X-Ray of a Fractured Hip

II. Hip Dislocation
   A. Posterior hip dislocations occur commonly after car accidents
      1. Physical exam: shortened, internally rotated leg
      2. Complication: sciatic nerve injury, femoral artery injury
   B. Anterior hip dislocations are rare
      1. Physical exam: shortened, externally rotated leg
      2. Complication: obturator nerve injury, femoral artery injury
   C. Treatment: closed reduction, bracing, follow-up CT scan

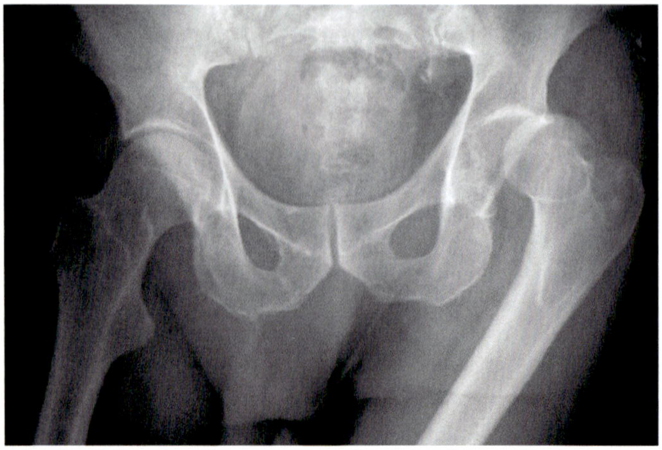

FIGURE 21.7.17 - X-Ray of a Dislocated Hip

III. Femur Shaft Fracture
   A. Etiology: trauma
   B. Presentation: shortened, painful extremity with a limited range of motion and inability to bear weight
   C. Warrants evaluation for concomitant femoral neck fracture
   D. Diagnosis: X-ray of the femur, hip, and knee
   E. Treatment: open reduction, internal fixation within 48 hours of injury
   F. Complications: hemorrhagic shock, fat embolism syndrome

IV. Fat Embolism Syndrome
   A. Etiology: fracture of long bones, orthopedic procedures, pancreatitis
   B. Pathophysiology: embolization of fat from the bone marrow into the circulation
   C. Classic presentation: respiratory symptoms, neurological changes, and a reddish-brown petechial rash within 24-72 hours of the inciting event
   D. Diagnosis is clinical
   E. Treatment is supportive (e.g. ventilatory support, fracture treatment)

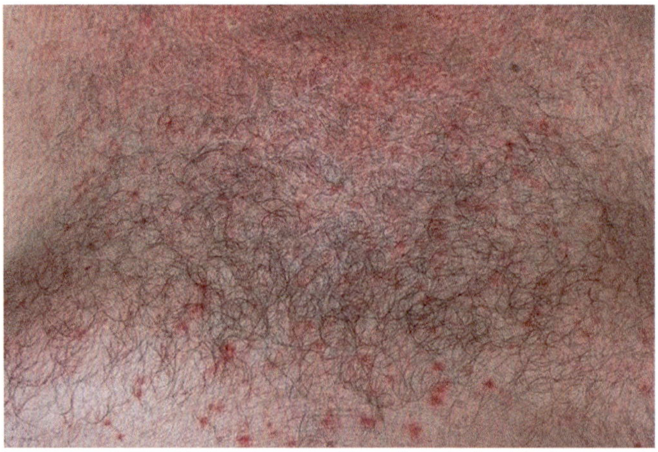

FIGURE 21.7.18 - Petechial Rash in Fat Embolism Syndrome

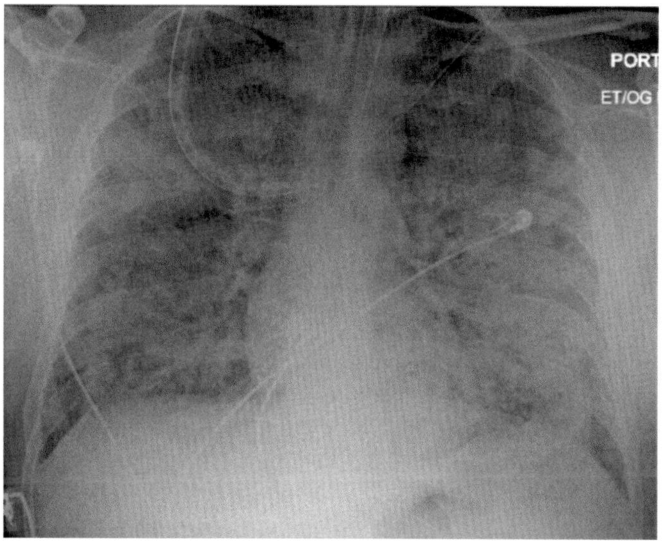

FIGURE 21.7.19 - Chest X-Ray Showing Fat Embolism Syndrome

V. Greater Trochanteric Pain Syndrome
   A. Pathophysiology: overuse of gluteus medius and minimus tendons as they pass over the greater trochanter
   B. Risk factors: age, female sex, obesity, osteoarthritis
   C. Presentation: pain in lateral hip that worsens with direct pressure over the greater trochanter and repeated hip flexion
   D. Diagnosis: clinical, ultrasound, X-ray
   E. Treatment: conservative, local corticosteroid injections

VI. Iliotibial Band Syndrome
   A. Overuse syndrome of the iliotibial band as it passes over the lateral femoral epicondyle
   B. Risk factors: intense exercise (e.g. runners, cyclists)
   C. Presentation: pain in lateral knee that worsens with exercise and direct palpation over the lateral femoral epicondyle
   D. Diagnosis: clinical
   E. Treatment: conservative

Injury	Key Feature(s)	Key Management
Hip fracture	- Externally rotated and shortened leg, fracture on X-ray	- VTE prophylaxis and open reduction, internal fixation
Hip dislocation	- Anterior (rare): shortened, externally rotated leg - Posterior (common): shortened, internally rotated leg	- Closed reduction, bracing, follow-up CT scan
Femur shaft fracture	- Associated with fat embolism syndrome and hemorrhagic shock	- Open reduction, internal fixation within 48 hours of injury
Greater trochanteric pain syndrome	- Pain in lateral hip, worse with palpation of greater trochanter	- Conservative, corticosteroid injections
Iliotibial band syndrome	- Pain in lateral knee, worse with palpation of lateral femoral epicondyle	- Conservative

TABLE 21.7.2 - Common Adult Orthopedic Injuries of the Hip

REVIEW QUESTIONS

1. A 75-year-old woman is brought to the emergency department following a ground-level fall 3 hours ago. She appears in pain. Physical examination shows bruising of the left hip and a shortened, externally rotated left lower extremity. What is the cause of this patient's physical examination findings?

- **The diagnosis is a left hip fracture.**
- Generally speaking, hip fractures are particularly common among elderly patients following ground-level falls because osteopenia or osteoporosis are particularly common in the elderly.
- On physical examination, hip fractures commonly present as a painful, shortened, externally rotated lower extremity.
- Though an anterior hip dislocation may also present as a shortened, externally rotated lower extremity, anterior hip dislocations are rare and do not typically occur following ground-level falls.
- Lastly, a posterior hip dislocation would be unlikely because it typically presents as a shortened, internally rotated lower extremity, rather than externally rotated lower extremity.

2. A 38-year-old woman comes to the emergency department via ambulance following a motor vehicle accident. She was hysterical in the ambulance due to pain in her lower extremity, but now is complaining of shortness of breath. As she is being evaluated, it is clear that she is confused and asks where she is several times. She often pauses while talking to catch her breath. Physical examination shows the right lower extremity injury and a red-brown petechial rash across her chest. Based on this patient's presentation, what is the most likely diagnosis?

A. IT band tear
B. Hip fracture
C. Femoral shaft fracture
D. Hip dislocation

- **The correct answer is option C.**
- This patient comes after a motor vehicle accident.
- She has pain in her lower extremity along with shortness of breath, confusion, and a red-brown petechial rash on her chest.
- These symptoms, coupled with the presence of a traumatic injury, point to fat embolism syndrome.
- Option A is incorrect because an IT band tear would not lead to fat embolization syndrome.
- Option B is incorrect because a hip fracture is more commonly associated with worry for tromboembolism rather than fat embolism.
- Option D is incorrect because a hip dislocation would not typically lead to fat embolization.

MSK | Section 3: Common Adult Orthopedic Injuries of the Knee

I. Knee Dislocation
   A. Etiology: direct blow to tibia
   B. Treatment: immediate reduction of the dislocated knee with a careful neurovascular exam of the extremity
   C. Complications
      1. Popliteal artery injury: check pulses, measure ankle-brachial index
      2. Peroneal nerve injury: neuro exam, nerve conduction studies

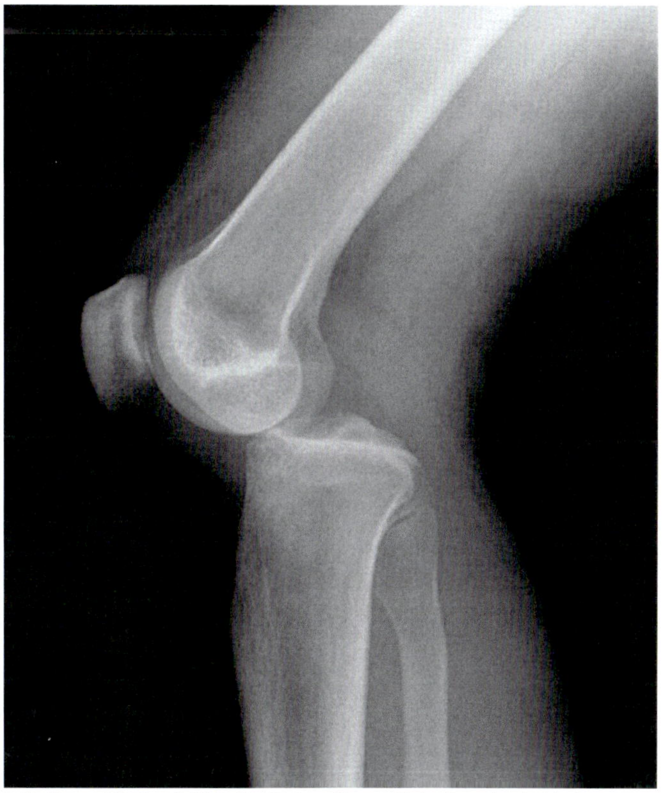

FIGURE 21.7.20 - X-Ray Depicting a Posterior Knee Dislocation

II. Patellar Dislocation
   A. Etiology: rapid lateral movement of a flexed knee
   B. Risk factors: competitive sports (e.g. gymnasts, soccer players)
   C. Patients report a "popping" noise at the time of injury
   D. Physical exam: dislocated patella and decreased knee extension
   E. Diagnosis: clinical or X-ray
   F. Treatment: closed reduction, splinting, physical therapy

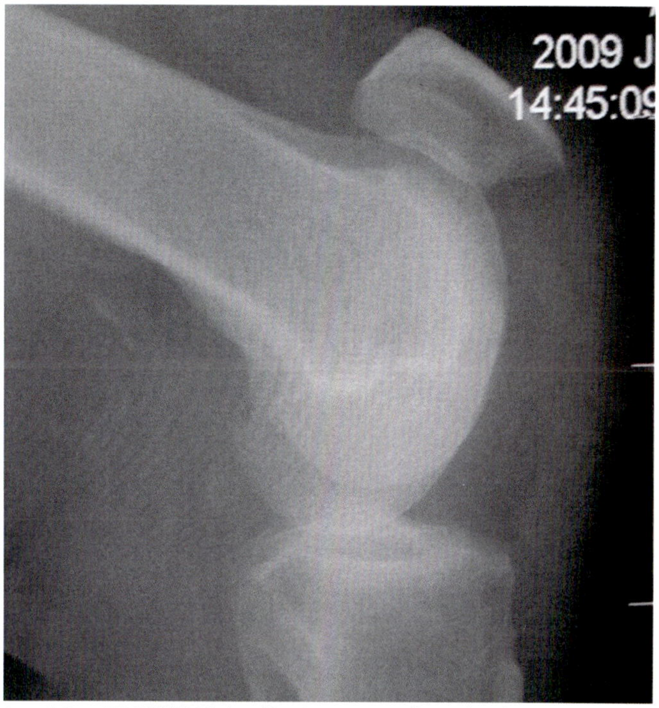

FIGURE 21.7.21 - X-Ray Depicting a Superiorly Dislocated Patella

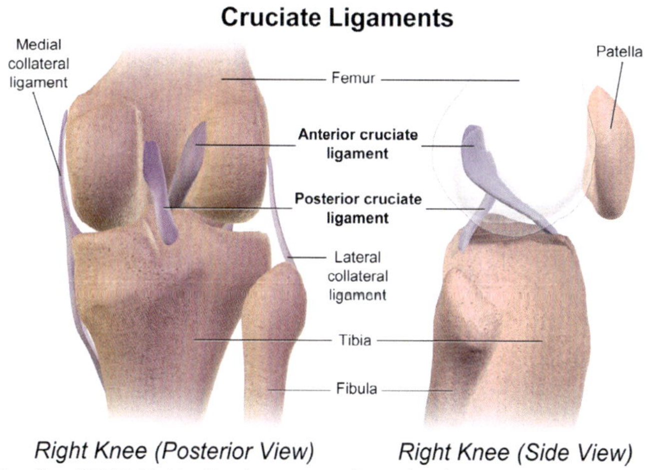

FIGURE 21.7.22 - Knee Ligaments Illustration

III. Knee Injuries: ACL
   A. Mechanisms of injury: abrupt deceleration, sudden direction change, or pivoting on the leg with the foot planted
   B. Physical exam: joint effusion, positive anterior drawer or lachman tests
   C. Diagnosis: knee MRI is the gold standard
   D. Treatment
      1. Physically active patients: surgery to reconstruct ACL
      2. Physically passive patients: conservative measures

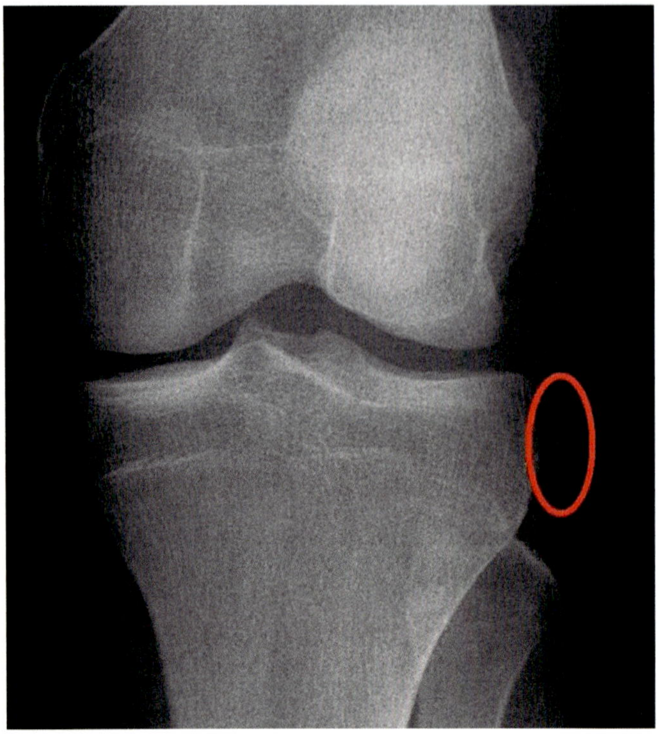

Ellisbjohns, Public domain, via Wikimedia Commons

FIGURE 21.7.23 - X-Ray Depicting a Segond Fracture

IV. Knee Injuries: PCL
   A. Mechanism of injury: force applied posteriorly on a flexed knee
   B. Physical exam: joint effusion, positive posterior drawer test
   C. Diagnosis: knee MRI is the gold standard
   D. Treatment: rest, ice, compression, elevation
      1. Physically active patients: surgery to reconstruct PCL
      2. Physically passive patients: conservative measures

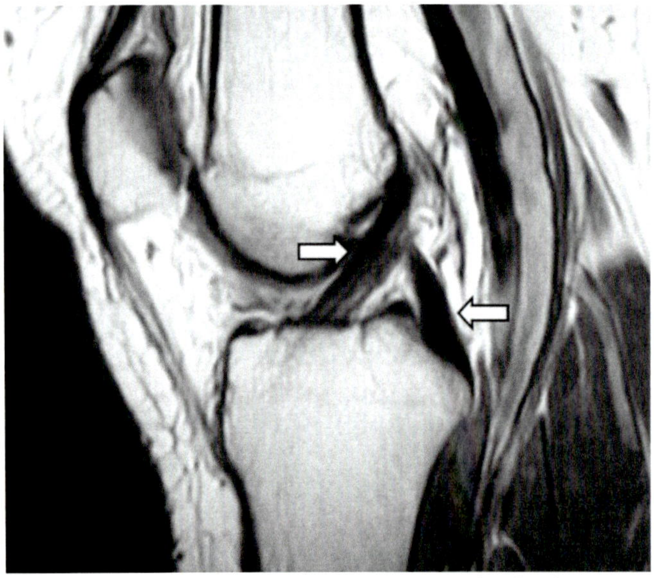

Marios G Lykissas, George I Mataliotakis, Nikolaos Paschos, Christos Panovrakos, Alexandros E Beris and Christos D Papageorgiou, CC BY-SA 2.0 <https://creativecommons.org/licenses/by-sa/2.0>, via Wikimedia Commons

FIGURE 21.7.24 - MRI of a Normal Knee Joint

V. Knee Injuries: MCL and LCL
   A. Mechanism of injury: direct trauma
   B. Physical exam: joint line tenderness, ecchymosis, no joint effusion
      1. MCL injury: positive valgus (abduction) stress test
      2. LCL injury: positive varus (adduction) stress test
   C. Diagnosis: clinical (MRI reserved for surgical candidates)
   D. Treatment: activity modification, ice, compression, elevation, pain control, physical therapy

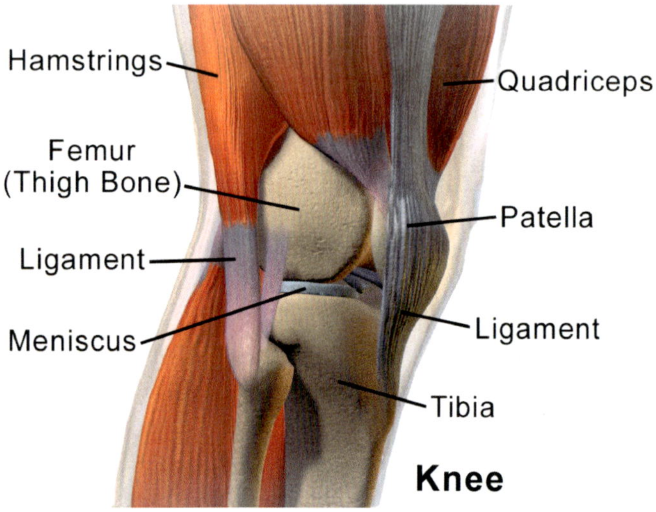

Blausen.com staff (2014). "Medical gallery of Blausen Medical 2014". WikiJournal of Medicine 1 (2). DOI:10.15347/wjm/2014.010. ISSN 2002-4436., CC BY 3.0 <https://creativecommons.org/licenses/by/3.0>, via Wikimedia Commons

FIGURE 21.7.25 - Illustration of the Knee

VI. Knee Injuries: Meniscal Tears
   A. Mechanism of injury: acute twisting force or chronic wear and tear
   B. Patients report "locking" or "catching" with motion of the affected knee
   C. Physical exam: joint line tenderness, positive McMurray test
   D. Diagnosis: knee MRI is the gold standard
   E. Treatment: conservative
      1. Surgery reserved for young, physically active patients or older patients who do not respond to conservative measures

Injury	Key Feature(s)	Key Management
Knee dislocation	- Associated with popliteal artery and peroneal nerve injury	- Closed reduction, careful neurovascular exam
Patellar dislocation	- Dislocated patella and decreased knee extension on exam	- Closed reduction, splinting, physical therapy
ACL, PCL injury	- ACL: positive anterior drawer or Lachman test - PCL: positive posterior drawer test	- Athletes/young patients: surgery to reconstruct ligament - Others: conservative
MCL, LCL injury	- MCL: positive valgus (abduction) stress test - LCL: positive varus (adduction) stress test	- Conservative
Meniscal injury	- "Locking" or "catching" sensation, positive McMurray test	- Physically active: surgery - Others: conservative

TABLE 21.7.3 - Common Adult Orthopedic Injuries of the Knee

REVIEW QUESTIONS

1. A 19-year-old man comes to an urgent care clinic because of left knee pain following an injury during a basketball game 2 hours ago. Physical examination shows a large joint effusion and increased laxity with anterior translation of the tibia relative to the femur. What is the most likely diagnosis?

- **The most likely diagnosis in this case is injury to the anterior cruciate ligament.**
- The increased laxity of the joint with anterior translation of the tibia relative to the femur is consistent with a positive anterior drawer test of the knee.
- Recall, the knee ligament responsible for resisting the anterior motion of tibia on the femur is the anterior cruciate ligament.

2. A 16-year-old man comes to the emergency department because of an injury to his right knee 30 minutes ago during a soccer game. He was playing in his high school soccer match when the injury occurred. The patient reports that he feels like his knee is "locking" when he moves it. The physician places his hand over the knee joint and fully flexes the knee. As they externally rotate the tibia, and use valgus force on the joint, while extending the knee, the pain is reproduced. Diagnosis is confirmed with an MRI. Based on this patient's likely diagnosis, what is the mechanism that caused this injury?

   A. Direct trauma to lateral knee
   B. Abrupt deceleration
   C. Acute twisting
   D. Blow to the tibia

- **The correct answer is option C.**
- The 16-year-old man presents with an injury to his right knee after a soccer match.
- The patient reports it feels like his knee is "locking" as he moves it.
- The maneuver the physician applies to the knee joint is known as the McMurray test to assess the integrity of the medial meniscus.
- Based on the recreation of the patient's pain, he most likely has an injury to his right medial meniscus.
- Meniscus injury is most often caused by an acute twisting injury in a young patient or chronic wear and tear in an older patient.
- Option A is incorrect because direct trauma to the lateral knee is the mechanism for an LCL injury.
- Option B is incorrect because abrupt deceleration is the mechanism for ACL injury.
- Option D is incorrect because a blow to the tibia is the mechanism for knee dislocation.

MSK | Section 4: Common Adult Orthopedic Injuries of the Shin

I. Popliteal (Baker) Cyst
   A. Swelling in popliteal fossa due to accumulation of synovial fluid in the bursa that lies between gastrocnemius and semimembranosus
   B. Risk factors: knee arthritis or repeated inflammation/ injury
   C. Presentation: asymptomatic or swelling and pain in popliteal fossa/calf
      1. Ruptured cyst: severe pain, warmth, erythema, "crescent sign"
   D. Diagnosis: clinical, ultrasound to rule out DVT
   E. Treatment: conservative; arthrocentesis, steroid injections

II. Tibial Stress Fracture
   A. Etiology: repeated forces applied to the bone without sufficient rest
   B. Female athlete triad: low bone density, hypomenorrhea, poor nutrition
   C. Presentation: dull, aching pain in anterior shin
   D. Physical exam: focal tenderness to palpation at fracture site
   E. Diagnosis: clinical, x-ray
   F. Treatment: conservative (reduce weight bearing, pain medications)
      1. Surgery if fracture is at high risk for nonunion

III. Medial Tibial Stress Syndrome
   A. Also known as shin splints
   B. Commonly seen in casual runners who are overweight
   C. Presentation: pain in the shin
   D. Physical exam: diffuse tenderness to palpation over anterior leg
   E. Diagnosis: clinical
   F. Treatment: reduce intensity of exercise

Injury	Key Feature(s)	Key Management
Popliteal (Baker) Cyst	- Popliteal fossa swelling, "crescent sign" - Associated with knee arthritis and repeated inflammation	- Asymptomatic: conservative - Symptomatic: r/o DVT, arthrocentesis, steroid injections
Tibial stress fracture	- "Female athlete triad," focal tenderness to palpation	- Surgery if fracture is high risk for nonunion, otherwise conservative
Medial tibial stress syndrome	- Shin splints, diffuse tenderness to palpation	- Reduce exercise intensity

TABLE 21.7.4 - Injuries of the Shin

REVIEW QUESTIONS

1. A 45-year-old male presents to his primary care provider due to worsening pain in the left leg over the past several weeks. About a month ago, he started preparing for a local half-marathon in an attempt to lose weight and improve his overall health. Past medical history is notable for hypertension, hyperlipidemia, and type 2 diabetes mellitus, for which he takes lisinopril, atorvastatin, and metformin, respectively. Blood pressure is 130/80 mmHg, pulse is 71 beats/minutes, and temperature is 37.3 °C. BMI is 32 kg/m2. Physical examination of the lower extremities is notable for diffuse tenderness to palpation over the anterior aspect of the left lower leg. The remainder of the examination is within normal limits. Which of the following is the most likely diagnosis?

   A. Tibial stress fracture
   B. Medial tibial stress syndrome
   C. Meralgia paresthetica
   D. Iliotibial band syndrome

- **The correct answer is B.**
- This is a case of a 45-year-old male with a BMI of 32 who is presenting with pain in the left leg that started soon after he started preparing for a half-marathon.
- His physical examination is largely within normal limits with the exception of diffuse tenderness to palpation over the anterior aspect of the left lower leg, that is his shin.
- This clinical picture is classic for medial tibial stress syndrome or shin splints.
- Option A, tibial stress fracture, is incorrect because it typically presents with point tenderness to palpation, rather than diffuse tenderness to palpation over the shin. This diagnosis is also more commonly seen in patients with the female athlete triad, that is low bone density, hypomenorrhea, and poor nutrition. This is certainly not the case in an obese male patient.
- Option C, meralgia paresthetica, is incorrect because it typically presents with paresthesia over the lateral thigh due to compression of the lateral femoral cutaneous nerve. This patient does not have any symptoms to suggest this diagnosis.
- Lastly, option D, iliotibial band syndrome, is incorrect because it typically presents as pain over the lateral knee that worsens with exercise.
- Even though iliotibial band syndrome can develop with intense exercise, such as in people preparing for a half-marathon, it wouldn't lead to pain over the shin as is the case with this patient.

MSK | Section 5: Common Adult Orthopedic Injuries of Ankle and Foot

I. Ankle Injury: Definition
   A. Ankle sprain: injury to ankle ligaments
      1. Anterior talofibular ligament (most common)
      2. Calcaneofibular ligament (second most common)
      3. Deltoid ligament
   B. Ankle fracture: injury to ankle bones

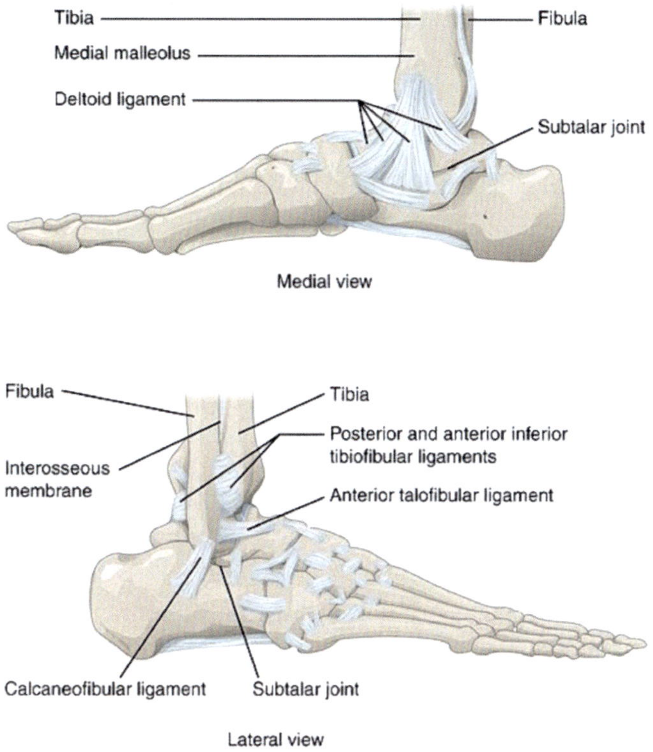

FIGURE 21.7.26 - Medial and Lateral View of Ankle

II. Ankle Sprain: Mechanism of Injury
   A. Anterior talofibular ligament
      1. Forceful plantar flexion and inversion of the foot
   B. Calcaneofibular ligament
      1. Forceful dorsiflexion and inversion of the foot
   C. Deltoid ligament
      1. Forceful eversion of the foot

III. Ankle Sprain: Risk Factors
   A. Professional dancing
   B. Indoor court sports (e.g. basketball)

IV. Ankle Sprain: Clinical Presentation
   A. Pain with weight bearing
   B. Physical examination
      1. Tenderness to palpation and swelling over injured ligaments
      2. Positive anterior drawer test

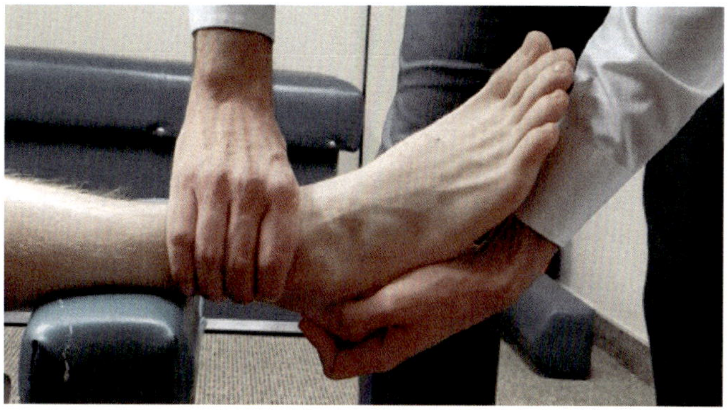

FIGURE 21.7.27 - Anterior Drawer Test

V. Ankle Injury: Diagnosis
   A. Ankle sprains: clinical diagnosis, imaging not warranted
   B. Ankle fractures: imaging warranted
   C. Ottawa ankle rules: effective in ruling out ankle fractures based on physical examination alone

VI. Ankle Injury: Ottawa Ankle Rules
   A. Obtain X-ray of the ankle if physical examination reveals pain in the malleolar zone along with either one of the following
      1. Tenderness to palpation along the distal 6 cm of the posterior edge of tibia or tip of medial malleolus
      2. Tenderness to palpation along the distal 6 cm of the posterior edge of fibula or tip of lateral malleolus
      3. Inability to bear weight for 4 steps (2 steps on each foot)
   B. Obtain X-ray of the foot if physical examination reveals pain in the midfoot zone along with either one of the following
      1. Tenderness to palpation at the navicular bone
      2. Tenderness to palpation at the base of the 5th metatarsal bone
      3. Inability to bear weight for 4 steps (2 steps on each foot)

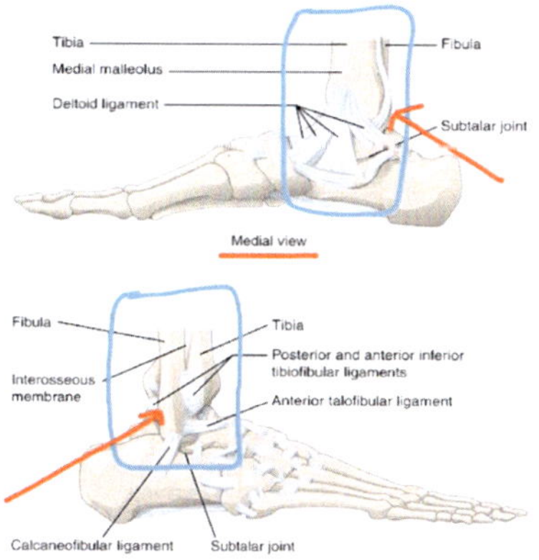

FIGURE 21.7.28 - "Malleolar Zone" as Defined by Ottawa Ankle Rules

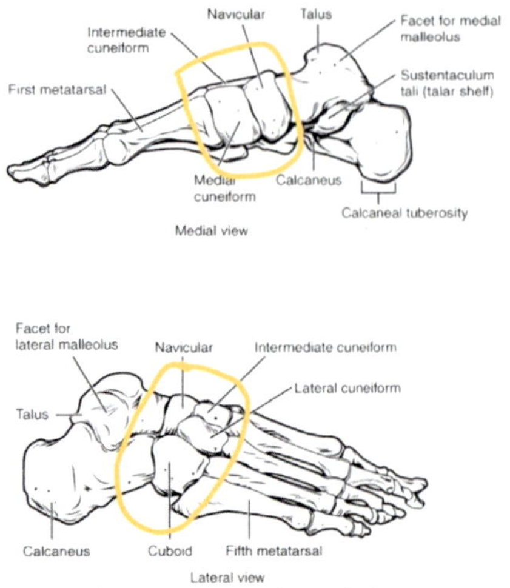

FIGURE 21.7.29 - "Midfoot Zone" as Defined by Ottawa Ankle Rules

VII. Ankle Injury: Management
  A. Ankle sprains
    1. Rest, ice, compression, elevation, physical therapy
    2. Surgery
  B. Ankle fractures
    1. Short leg walking cast
    2. Open reduction, internal fixation

VIII. Syndesmotic Injury
  A. Injury to syndesmotic structures of the ankle (e.g. interosseous membrane) leads to ankle instability
  B. Mechanism of injury: forceful dorsiflexion and eversion of the foot
  C. Physical examination: pain, swelling, positive "squeeze test"
  D. Diagnosis: X-ray of the ankle ("wide ankle mortise")
  E. Management: non-weight-bearing boot or cast for 2-3 weeks
    1. Surgery reserved for significant ankle instability or fractures

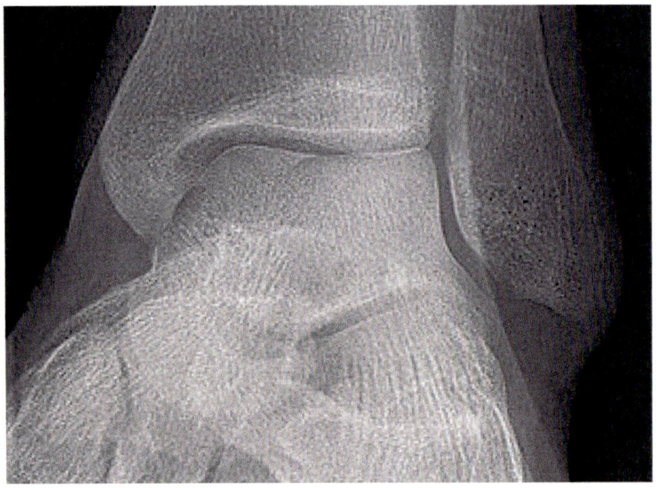

FIGURE 21.7.30 - X-Ray Depicting Normal Mortise View of Ankle

IX. Achilles Tendinopathy
  A. Pain at the insertion site of the Achilles tendon on the calcaneus
  B. Risk factors: age > 60, female sex, abrupt increase in physical activity, fluoroquinolones, corticosteroids
  C. Physical examination: tenderness to palpation, warmth and swelling at posterior heel
  D. Diagnosis: clinical, ultrasound, MRI
  E. Management: rest, ice, pain control, eccentric resistance exercises

X. Achilles Tendon Rupture
  A. Classic history: "weekend warrior" experiencing a sudden "popping" sensation and acute pain during a sports event (e.g. basketball)
  B. Risk factors: Achilles tendinopathy, athletic activity
  C. Physical examination: limited plantar flexion, positive Thompson test
  D. Diagnosis: clinical, ultrasound, MRI
  E. Treatment: surgery, long-leg cast for 6 weeks

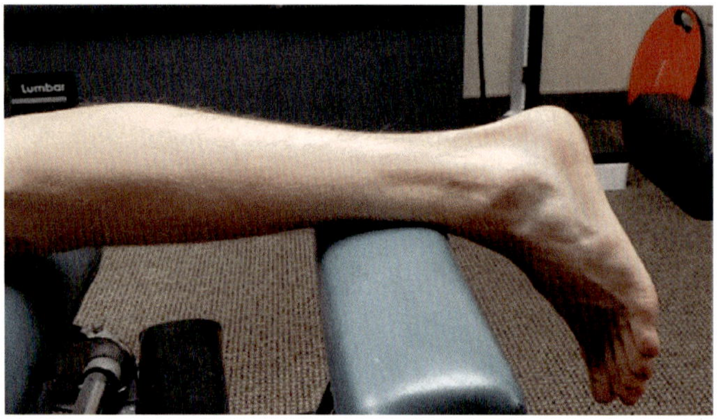

FIGURE 21.7.31 - Thompson Test

XI. Calcaneal Apophysitis (Sever Disease)
  A. Overuse injury of the calcaneal apophysis leading to bilateral heel pain that worsens with activity
  B. Risk factors: sports, footwear without heel padding, growth spurts
  C. Physical examination: tenderness to palpation at the base of the heel and a positive calcaneal compression test
  D. Diagnosis: clinical
  E. Management: conservative (e.g. rest, NSAIDs, heel cushioning)

XII. Plantar Fasciitis
  A. Overuse injury of the plantar aponeurosis leading to unilateral heel pain that worsens with toe dorsiflexion and weight bearing (especially with first steps after a long period of rest)
  B. Risk factors: obesity, flat feet, walking on hard surfaces
  C. Physical examination: focal tenderness over the plantar fascia
  D. Diagnosis: clinical (X-rays may reveal "heel spurs")
  E. Management: conservative (e.g. rest, NSAIDs, heel cushioning)

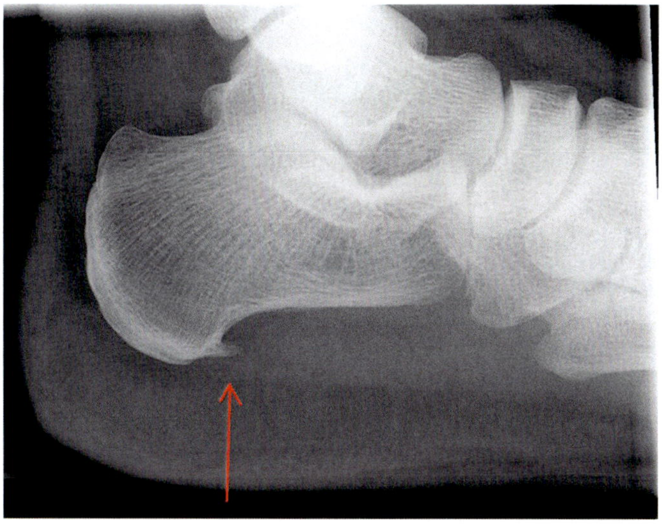

FIGURE 21.7.32 - X-Ray of Heel Spur in Plantar Fasciitis

XIII. Calcaneal Stress Fracture
   A. Unilateral heel pain that worsens with weight bearing (especially with first steps after a long period of rest)
   B. Risk factors: female sex, obesity, abrupt increase in exercise intensity, high-impact activities (e.g. running)
   C. Physical examination: positive calcaneal compression test
   D. Diagnosis: X-ray, MRI
   E. Management: conservative (e.g. reduction in weight bearing)

XIV. Tarsal Tunnel Syndrome
   A. Compression of the posterior tibial nerve as it passes through the tarsal tunnel, leading to paresthesias in medial ankle and foot
   B. Mechanism of injury: trauma, overuse, inflammation
   C. Physical examination: positive Tinel test
   D. Diagnosis: clinical, nerve conduction studies
   E. Management: conservative (e.g. rest, orthotics, steroid injections)
      1. Surgery reserved for refractory cases

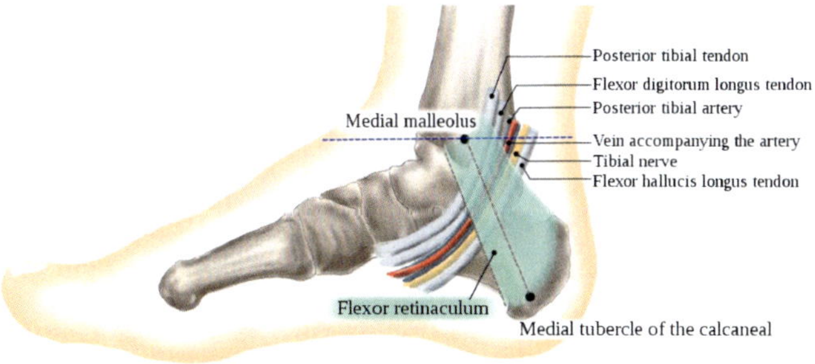

FIGURE 21.7.33 - Tarsal Tunnel

Injury	Key Feature(s)	Key Management
Ankle injury	- Ankle sprain: injury to ankle ligaments (ATFL, CFL) - Ankle fracture: injury to ankle bones	- Ottawa ankle rules to decide if imaging is warranted
Syndesmotic injury	- Mechanism: forceful dorsiflexion and eversion - Positive "squeeze test," wide ankle mortise on X-ray	- Non-weight-bearing boot/cast for 2-3 weeks
Achilles tendinopathy	- Risk factors: abrupt increase in physical activity, fluoroquinolones corticosteroids	- Eccentric resistance exercises
Achilles tendon rupture	- Classic patient: "weekend warrior" playing basketball - Positive Thompson test	- Surgery, long leg cast for 6 weeks
Calcaneal apophysitis (Sever disease)	- Bilateral heel pain, worse with activity and compression of calcaneus, common during growth spurts	- Rest, NSAIDs, heel cushioning
Plantar fasciitis	- Unilateral heel pain, worse with toe dorsiflexion and weight bearing, especially first steps after long rest - Focal tenderness over plantar fascia - "Heel spurs" on X-ray	- Rest, NSAIDs, heel cushioning
Calcaneal stress fracture	- Unilateral heel pain, worse with weight bearing, especially first steps after long rest - Positive calcaneal compression test - Does not worsen with toe dorsiflexion	- Heel cushioning, reduction in weight bearing
Tarsal tunnel syndrome	- Paresthesias in medial ankle and foot - Positive Tinel test over tarsal tunnel	- Rest, orthotics, steroid injections

TABLE 21.7.5 - Summary of Ankle and Foot Injuries

REVIEW QUESTIONS

1. A 16-year-old boy is brought to his pediatrician because of right ankle pain which he sustained during his highschool basketball game yesterday. Physical examination shows an edematous right ankle. There is no focal tenderness over the malleoli or the posterior ankle. He is able to bear weight for 8 steps, although he is somewhat limited by pain. What is the next best step in management?
   - **The next step in management would be to treat the ankle sprain with conservative measures, such as rest, ice, compression, elevation, and potentially physical therapy.**
   - This is a classic presentation of an ankle sprain.
   - Since there is no tenderness to palpation over the malleolar tips or the distal 6 cm of the posterior edge of the tibia or fibula, and he is able to bear weight for more than 4 steps, an ankle fracture is unlikely and imaging is not warranted.

2. A 65-year-old woman returns to her primary care provider a week after starting ciprofloxacin for a urinary tract infection because of right heel pain. Physical examination shows tenderness to palpation and warmth at the right posterior heel. What is the most likely diagnosis?
   - **The most likely diagnosis is achilles tendinopathy.**
   - Use of both fluoroquinolones and corticosteroids has been associated with increased risk for Achilles tendinopathy and rupture.
   - Fluoroquinolones are known to cause collagen fiber dysplasia, leading to decreased tensile strength of the tendon.
   - Corticosteroids, on the other hand, predispose patients to injury by masking the pain of overexertion, leading to overuse and subsequent weakening of the tendon.

3. A 13-year-old boy is brought to his pediatrician because of heel pain for 2 days. The boy states that he first noticed the heel pain after playing basketball with his little brother. His father says he is now complaining of heel pain when running around the house barefoot. Physical examination shows tenderness to palpation of the heel bilaterally. What is the most likely diagnosis?
   - **The most likely diagnosis is calcaneal apophysitis.**
   - The case describes a young boy experiencing bilateral heel pain when playing basketball or when running around the house.
   - Bilateral heel pain that worsens with activity in a young patient undergoing a growth spurt should always prompt suspicion of calcaneal apophysitis.
   - Plantar fasciitis can be considered on the differential because the boy runs a lot barefoot.
   - However, it is less likely in this scenario because it typically presents as unilateral heel pain, rather than bilateral heel pain.
   - Furthermore, plantar fasciitis is typically worst when first stepping out of bed, which isn't the case in this question.

REVIEW QUESTIONS

4. A 25-year-old otherwise healthy woman comes to her general practitioner because of left foot pain that she first noticed 3 weeks ago when she started preparing for an Ironman Triathlon. She says the pain is at its worst during exercise, particularly if she goes running first thing in the morning. Review of systems is otherwise negative. She doesn't take any medications and does not use alcohol or tobacco products. Vital signs are within normal limits and her BMI is 27 kg/m^2. Physical examination shows bilateral pes planus and tenderness to palpation over the sole of the left foot that is exacerbated with toe dorsiflexion. Range of motion, strength, and sensation are intact in both feet. Which of the following is the most likely diagnosis?

   A. Achilles tendinopathy
   B. Plantar fasciitis
   C. Calcaneal stress fracture
   D. Calcaneal apophysitis
   E. Tarsal tunnel syndrome

- **The correct answer is option B.**
- This patient is a young, overweight woman who recently started preparing for a challenging triathlon and now presents with unilateral foot pain.
- Notably, her pain is at its worst with activity, especially first thing in the morning, which is the classic pattern of pain observed in plantar fasciitis.
- Furthermore, her physical exam reveals bilateral pes planus, or flat foot, along with tenderness over the sole of her left foot that worsens with toe dorsiflexion, which is also consistent with a diagnosis of plantar fasciitis.
- Option A is incorrect because Achilles tendinopathy is more likely to present with ankle pain rather than foot pain. That being said, it wouldn't be unreasonable to consider Achilles tendinopathy on the differential, as an abrupt increase in exercise intensity is a notable risk factor for it.
- Option C is incorrect because a calcaneal stress fracture is not supported by the physical examination described in the vignette. Additionally, it would be more likely in a case of female athlete triad rather than in a woman with a BMI of 27. As a reminder, the female athlete triad is low bone mineral density, poor caloric intake, and hypo- or oligomenorrhea.
- Option D is incorrect because calcaneal apophysitis typically presents as bilateral heel pain, rather than unilateral heel pain, and it more commonly occurs in children during growth spurts rather than adult women.
- Option E is incorrect because tarsal tunnel syndrome tends to manifest in the form of neuropathic pain localizing to the medial ankle, which isn't the case with this patient.

PULMONOLOGY

Pulmonology | Section 1: Lung Neoplasms

Type		Location	Key Features	Paraneoplastic Syndrome
NSCLC	Adenocarcinoma	- Peripheral	- Most common type - More common in women and nonsmokers - Imaging: resembles pneumonia	- Hypertrophic osteoarthropathy (clubbing)
	Squamous cell carcinoma	- Central	- High association with smoking - Imaging: cavitary lesions - Histology: keratin pearls, intercellular bridges	- PTHrP: hypercalcemia
	Large cell carcinoma	- Peripheral	- Highly undifferentiated; poor prognosis	- β-HCG: gynecomastia
	Bronchial carcinoid tumor	- Central/ peripheral	- Neuroendocrine tumor - Causes mass effect - Good prognosis	- Carcinoid syndrome (flushing, wheezing, diarrhea)
SCLC		- Central	- Neuroendocrine tumor - Chromogranin A + - Poor prognosis	- ACTH: Cushing syndrome - SIADH - Antibodies against presynaptic Ca^{2+} channels: Lambert-Eaton syndrome

TABLE 21.8.1 - Types of Lung Cancer

I. Primary Lung Cancer: Classification
   A. Leading cause of cancer-related death in the US
   B. Non-small cell lung cancer (NSCLC)
   C. Small-cell lung cancer (SCLC)

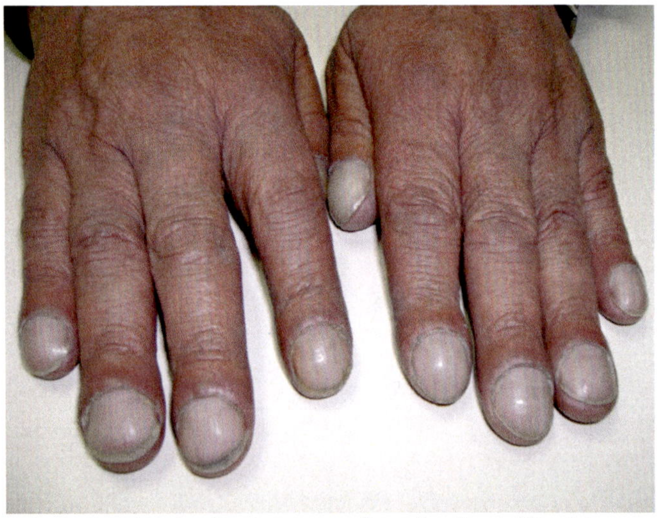

FIGURE 21.8.1 - Digital Clubbing

II. Primary Lung Cancer: Risk Factors
      a. Smoking; most important factor
   A. Environmental exposures (e.g. asbestos, radon)
   B. Genetic (e.g. mutations in *EGFR, ALK, KRAS genes*)

III. Primary Lung Cancer: Clinical Features
   A. General symptoms include cough, hemoptysis, chest pain, dyspnea, and weight loss
   B. Specific symptoms include
      1. Local invasion or compression: SVC syndrome, hoarseness, diaphragm paralysis, pancoast syndrome, pleural effusions
      2. Metastasis: liver, adrenals, bone, brain
      3. Paraneoplastic syndromes

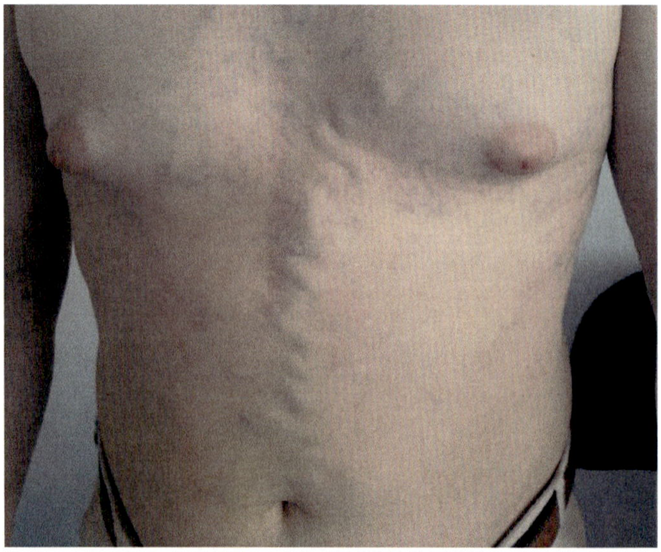

FIGURE 21.8.2 - Dilated Superficial Veins of the Chest in SVC Syndrome

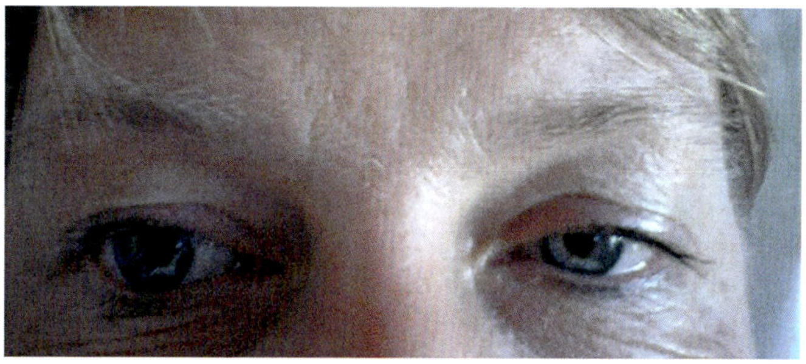

FIGURE 21.8.3 - Miosis and Ptosis in Horner Syndrome

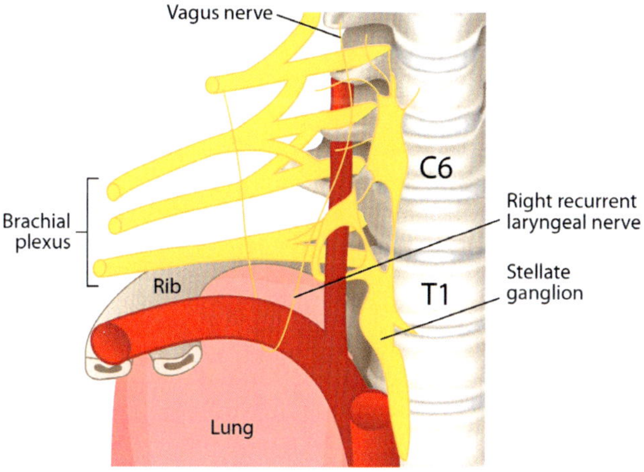

FIGURE 21.8.4 - Brachial Plexus and Apex of Lung

IV. Primary Lung Cancer: Diagnosis
   A. History and physical exam
      1. Neurologic symptoms can be a sign of brain and spinal cord metastasis
   B. Chest X-ray
      1. Infiltrates mimicking pneumonia
      2. Cavitations (squamous cell carcinoma)
      3. Mediastinal widening
   C. CT scan (with IV contrast)
      1. For all patients suspected with lung cancer
      2. Staging (LN involvement, metastasis)
   D. Labs including CBC, electrolytes (Na^+, Ca^{2+}), liver panel (ALP, AST, ALT)
   E. Biopsy
   F. Full body PET scan or MRI

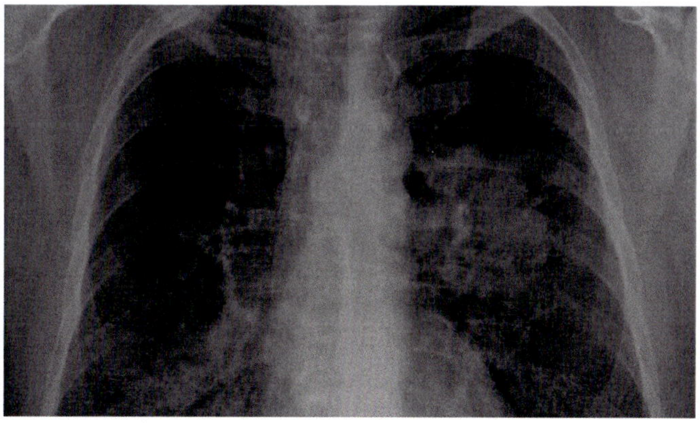

FIGURE 21.8.5 - Chest X-Ray: Left-Sided Lesion of Lung Cancer

V. Primary Lung Cancer: Management
   A. Non-small cell lung cancer (NSCLC)
      1. Surgery + / - adjuvant chemotherapy (stages 1B-3)
      2. Non-surgical candidate: radiation therapy
      3. Targeted therapy: EGFR, ALK, KRAS mutations
   B. Small cell lung cancer (SCLC)
      1. Chemotherapy (+ / - radiotherapy)

VI. Solitary Pulmonary Nodule: General Information
   A. Well-defined solitary mass with no associated LN involvement
   B. Usually small (≤ 30mm)
   C. Discovered incidentally on imaging
   D. Differential diagnosis is wide
      1. Benign etiologies: granuloma, hamartoma, adenoma
      2. Malignant etiologies: lung carcinoma, metastasis, carcinoid tumor

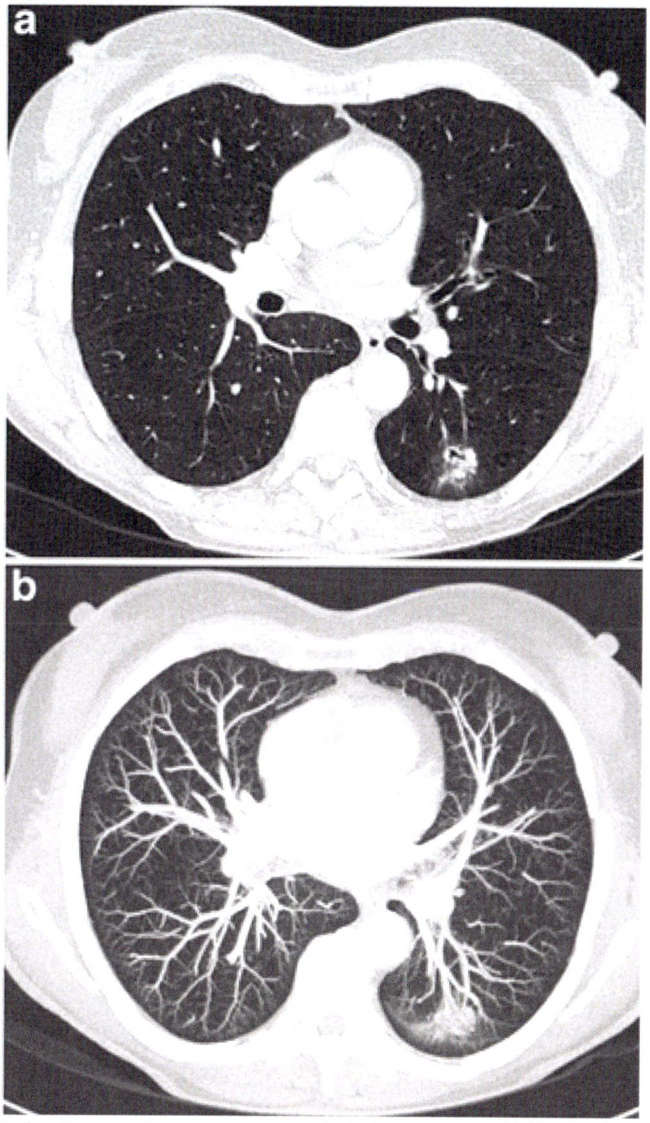

FIGURE 21.8.6 - CT Scan of Chest: Solitary Nodule of Lower Lobe of the Left Lung

VII. Solitary Pulmonary Nodule: Diagnostic Workup
   A. Clinical risk assessment for malignancy
   B. Obtain imaging
      1. Usually a CT scan
   C. Imaging risk assessment
      1. Compare to previous images

VIII. Solitary Pulmonary Nodule: Risk Assessment
   A. Clinical risk assessment for malignancy
      1. Age > 35
      2. Smoking status
      3. Associated symptoms (e.g. hemoptysis, weight loss, chronic cough)
   B. Imaging risk assessment for malignancy
      1. Large size (> 2cm)
      2. Irregular borders
      3. Absence of calcification
      4. Growth

IX. Solitary Pulmonary Nodule: Management
   A. Localized disease
      1. Very individualized depending on risk assessment
      2. No change in size in 2 or more years: yearly follow-up
      3. Suspicion of malignancy on imaging: biopsy or resection

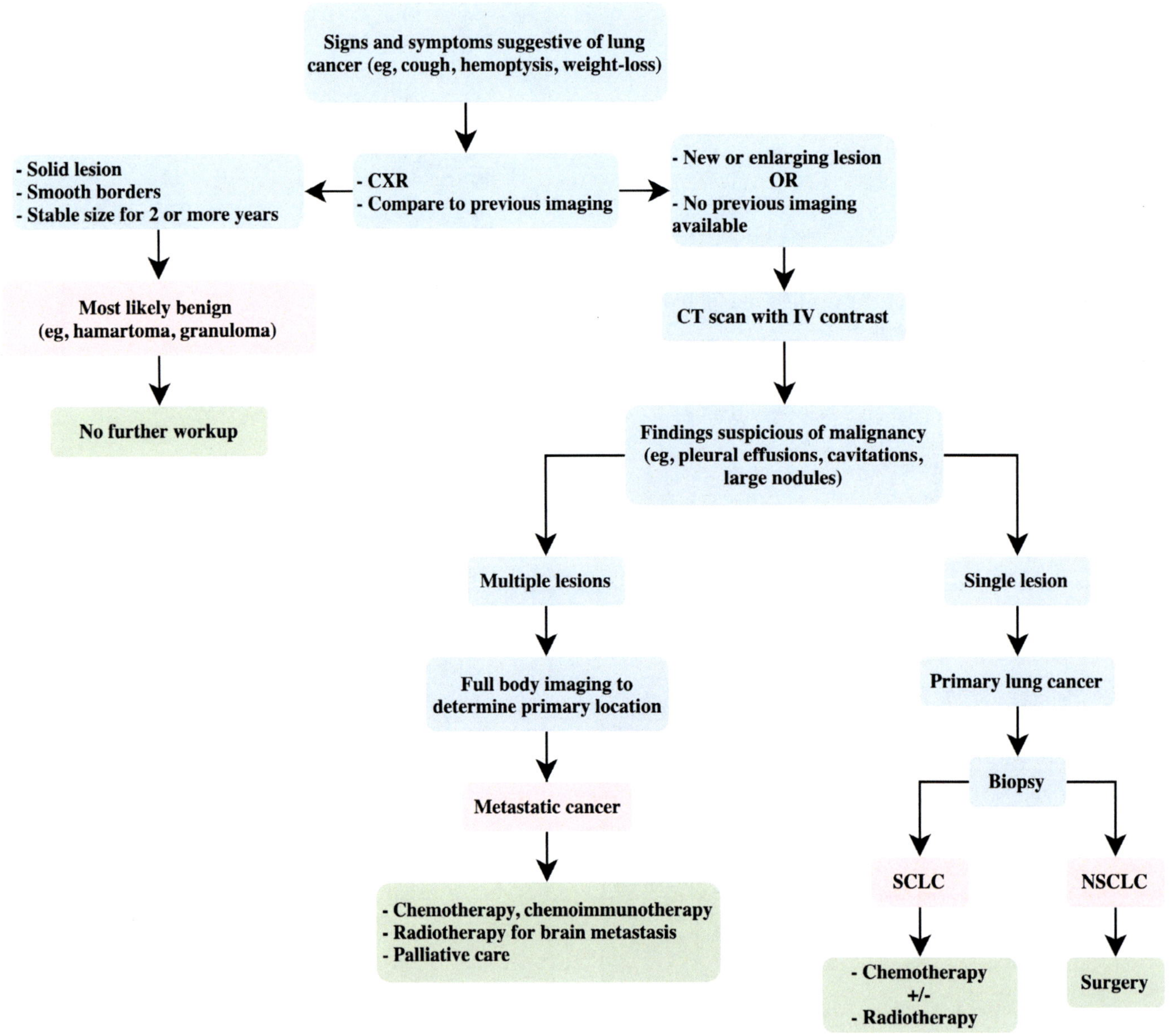

FIGURE 21.8.7 - Evaluation and Management of Lung Cancer

Location		Masses	Clinical Presentation
Superior mediastinum		- Thymoma - Lymphoma	
Inferior mediastinum	Anterior mediastinum	4 T's - **T**hyroid tumors - **T**hymoma - Lymphoma ('**t**errible') - **T**eratoma	
	Middle mediastinum	- Lung cancer - Lymphadenopathy - Aneurysm - Mediastinal hernia	- Asymptomatic - Compression of major structures (e.g. cough, dyspnea, hemoptysis, chest pain - Nerve affection causing hoarseness (recurrent laryngeal), Horner syndrome (sympathetic ganglia), paralysis of diaphragm (phrenic nerve)
	Posterior mediastinum	- Neurogenic tumors (e.g. neuroblastoma) - Esophageal cancer - Lung cancer	

TABLE 21.8.2 - Mediastinal Masses

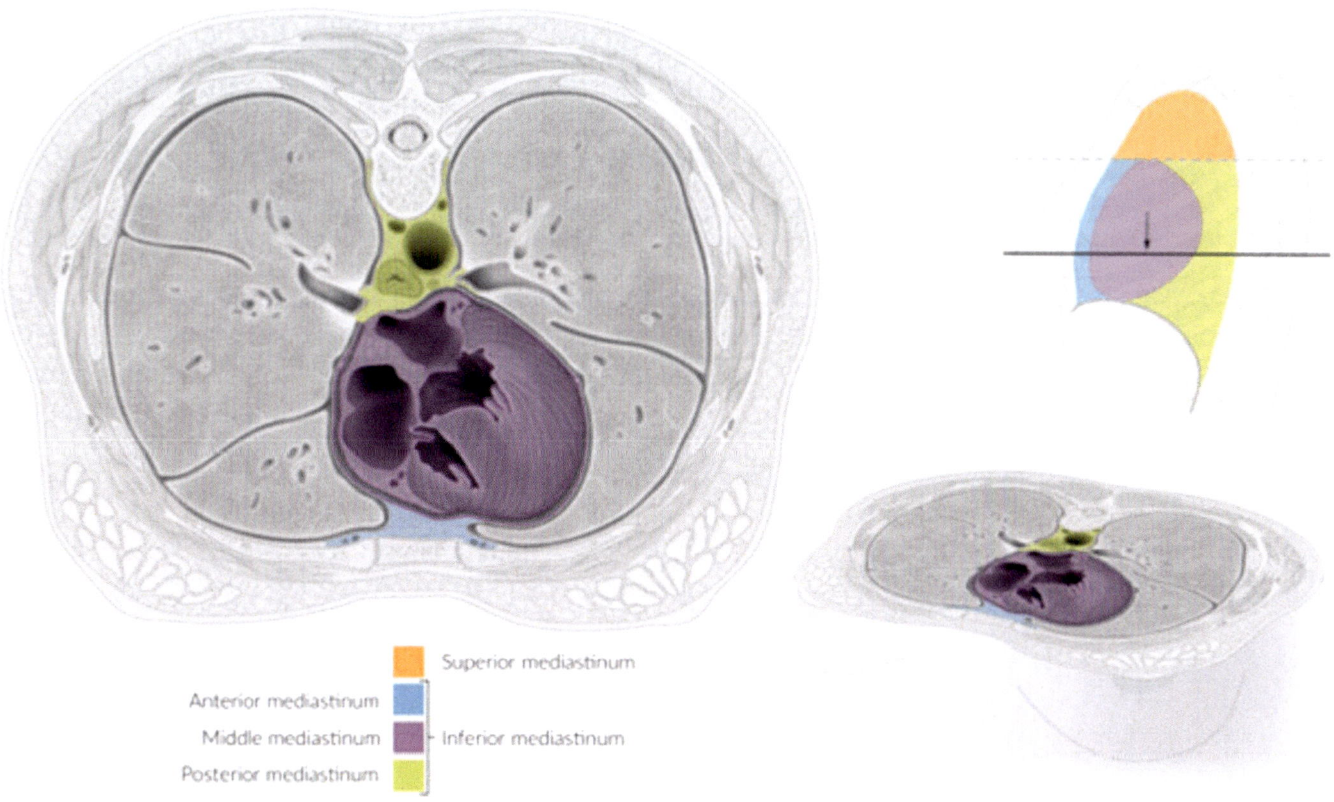

FIGURE 21.8.8 - Mediastinum

X. Lung Cancer Screening
   A. Low-dose chest CT annually without IV contrast
   B. 55-80 years old
   C. History of ≥ 20 pack-year smoking
   D. Current smokers or stopped within the past 15 years
   E. Stop screening if cessation period is 15 years or more or limited life expectancy

REVIEW QUESTIONS

1. A 57-year-old man comes to the physician due to worsening weakness in his shoulders and hips for the last 6-weeks. The weakness is noted to be worst while trying to get up from his rocking chair. He states it takes him several attempts to rise from his chair. He has a 40-pack-year smoking history and endorses a chronic cough. The patient also notes recent erectile dysfunction and increasingly dry mouth. What is the most likely underlying cause of this patient's current condition?
    - **The most likely cause of this patient's condition is Lambert-Eaton myasthenic syndrome, secondary to small cell lung cancer.**
    - The patient presents with worsening weakness in his proximal muscles, particularly in his shoulders and hips.
    - The patient has a long smoking history, along with associated chronic cough.
    - Lung cancer should be high on the differential.
    - This presentation is classic for Lambert-Eaton myasthenic syndrome (LEMS), a paraneoplastic disorder caused by small cell lung cancer.
    - LEMS is caused by antibodies against presynaptic calcium channels.
    - Calcium is necessary in the presynaptic terminal in order for acetylcholine exocytosis to occur. Antibodies decrease calcium entry in the neuron and, therefore, acetylcholine release is decreased, leading to muscle weakness.
    - LEMS mostly involves large proximal muscles in contrast to myasthenia gravis, which involves small muscles such as extraocular muscles.
    - LEMS, in contrast to myasthenia gravis, is also characterized by autonomic symptoms like dry mouth and erectile dysfunction because acetylcholine is necessary for both saliva production and erection.

2. A 55-year-old woman was found to have a 1.5cm solitary pulmonary nodule on a chest X-ray. She is a nonsmoker. Previous chest X-ray from 5 years ago shows the solitary pulmonary nodule to be 1 cm. CT scan is performed and shows the nodule with smooth borders and no spiculations, calcifications, or lymphatic invasion. What is the best next step in management of this patient?
    - **The best next step in the management of this patient is serial CT scans to track the size and features of the solitary pulmonary nodule.**
    - This patient presents with an incidentally discovered solitary pulmonary nodule of 1.5 cm in diameter.
    - Chest X-ray performed 5 years ago showed this nodule to be 1 cm.
    - This means that the nodule is growing in size which is why she underwent CT scan.
    - CT scan shows the features of a benign nodule. Smooth borders, no spiculations, calcifications, or lymphatic invasion.
    - According to these findings along with her non smoking status, relatively slow growth of the mass, her pretest probability of having lung cancer is low.

REVIEW QUESTIONS

3. An 82-year-old woman comes to the physician because of increased urinary frequency for the past 6-months. She currently uses the bathroom 8 times per day. She denies dysuria. She also mentions that she is more constipated than usual. She has a past medical history of an ischemic stroke 5-years ago complicated with oropharyngeal dysphagia. She also suffered from a kidney stone treated with shock wave lithotripsy 6-months ago and right lower lobe pneumonia 3-weeks ago. She has smoked 2-packs of cigarettes per day for 60 years. Physical exam shows a dehydrated woman with a flat affect. Serum calcium is 15 mg/dL (8.4-10.2 mg/dL) and parathyroid hormone is 100 pg/mL (N=230 to 630 pg/mL). A chest X-ray is performed and shows a left hilar cavity. Which of the following is the most likely diagnosis in this patient?

   A. Squamous cell carcinoma
   B. Small cell lung cancer
   C. Lung abscess
   D. Post-pneumonia bronchogenic cyst

- **The correct answer is option A.**
- The patient presents with increased urinary frequency and constipation,
- Examination and serum studies show flat affect, dehydration, and elevated serum calcium with low parathyroid hormone.
- All these features together are the classic manifestations of hypercalcemia remembered by mnemonic "Stones, bones, groans, thrones, psychiatric overtones."
- This patient has an extensive smoking history and she also has a left hilar cavity on her chest X-ray.
- All these findings point towards squamous cell carcinoma of the lungs which is associated with paraneoplastic PTH-independent hypercalcemia. It is also associated more commonly with cavitary lesions.
- Option B is possible in this patient with an extensive smoking history and a central, hilar mass on the chest X-ray. However, SCLC is characterized by paraneoplastic syndromes such as ectopic ACTH-dependent Cushing syndrome, SIADH, and Lambert-eaton myasthenic syndrome. SCLC has not been shown to cause PTH-independent hypercalcemia.
- Option C is possible in this patient with stroke-induced oropharyngeal dysphagia and a history of recent pneumonia. However, lung abscess usually shows air-fluid levels in addition to the cavity. This patient, on the other hand, had only a cavity on chest X-ray.
- Option D is possible in this patient with a recent history of right lower lobe pneumonia. However, bronchogenic cyst usually appears in the lobe previously affected by pneumonia.
- Also, none of the above mentioned conditions would explain hypercalcemia with low PTH levels.
- This patient had the cavity in the left, rather than the right, hilum.

Pulmonology | Section 2: Pleural Effusion and Pleurisy

I. Pleural Effusion: Definition
   A. Increased pleural fluid in the pleural cavity
      1. Transudate
      2. Exudate

II. Pleural Effusion: Pathophysiology
   A. Increased accumulation of fluid in the pleural space secondary to changes in hydrostatic pressure, oncotic pressure and/or capillary permeability

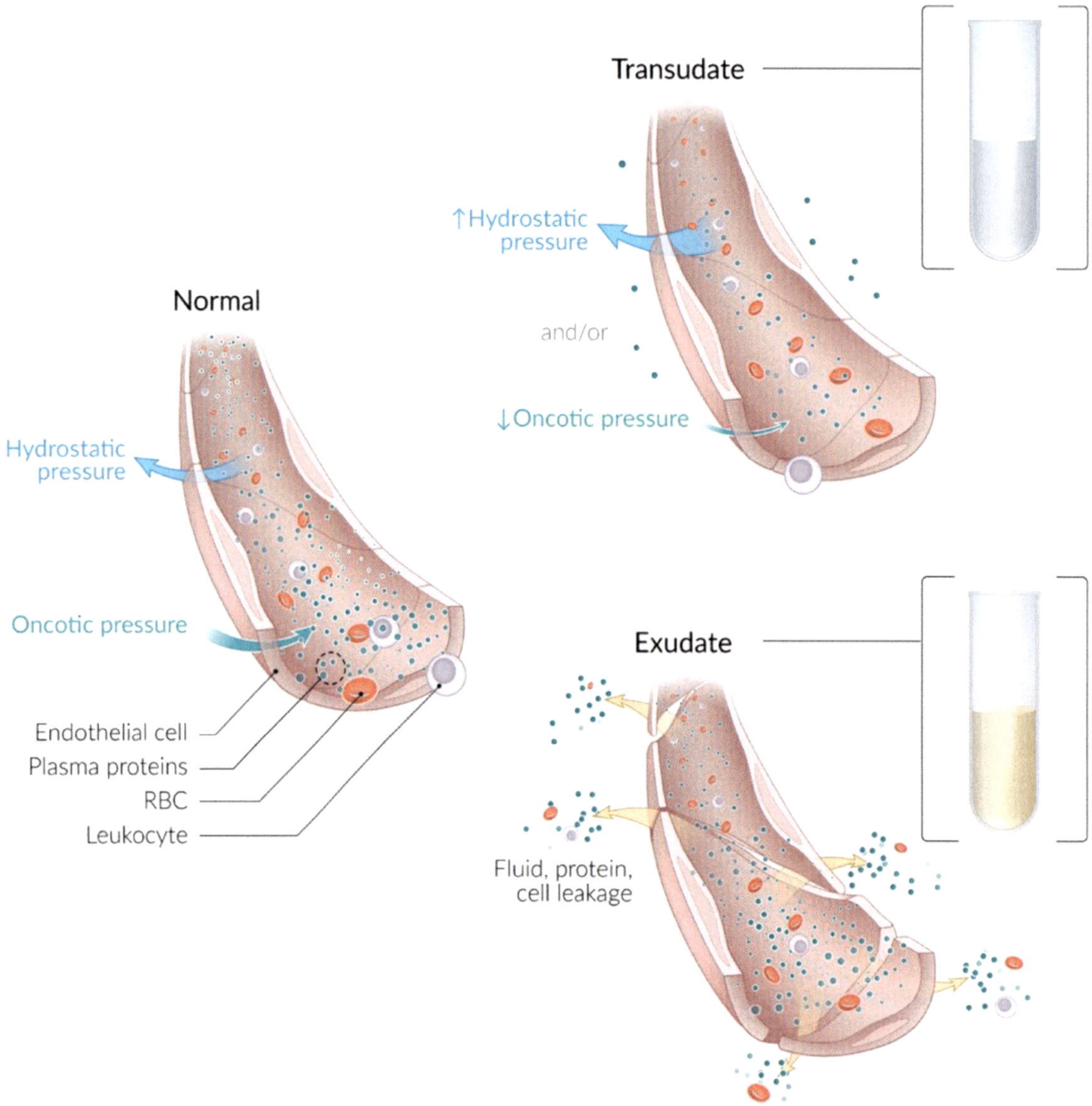

FIGURE 21.8.9 - The Pathophysiology of Transudative and Exudative Pleural Effusions

I. Pleural Effusion: Etiology
   A. Transudate
      1. Examples include CHF, cirrhosis, nephrotic syndrome, PE
   B. Exudate
      1. Examples include infections (pneumonia, TB), malignancy, autoimmune diseases (SLE, RA), chylothorax, hemothorax, PE

II. Pleural Effusion: Clinical Presentation
   A. Asymptomatic (small effusions < 300 mL)
   B. Pleuritic chest pain
   C. Dyspnea
   D. Symptoms associated with the underlying disease (e.g. edema in CHF)

III. Pleural Effusion: Diagnosis
   A. History and physical exam
      1. ↓ breath sounds, dull percussion, ↓ tactile fremitus

B. Imaging
   1. CXR (best initial step): detects as small as 250-300 mL; costophrenic angle blunting; lung opacification, tracheal deviation (large effusion)
   2. US: used in trauma (FAST); sensitive
C. Thoracentesis (best next step after CXR); diagnostic and therapeutic
   1. Indications: new unilateral effusion that is > 1 cm
   2. Not done in bilateral effusions or if there are clinical features of CHF
   3. Complication: pneumothorax
D. Pleural fluid analysis
   1. Determines transudative or exudative
   2. Measure: LDH, pH, triglycerides, glucose, amylase
   3. Cytology, microbiology, cell count and differential
E. Light's criteria: presence of any of these makes it an exudate
   1. Pleural protein / serum protein ratio > 0.5
   2. Pleural LDH / serum LDH ratio > 0.6
   3. LDH > ⅔ the upper limit of normal serum LDH

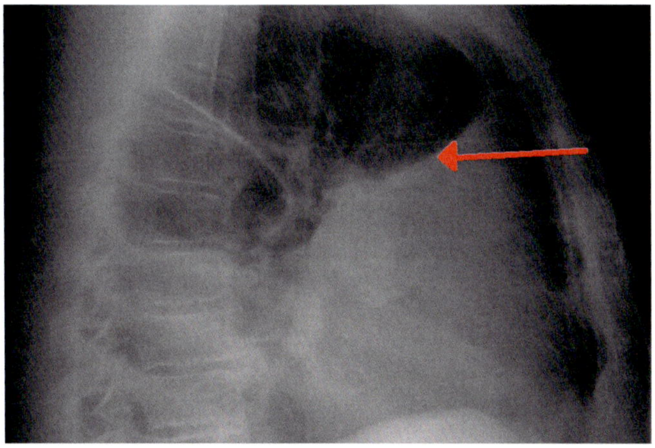

FIGURE 21.8.10 - Chest X-Ray of Pleural Effusion

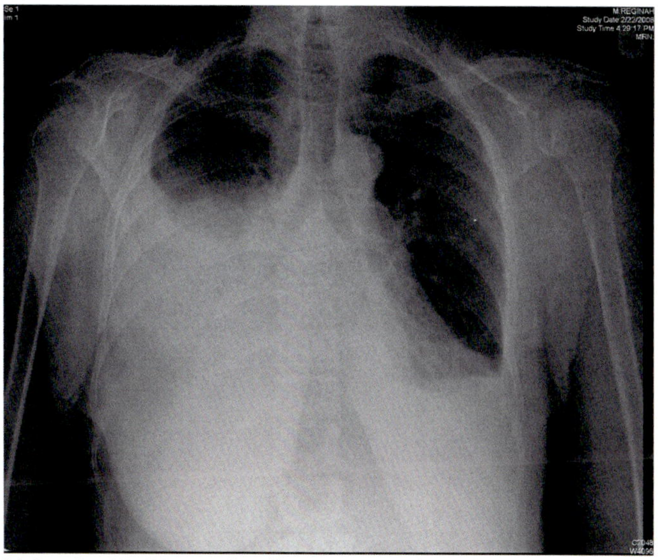

FIGURE 21.8.11 - Chest X-Ray of Pleural Effusions due to Metastatic Breast Carcinoma

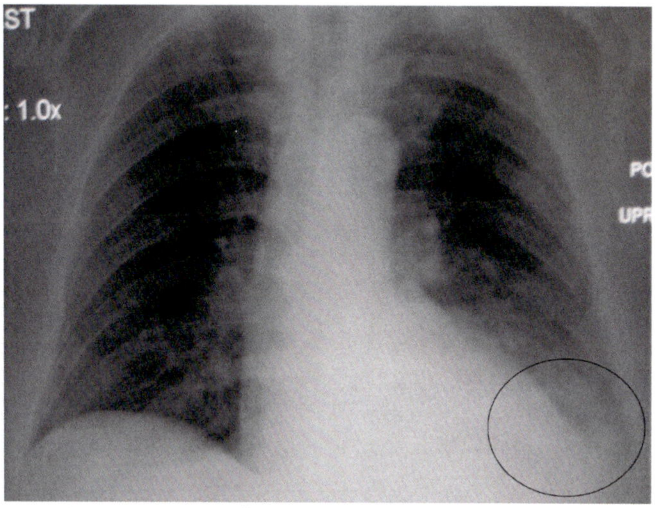

FIGURE 21.8.12 - Chest X-Ray of Pleural Effusion due to Left Lower Lobe Pneumonia

		Transudate	Exudate
Light's criteria	Pleural protein/serum protein ratio	≤ 0.5	> 0.5
	Pleural LDH/serum LDH ratio	≤ 0.6	> 0.6
	Pleural fluid LDH	< ⅔ the upper limit of normal serum LDH	> ⅔ the upper limit of normal serum LDH
Gross appearance		- Clear	- Milky (e.g. chylothorax) - Bloody (e.g. hemothorax, malignant) - Purulent (e.g. empyema)
pH (N=7.6)		- 7.4-7.55	- < 7.30-7.45
Glucose		- ≥ 60 mg/dL	- < 60 mg/dL
LDH (N=45-200 U/L)		- < 200 U/L	- > 200 U/L

TABLE 21.8.3 - Comparison of Transudates and Exudates

IV. Exudative Pleural Effusion: Exudative Effusions
   A. Hemothorax
   B. Chylothorax
   C. Malignant effusions

V. Exudative Pleural Effusion: Diagnosis
   A. Hemothorax
      1. Traumatic or non-traumatic (e.g. pneumothorax, malignancy)
      2. Key features: symptoms of underlying disorder; shock (hypotension, tachycardia)
      3. Pleural fluid analysis: bloody, RBC count > 5,000 cells/μL
      4. Lab: ↓ hematocrit
      5. Always drained
   B. Chylothorax
      1. Lymphatic fluid in the pleural cavity
      2. Trauma (to thoracic duct), malignancy
      3. Key features: absent fever and chest pain
      4. Pleural fluid analysis: milky, high lipid content (e.g. triglycerides, cholesterol)
      5. Triglycerides > 110 mg/dL
   C. Malignant effusions: cancer-related destruction of capillary walls
      1. Lung cancer, breast cancer, mesothelioma
      2. Key features: symptoms of underlying cancer; cachexia
      3. Pleural fluid analysis: cloudy-bloody fluid with tumor cells; low glucose (< 60 mg/dL), high LDH

VI. Pleural Effusion: Complications
   A. Parapneumonic effusions
   B. Empyema
   C. Recurrent effusions
   D. Parapneumonic effusions: exudative pleural fluid in response to pneumonia
      1. Uncomplicated (no bacterial invasion) or complicated (infection extends to pleural cavity)
      2. Key features: systemic signs of infection (e.g. fever, chills), cough
      3. Pleural fluid analysis: clear or cloudy; ↑ WBC count; negative gram stain and culture
      4. Pleural fluid analysis
         a) Complicated: pH < 7.2, ↓ glucose (< 60 mg/dL)
      5. Treatment: systemic antibiotics ± chest tube drainage (thoracostomy) in complicated effusions
   E. Empyema: pus in the pleural cavity (infected pleural effusion)
      1. Pneumonia, infected hemothorax
      2. Key features: fever, chills
      3. Pleural fluid analysis: pH < 7.2, very low glucose (< 30-60 mg/dL), positive gram stain and culture
      4. Treatment: systemic antibiotics and chest tube (thoracostomy) drainage

VII. Pleural Effusion: Management
   A. Treat underlying cause (e.g. treat pneumonia, CHF)
   B. Stabilize the patient in case of severe respiratory distress
   C. Therapeutic thoracentesis
   D. Surgical
      1. Tube thoracostomy: for emergent cases (e.g. penetrating trauma)
      2. Pleurodesis: used for recurrent and treatment non-responsive effusions

VIII. Pleurisy
   A. Pleuritis or inflammation of the pleura
   B. Etiology: most commonly viral (e.g. coxsackieviruses, adenovirus, influenza virus), inflammatory diseases (e.g. SLE, RA), drugs (e.g. amiodarone, bleomycin)
   C. Clinical features: sharp, pleuritic chest pain, pleural friction rub
   D. Diagnosis: clinical; X-ray usually normal or signs of underlying disease
   E. Treatment: painkillers; NSAIDs (first line)

	Uncomplicated Parapneumonic Effusion	Complicated Parapneumonic Effusion	Empyema
Definition	- Pleural effusion secondary to pneumonia; non-infected	- Extension of infection to pleural cavity	- Infected bacterial effusion
Gross appearance	- Clear or cloudy	- Cloudy	- Purulent
Pleural fluid analysis	- pH > 7.2 - Normal or ↓ glucose	- pH < 7.2 - ↓ glucose	- pH < 7.2 - ↓ ↓ glucose
Gram stain and culture	- Negative	- Negative	- Positive
Management	- Systemic antibiotics	- Systemic antibiotics and chest tube drainage	- Systemic antibiotics and chest tube drainage

TABLE 21.8.4 - Comparison of Uncomplicated and Complicated Parapneumonic Effusions and Empyema

REVIEW QUESTIONS

1. A 61-year-old man comes to the physician due to increasing shortness of breath for the past 1-month. He has had a chronic cough and fatigue for the past year. He states he thinks he has lost 15 lbs over the past 5 months. He has smoked 3-packs of cigarettes daily for the past 35 years. Physical examination shows a thin, pale man. Lung exam shows decreased breath sounds, dullness to percussion, and decreased tactile fremitus at the right lung base. A chest X-ray is performed and shows a right central lung mass, blunting of the right costophrenic angle, as well as opacification of the right lower lobe of the lung. What is the next best step in the diagnosis of this patient?
   - **The next best step in the diagnosis of this patient is a thoracentesis.**
   - The patient presents increasing shortness of breath, chronic cough and fatigue.
   - Physical examination shows a thin, pale man with decreased breath sounds, dullness to percussion, and decreased tactile fremitus on the right lung base which is classic for pleural effusion.
   - Imaging shows a central lung mass in the right lung with associated pleural effusion.
   - A thoracentesis should be performed for pleural fluid analysis.

2. A 60-year-old man is brought to the emergency department by his son due to malaise and altered mental status for the past 3-hours. The son states that the patient has had a productive cough and fever for the past 4-days. He was treated with antibiotics, but his condition has continued to worsen. Lung examination shows decreased breath sounds, crackles, and decreased percussion over the right lung base. A chest X-ray is performed and shows a right-sided pleural effusion. Pleural fluid analysis shows cloudy fluid with a pH of 7.3, glucose of 45 mg/dL, and a LDH of 245 U/L. What is the most likely underlying cause of this patient's condition?
   - **The most likely underlying cause of this patient's condition is pneumonia.**
   - The patient presents with altered mental status and systemic signs of infection after recent illness not controlled by antibiotics.
   - Lung examination shows decreased breath sounds, crackles, and decreased percussion over the right lung base.
   - Pleural fluid analysis with a pH of 7.3, glucose of 45 mg/dL, and an LDH of 245 U/L indicates an exudative pleural effusion via light's criteria.
   - Exudative pleural effusions typically have pH of < 7.30-7.45, a glucose of < 60 mg/dL, and an LDH level of > 200 U/L.
   - Parapneumonic effusions are exudative and occur in response to pneumonia and is most likely the cause of this patient's condition.

3. A 26-year-old woman comes to the physician because of chest pain for the past 1-week. She says the pain is worse on deep inspiration or when she coughs. 4-days ago she had a flu which resolved. Physical examination shows chest pain that improves with sitting up and leaning forward and worsens on deep inspiration. On auscultation of the lungs a pleuritic friction rub is heard. D-dimer result is within normal limits. What is the most likely cause of this patient's condition?
   - **The most likely cause of this patient's condition is a recent infection.**
   - Pleurisy is a clinical diagnosis and is typically suspected in patients with classical pleuritic chest pain, pleuritic friction rub, and a supportive history.
   - Remember that pleurisy is most commonly associated with viral infections, but can be caused by inflammatory diseases such (ie. SLE and RA) as well as drugs (ie. amiodarone and bleomycin)

Pulmonology | Section 3: Pneumothorax

I. Pneumothorax: Definition
   A. Air within the pleural space
   B. Types
      1. Spontaneous pneumothorax: primary or secondary
      2. Traumatic pneumothorax
      3. Tension pneumothorax

II. Pneumothorax: Pathophysiology
   A. Loss of negative intrapleural pressure → pulmonary collapse

III. Spontaneous Pneumothorax
   A. Primary or secondary
   B. Primary
      1. Also called "simple" pneumothorax
      2. In healthy individuals (no underlying disease)
      3. Mostly affects tall, young men
      4. Usually not life-threatening
   C. Secondary
      1. Due to an underlying disease (e.g. COPD, cancer, TB)
      2. More life-threatening

IV. Traumatic Pneumothorax
   A. Caused by trauma
   B. Iatrogenic (chest tube insertions, PEEP)
   C. Penetrating and blunt trauma
   D. Open or closed pneumothorax

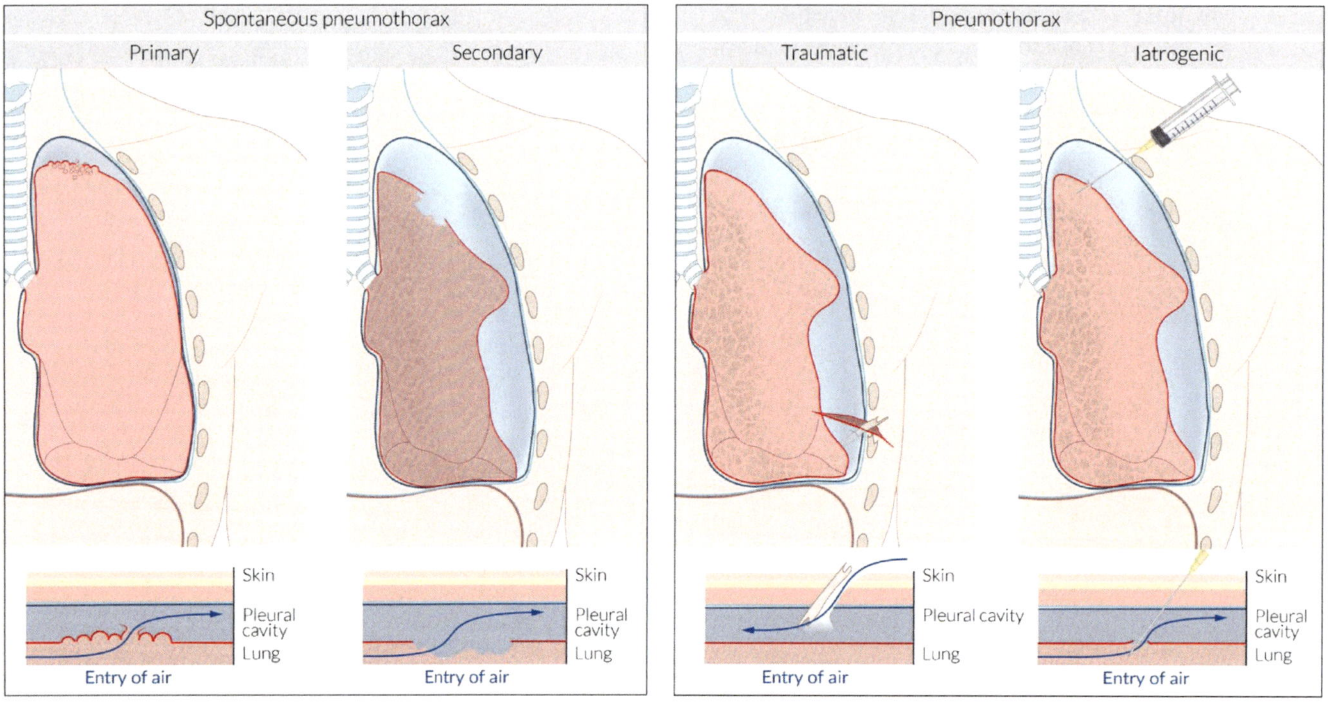

FIGURE 21.8.13 - Types of Pneumothorax

V. Tension Pneumothorax
   A. A condition where air enters the pleural space but cannot go out
   B. Pushes on contralateral lung, heart, and major structures
   C. Impedes venous return and cardiac output
   D. Life-threatening; can lead to hemodynamic instability and collapse
   E. Risk factors
      1. Mechanical ventilation (e.g. PEEP, PPV)
      2. Trauma
      3. CPR

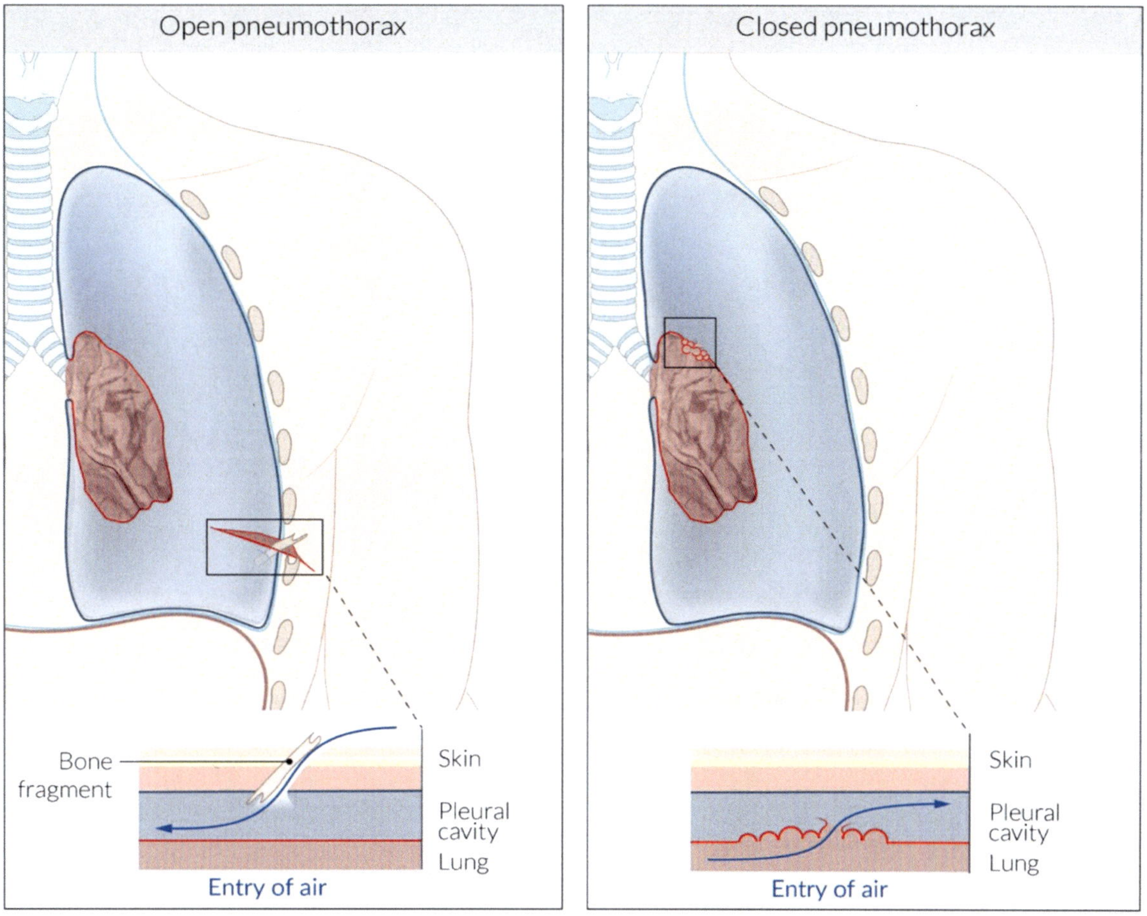

(c) AMBOSS Used under special agreement. Accessed December 21, 2021

FIGURE 21.8.14 - Open Pneumothorax vs. Closed Pneumothorax

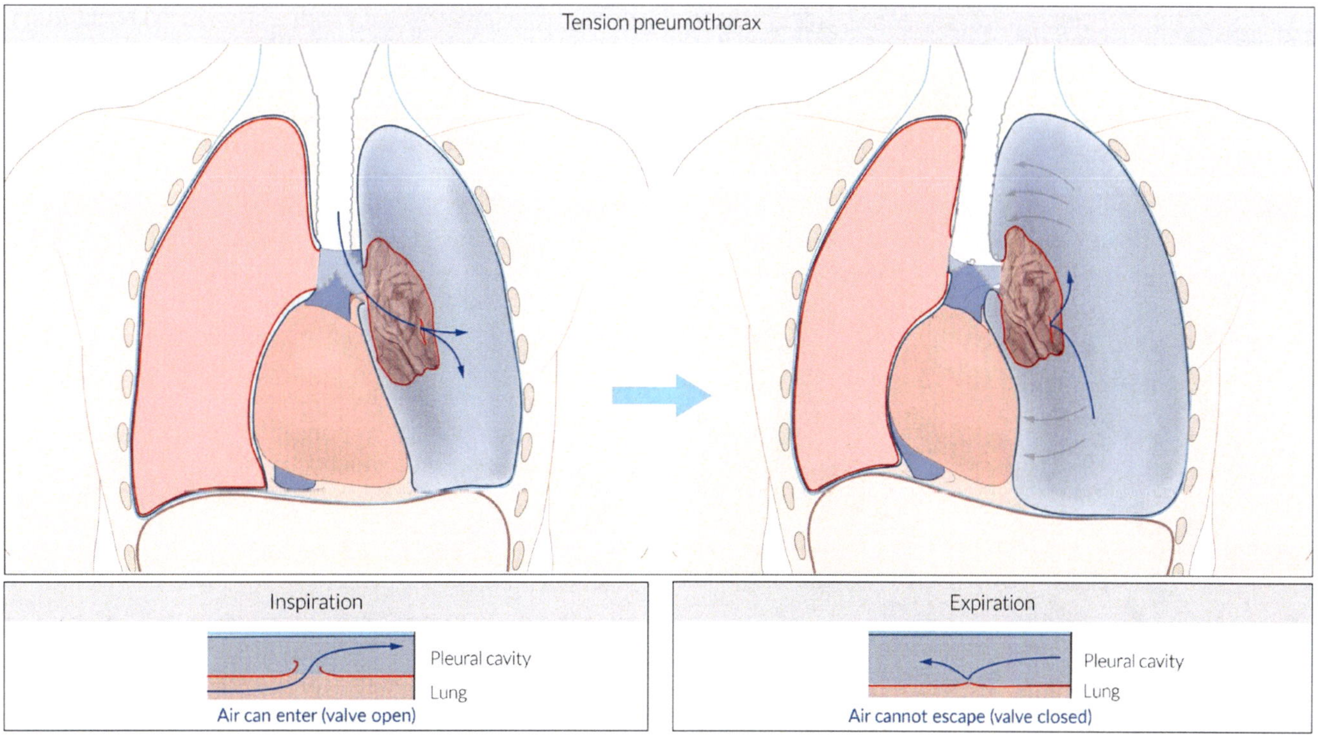

(c) AMBOSS Used under special agreement. Accessed December 21, 2021

FIGURE 21.8.15 - Tension Pneumothorax

VI. Pneumothorax: Clinical Presentation
   A. Acute, severe, pleuritic chest pain
   B. Mostly unilateral
   C. Dyspnea
   D. Tension pneumothorax: hemodynamic instability (e.g. hypotension, respiratory distress, hypoxia)

VII. Pneumothorax: Diagnosis
   A. History and physical exam
      1. ↓ or absent breath sounds, hyperresonance, ↓ tactile fremitus
      2. Distended neck veins (JVD)
      3. Subcutaneous emphysema
   B. Imaging
      1. CXR: confirms the diagnosis; ↓ lung markings, lucency changes
         a) Tension pneumothorax: tracheal and mediastinal deviation towards the normal side; diaphragmatic flattening ipsilaterally
   C. US: used in trauma (FAST)
   D. CT scan

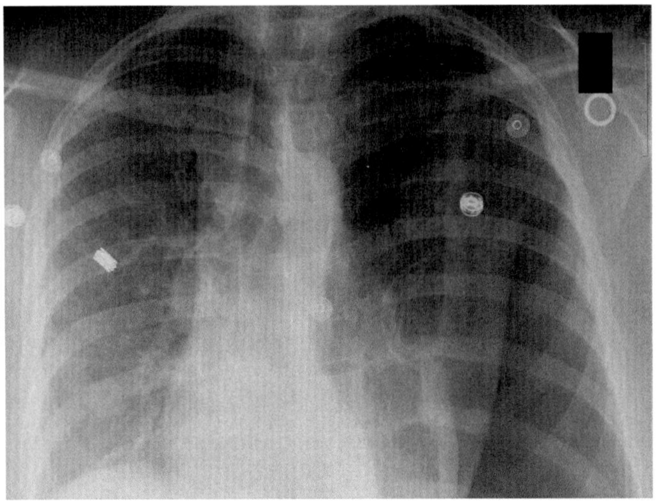

FIGURE 21.8.16 - Chest X-Ray: Left-Sided Pneumothorax

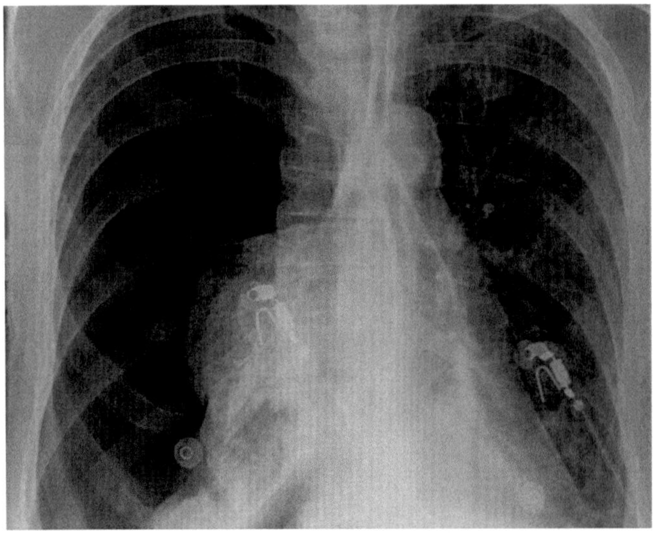

FIGURE 21.8.17 - Chest X-Ray: Right-Sided Pneumothorax

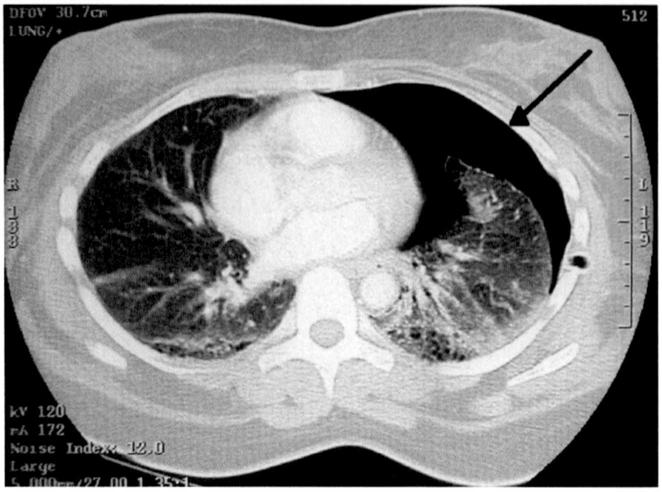

FIGURE 21.8.18 - CT Scan of Chest: Left-Sided Pneumothorax

VIII. Pneumothorax: Management
   A. General management
      1. Assess whether the patient is stable
      2. Manage symptoms of respiratory distress and dyspnea
         a) Airway management, supplemental O_2
      3. Immediate tube thoracostomy for patients who require mechanical ventilation
      4. Identify type of pneumothorax and manage accordingly
   B. Primary spontaneous pneumothorax
      1. Patients usually stable
      2. Small < 2 cm: observation; resolves spontaneously within 10 days; follow-up with CXR
      3. Large: supplemental O_2, chest tube (or needle aspiration); conservative treatment if asymptomatic
   C. Secondary spontaneous pneumothorax
   D. Observation if small, stable and asymptomatic
   E. Chest tube (tube thoracostomy) if unstable and symptomatic
      1. Open pneumothorax
      2. Assess hemodynamic stability
      3. Control bleeding if present; consult cardiothoracic surgery
      4. Dressing to occlude opening → thoracostomy
   F. Tension pneumothorax: medical emergency
      1. Emergent needle thoracostomy → chest tube placement
      2. Needle thoracostomy: 2nd intercostal, midclavicular line
      3. Chest X-ray is always required after chest tube placement to ensure correct positioning
   G. Bilateral pneumothorax or unstable patients: chest tube placement for emergent chest decompression

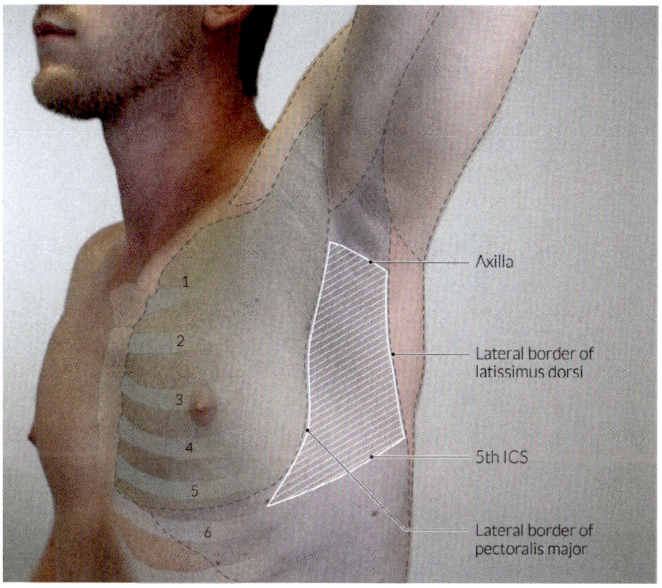

FIGURE 21.8.19 - "Safe Triangle" for Chest Tube Insertion

REVIEW QUESTIONS

1. A 23-year-old man is brought to the emergency department after sustaining injuries to his chest during a high-speed motor vehicle accident. On the way to the hospital, he complained of severe chest pain and dyspnea. Vitals signs show he is hypotensive. The patient now becomes unresponsive. Pulse oximetry shows an oxygen saturation of 89%. Distended neck veins are noted. Lung examination shows decreased breath sounds and hyperresonance on the right. What is the best next step in management?
   - **The best next step in management is needle thoracostomy.**
   - The patient presents with hemodynamic instability after a motor vehicle accident.
   - Physical examination shows decreased breath sounds and hyperresonance on the right which supports the diagnosis of pneumothorax.
   - His low oxygen saturation along with his distended neck veins should raise suspicion of tension pneumothorax. Immediate decompression is needed and should not be delayed by imaging.

Pulmonology | Section 4: Malignant Mesothelioma

I. Malignant Mesothelioma: General Characteristics
   A. Malignant tumor from mesothelial cells
   B. Etiology: asbestos exposure
   C. Plumbers, carpenters, electrician, and insulation workers at risk
   D. Clinical features
      1. Dyspnea, cough, weight loss
      2. Pleural effusions (bloody)

II. Malignant Mesothelioma: Diagnosis
   A. History of asbestos exposure
   B. Imaging: pleural thickening on CXR and CT scan
   C. Pleurocentesis: bloody exudate
   D. Biopsy: mesothelial cells, asbestos bodies, psammoma bodies, calretinin positive

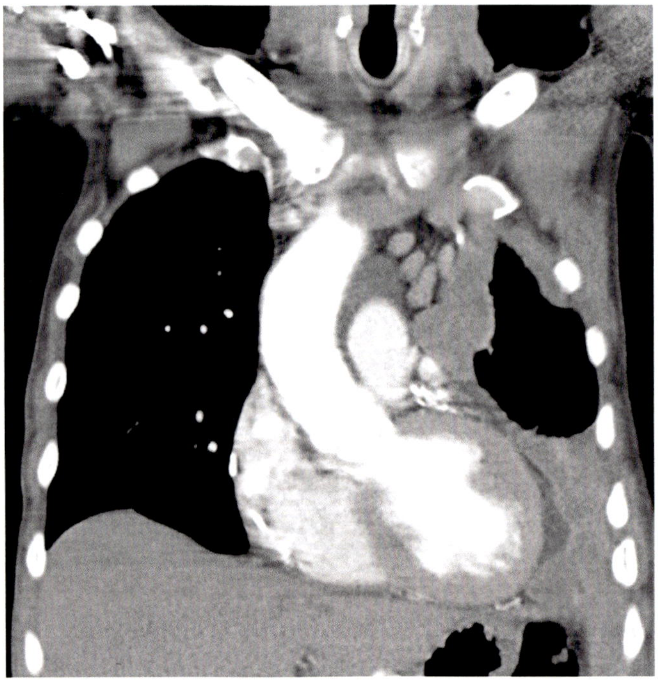

FIGURE 21.8.20 - CT Scan of Chest Showing Left Sided Mesothelioma

III. Malignant Mesothelioma: Treatment
   A. Radiation ± chemotherapy
   B. Surgery: pleurectomy

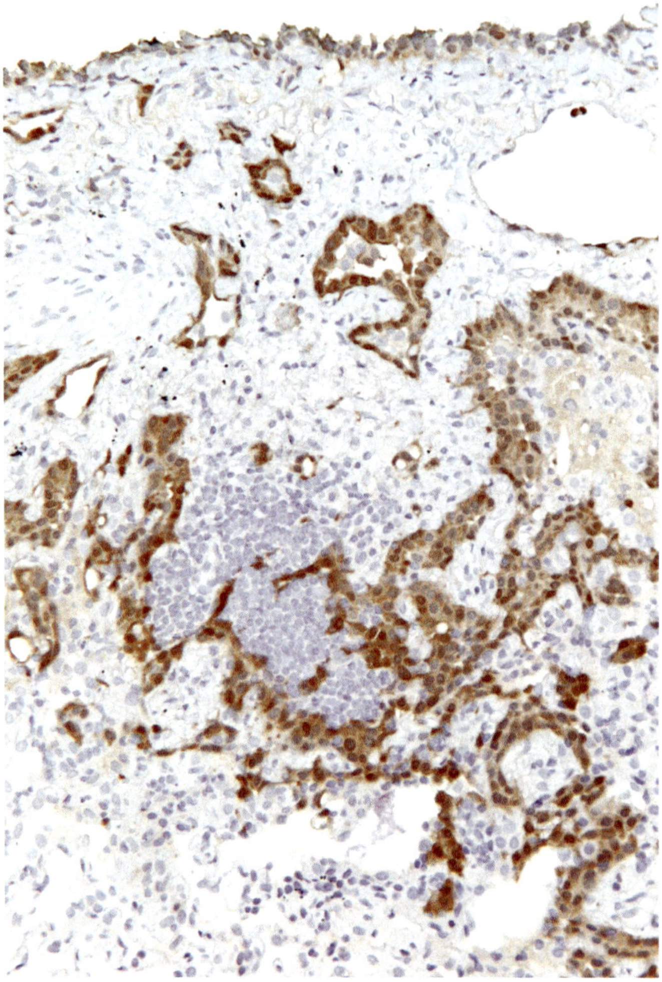

FIGURE 21.8.21 - Claretinin-Positive Cells in Mesothelioma

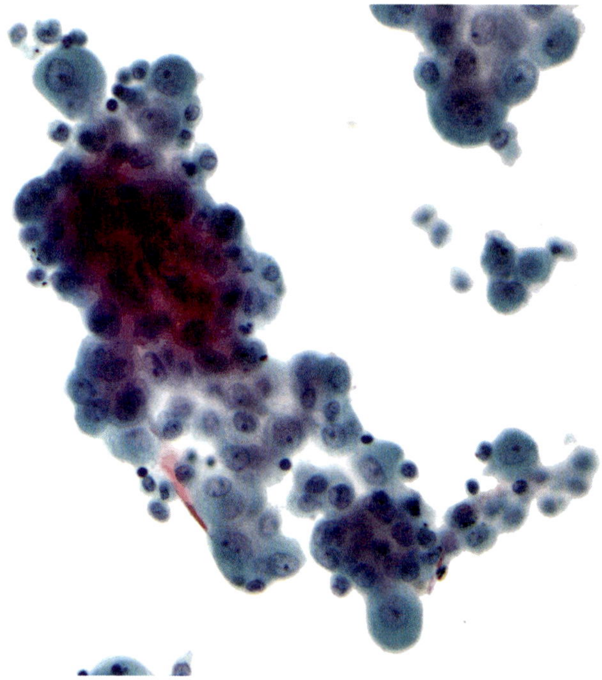

FIGURE 21.8.22 - Malignant Mesothelial Cells in Pleural Fluid

REVIEW QUESTIONS

1. A 69-year-old man comes to the physician because of worsening shortness of breath after working in the yard over the last 6-months. He does not have any significant cough or unintentional weight loss. He has never smoked and will occasionally have a beer on the weekends. He has worked as an electrician all of his life and recently retired. Based on this patient's most likely condition, what is the expected finding if a CT chest was performed?

- **Pleural plaques would be expected to be found if a chest CT were to be performed.**
- This patient has most likely been exposed to asbestos due to his work as an electrician for all of his life.
- Since this patient denies significant coughing and unintentional weight loss, he is unlikely to have a neoplasm of lungs such as malignant mesothelioma.
- It is important to know that the most common manifestation of asbestos exposure is benign pleural plaques, which are lesions of scar tissue that may be calcified. These pleural plaques can be detected on imaging such as CT.
- They are usually found as patches on the lining of the rib cage or on the diaphragm.
- Most patients with asbestosis are asymptomatic for long periods of time, and eventually present with exertional dyspnea.
- Patients with a history of exposure to asbestos are more likely to develop benign pleural nodules than malignant mesothelioma.

2. A 68-year-old man comes to the physician because of progressive shortness of breath during normal daily activities for the past 3-months. He states he has had a constant coughing for about 6-months and has lost 15lbs within the last 2-months. The patient mentions that he worked as a carpenter for 45 years and recently retired. A CT chest scan shows extensive pleural thickening. A biopsy of these lesions would most likely stain positive for which of the following?

   A. Calcitonin
   B. Calretinin
   C. Synaptophysin
   D. Chromogranin

- **The correct answer is B.**
- The patient presents with progressive dyspnea associated with a constant cough and recent unintentional weight loss.
- He worked as a carpenter for 45 years, indicating he had significant risk for exposure to asbestos throughout his life.
- His CT chest scan shows extensive pleural thickening.
- Considering all this, it suggests the patient most likely has malignant mesothelioma.
- Mesothelioma is a malignant tumor that originates from mesothelial cells. A biopsy would stain positive for calretinin, a protein found in tissues of mesothelial origin.
- Answer choice A is incorrect because calcitonin is a hormone produced in the thyroid gland to oppose the actions of PTH and is not associated with mesothelioma.
- Answer choices C and D are incorrect because synaptophysin and chromogranin are markers of neuroendocrine cells that are associated with medullary thyroid cancer and small cell lung cancer, but not mesothelioma.

PEDIATRICS

Pediatrics | Section 1: Hypertrophic Pyloric Stenosis, Intussusception & Malrotation with Volvulus

I. Hypertrophic Pyloric Stenosis: Definition
   A. Thickening and lengthening of gastric pylorus ~ 2 - 6 weeks after birth
   B. Most common cause of gastric outlet obstruction in infants
   C. More common in firstborn males

II. Hypertrophic Pyloric Stenosis: Etiology
   A. Not completely understood
   B. Associated with macrolide exposure before or shortly after birth

III. Hypertrophic Pyloric Stenosis: Clinical Presentation
   A. Palpable olive-shaped epigastric mass
   B. Visible peristaltic waves
   C. Projectile vomiting

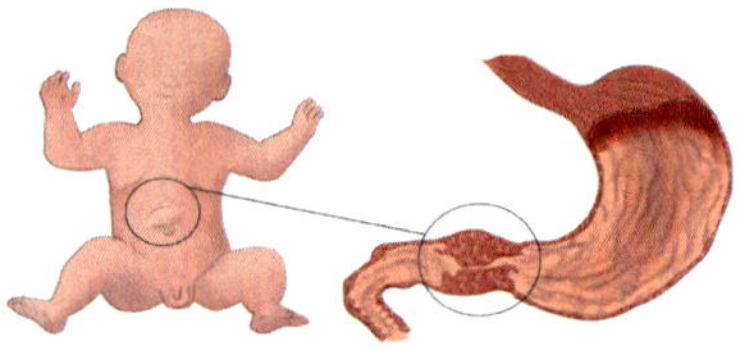

FIGURE 21.9.1 - Hypertrophic Pyloric Stenosis

IV. Hypertrophic Pyloric Stenosis: Diagnosis
   A. Hypokalemic hypochloremic metabolic alkalosis due to:
      1. Loss of gastric acid
      2. Volume contraction activating renin-angiotensin-aldosterone system
   B. Abdominal ultrasoun
      1. Thickened and lengthened pylorus
      2. Narrowed pyloric channel

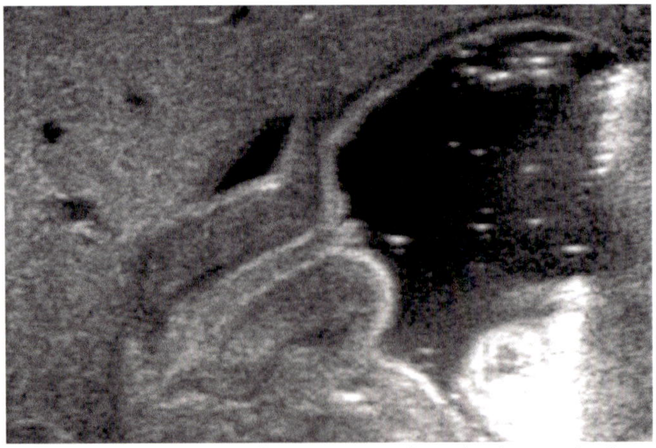

FIGURE 21.9.2 - Abdominal Ultrasound: Thickened Pyloric Walls and Narrowed Pyloric Channel in Hypertrophic Pyloric Stenosis

V. Hypertrophic Pyloric Stenosis: Management
   A. Volume resuscitation and electrolyte correction before surgery
   B. Surgical incision of pyloric muscles (pyloromyotomy)

VI. Intussusception: Definition
   A. Telescoping of proximal bowel segment into the distal bowel segment
   B. Most common at the ileocecal junction

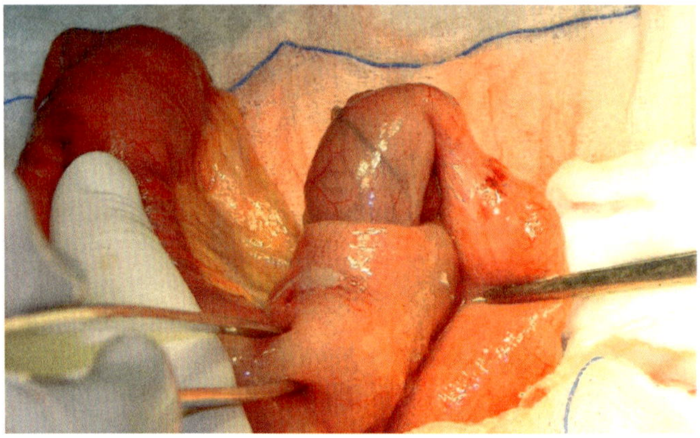

FIGURE 21.9.3 - Intussusception

VII. Intussusception: Etiology
   A. Most commonly idiopathic
   B. Due to lead point
      1. Meckel diverticulum (children)
      2. Intraluminal tumor (adults)
      3. Peyer patch hypertrophy due to:
         a) Henoch-Schonlein purpura
         b) Recent viral GI infection

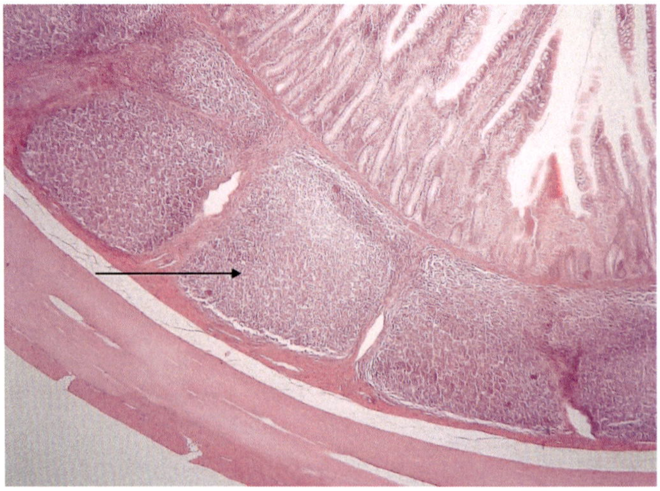

FIGURE 21.9.4 - Light Microscopy: Peyer Patches

VIII. Intussusception: Clinical Presentation
   A. Intermittent abdominal pain with "currant jelly" dark red stools due to ischemia and necrosis of proximal bowel segment
   B. Sausage-shaped mass in the right abdomen
   C. Drawing legs to chest relieves the pain (fetal position)

IX. Intussusception: Diagnosis
   A. Ultrasound or CT
      1. Target sign: concentric layers of telescoped proximal bowel

X. Intussusception: Management
   A. Water soluble contrast or air enema: diagnostic and therapeutic
   B. Laparotomy if enema is unsuccessful or there are signs of bowel perforation and necrosis
      1. Hypotension
      2. Lactic acidosis
      3. Rebound tenderness
      4. Abdominal rigidity

XI. Malrotation with Volvulus: Definition
   A. Malrotation
      1. Incomplete rotation of midgut around superior mesenteric artery during weeks 6 - 10 of gestation
   B. Volvulus
      1. Twisting of bowel around its mesentery

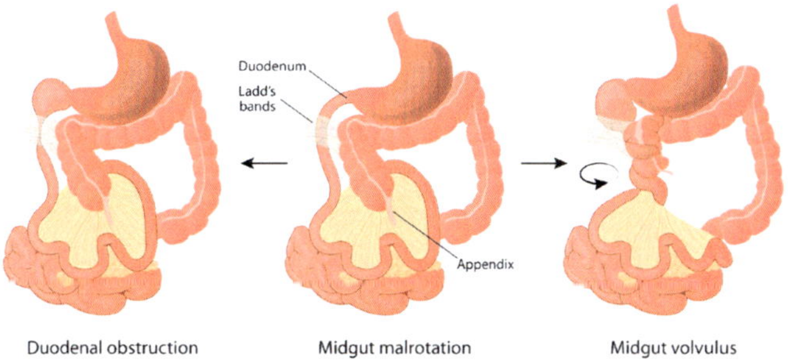

FIGURE 21.9.5 - Midgut Malrotation

XII. Malrotation with Volvulus: Etiology
   A. Malrotation: unknown
   B. Volvulus
      1. Malrotation (infants and children)
      2. Constipation (elderly)

XIII. Malrotation with Volvulus: Clinical Presentation
   A. Malrotation
      1. Mostly asymptomatic
      2. Constipation and bilious vomiting
   B. Volvulus
      1. Abdominal pain
      2. Obstipation (inability to pass stool and gas)
      3. Signs of peritonitis in case of bowel rupture (e.g. rigidity)

XIV. Malrotation with Volvulus: Diagnosis
   A. Malrotation
      1. Upper GI series with barium swallow: "corkscrew" bowel and right-sided ligament of Treitz
   B. Volvulus
      1. Abdominal X-ray: "coffee bean" sign directed to the left (midgut) or right (sigmoid) upper quadrant
      2. Midgut volvulus in children; sigmoid volvulus in elderly

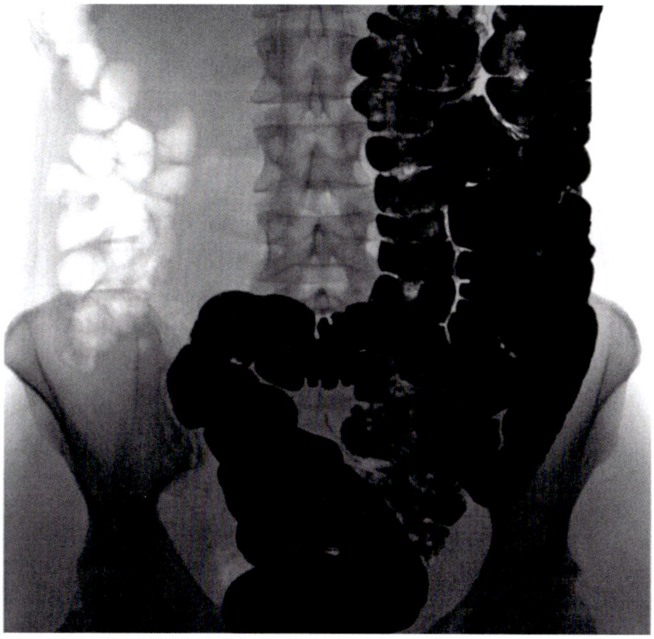

FIGURE 21.9.6 - Barium Enema: Intestinal Malrotation

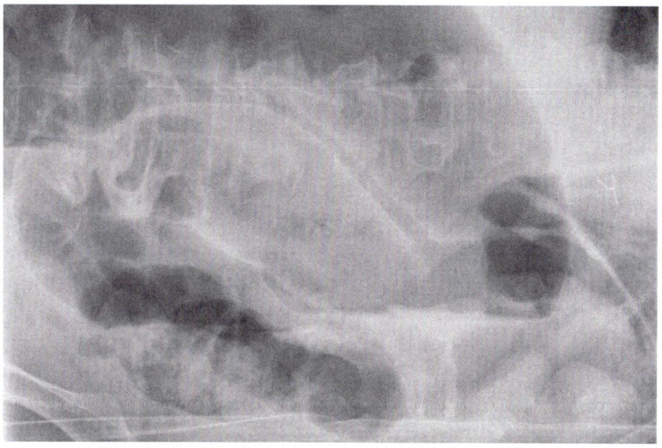

FIGURE 21.9.7 - X-ray of the Abdomen: "Coffee-Bean" Sign in Sigmoid Volvulus

XV. Malrotation with Volvulus: Management
   A. Malrotation
      1. Ladd procedure: surgical lysis of Ladd bands and bowel fixation in its normal location
   B. Volvulus
      1. Surgical detorsion

Condition	Etiology	Key Features
Hypertrophic pyloric stenosis	- More common in firstborn males - Associated with macrolide exposure of infant	- Palpable, olive-shaped epigastric mass - Visible peristaltic waves - Hypokalemic hypochloremic metabolic alkalosis - Medical treatment: correction of electrolyte imbalance and volume status before surgery - Surgical treatment: pyloromyotomy
Intussusception	- Telescoping of proximal bowel segment into distal bowel segment - Lead point: - Meckel diverticulum (children) - Intraluminal tumor (adults) - Peyer patch hypertrophy (e.g. Henoch-Schonlein purpura, viral GI infection)	- "Currant jelly" stools - "Target sign" on ultrasound/CT - Diagnosis and treatment: water soluble contrast or air enema - Laparotomy if enema is unsuccessful or there are signs of bowel perforation (e.g. rebound tenderness, rigidity)
Malrotation with volvulus	- Malrotation: incomplete rotation of midgut around SMA during 6-10 weeks of gestation - Volvulus: twisting of bowel around its mesentery	- Upper GI series with barium swallow: "corkscrew" bowel and right-sided ligament of Treitz in malrotation - Abdominal X-ray: coffee bean sign in volvulus - Midgut volvulus in children - Sigmoid volvulus in elderly - Treatment of malrotation: Ladd procedure (surgical lysis of Ladd bands) - Treatment of volvulus: surgical detorsion

TABLE 21.9.1 - Pediatric Gastrointestinal Diseases

REVIEW QUESTIONS

1. A 4-week-old boy is brought to his primary care physician because vomiting and weight loss for the past week. He is constantly hungry. The physical exam shows an olive-shaped epigastric mass, decreased skin turgor, and visible peristaltic waves. Laboratory findings are significant for hypokalemic hypochloremic metabolic alkalosis. What is the best initial treatment for this patient?

- **The best initial treatment for this patient is correction of volume and electrolyte status.**
- This patient presents with vomiting and weight loss for the past week.
- The physical exam shows an olive-shaped epigastric mass, decreased skin turgor, and visible peristaltic waves.
- These findings are consistent with the diagnosis of hypertrophic pyloric stenosis.
- Laboratory findings are significant for hypokalemic hypochloremic metabolic alkalosis.
- These electrolyte and acid-base abnormalities result from loss of gastric acid and the activation of the renin-angiotensin-aldosterone system by volume contraction.
- The best initial treatment for hypertrophic pyloric stenosis is correction of volume and electrolyte status before pyloromyotomy.

REVIEW QUESTIONS

2. A 3-year-old girl is brought to her primary care physician because of abdominal pain and dark red stools for the past day. She draws her knees to her chest to relieve the pain. She had multiple episodes of watery diarrhea and vomiting before her current complaints. The physical exam shows a sausage-shaped mass in the right lower quadrant. What will most likely be found on the ultrasound of this patient?

   - **The ultrasound of this patient will most likely show the target sign, which represents the concentric layers of the telescoped proximal bowel.**
   - This patient presents with abdominal pain and dark red stools for the past day. She draws her knees to her chest to relieve the pain.
   - The physical exam shows a sausage-shaped mass in the right lower quadrant.
   - These findings are consistent with the diagnosis of intussusception.
   - She had multiple episodes of watery diarrhea and vomiting before her current complaints. This is consistent with viral gastroenteritis. Viral gastroenteritis likely induced hypertrophy of Peyer patches which acted as the lead point for intussusception.

3. A 3-year-old girl is brought to her primary care physician because of constipation and intermittent bilious vomiting for the past week. Upper GI series with barium swallow show irregular narrowings of the small bowel and a right-sided ligament of Treitz. What is the most likely pathophysiology of this patient's underlying condition?

   - **The most likely pathophysiology of this patient's underlying condition is incomplete rotation of the midgut around the superior mesenteric artery during 6 to 10 weeks of gestation.**
   - This patient presents with constipation and intermittent bilious vomiting.
   - Upper GI series with barium swallow show irregular narrowings of the small bowel and the right-sided ligament of Treitz.
   - These findings confirm the diagnosis of malrotation, which is caused by incomplete rotation of the midgut around the superior mesenteric artery during 6 to 10 weeks of gestation.

4. A 4-year-old boy is brought to the physician by his parents because of abdominal pain and dark red stools for the past day. He has never had such symptoms before. He had two episodes of watery diarrhea and vomiting before his current complaints. His vital signs are normal. The physical exam shows a child in severe distress drawing his knees to his chest to relieve the pain. There is no rebound tenderness or abdominal rigidity. An abdominal ultrasound shows concentric layers of bowel in the right lower quadrant. Which of the following is the best initial step in the management of this patient?

   A. IV ampicillin
   B. Polyethylene glycol
   C. Water soluble enema
   D. Laparotomy

   - **The correct answer is option C.**
   - This 4-year-old boy presents with abdominal pain and dark red stools, also known as "currant jelly stools", for the past day. The physical exam shows a child in severe distress drawing his knees to his chest to relieve the pain.
   - An abdominal ultrasound shows concentric layers of bowel in the right lower quadrant. This description is consistent with the "target sign."
   - All these clues suggest the diagnosis of intussusception.
   - The best initial step in the management of a patient with intussusception is water soluble enema, which is both diagnostic and therapeutic.
   - Option A, intravenous (IV) ampicillin, is incorrect because antibiotics are not indicated in intussusception unless the patient has signs of infection.
   - Option B, polyethylene glycol, is incorrect because it is an osmotic laxative. Laxatives are contraindicated in intussusception due to potential for bowel obstruction at the ileocecal junction.
   - Option D, laparotomy, is incorrect because it is used when the enema is unsuccessful or the patient has signs of bowel perforation and necrosis. This patient has a benign abdominal exam with no rebound tenderness or abdominal rigidity.

Pediatrics | Section 2: Meckel Diverticulum, Hirschsprung Disease & Necrotizing Enterocolitis

I. Meckel Diverticulum: Definition
   A. True congenital diverticulum in the terminal ileum
   B. Most common congenital GI tract anomaly
   C. May contain heterotopic gastric mucosa and/or pancreatic tissue

II. Meckel Diverticulum: Etiology
   A. Incomplete resorption of proximal vitelline (omphalomesenteric) duct

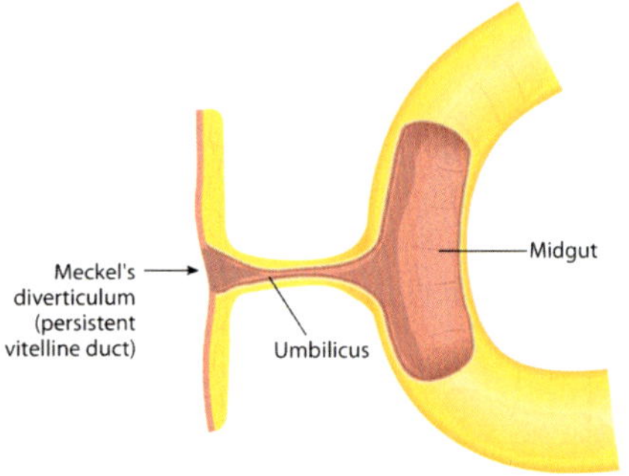

FIGURE 21.9.8 - Meckel's Diverticulum

III. Meckel Diverticulum: Clinical Presentation
   a. Most commonly asymptomatic
   A. Right lower quadrant pain
   B. Hematochezia or melena
   C. Intussusception

IV. Meckel Diverticulum: Diagnosis
   A. ^{99m}Tc-pertechnetate scan (Meckel scan)
      1. Signal from stomach and the terminal ileum

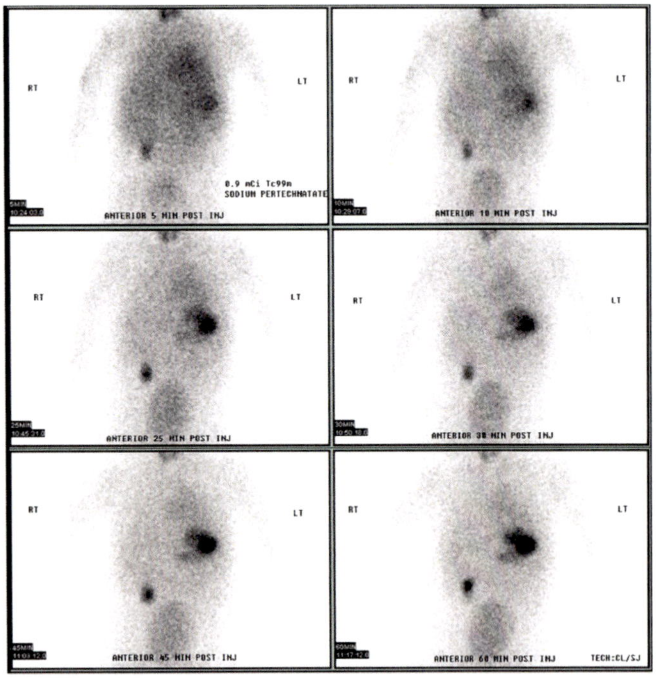

FIGURE 21.9.9 - Meckel Scan

V. Meckel Diverticulum: Management
   A. Observation if asymptomatic
   B. Surgical excision if symptomatic

VI. Hirschsprung Disease: Definition
   A. Absence of Auerbach and Meissner plexuses in the sigmoid colon and rectum

VII. Hirschsprung Disease: Etiology
   A. Congenital
      1. Failure of neural crest cell migration to the distal colon
      2. Loss of function mutation in *RET* gene
      3. Associated with Down syndrome
   B. Acquired
      1. Chagas disease by *Trypanosoma cruzi*

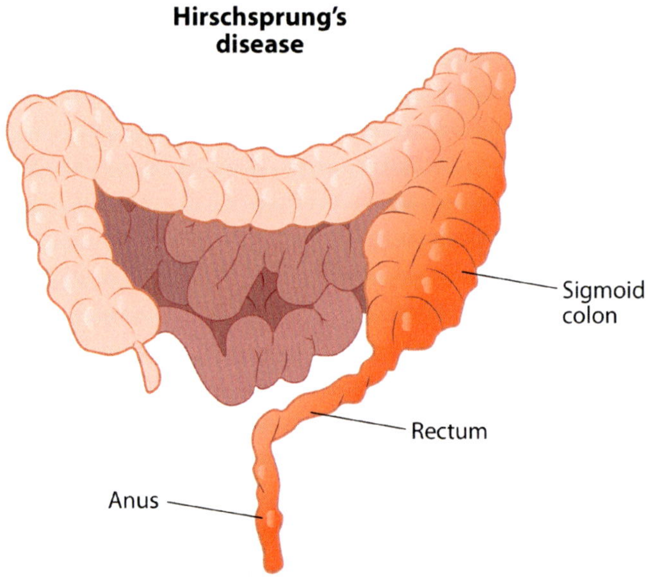

FIGURE 21.9.10 - Hirschsprung Disease

VIII. Hirschsprung Disease: Clinical Presentation
   A. Bilious vomiting
   B. Abdominal distension
   C. Delayed passage of meconium
   D. Chronic constipation

IX. Hirschsprung Disease: Diagnosis
   A. Squirt sign
      1. Explosive expulsion of feces on digital rectal exam
   B. Rectal manometry
      1. Increased pressure in rectum and sigmoid colon
   C. Rectal suction biopsy
      1. Absence of Auerbach and Meissner's plexus in colonic wall

X. Hirschsprung Disease: Management
   A. Surgical resection of aganglionic segment

XI. Necrotizing Enterocolitis: Definition
   A. Intestinal inflammation and necrosis in infants
   B. Most commonly affects the terminal ileum and cecum

XII. Necrotizing Enterocolitis: Etiology
   A. Invasion of GI mucosa by gas-producing bacteria → intestinal necrosis

XIII. Necrotizing Enterocolitis: Risk Factors
   A. Very low birth weight (< 1.5 kg)
   B. Prematurity
   C. Enteral feeding

XIV. Necrotizing Enterocolitis: Clinical Presentation
   A. Nonspecific signs
      1. Apnea, lethargy, fussiness
      2. Septic shock (hypotension, tachycardia, fever)
   B. Gastrointestinal signs
      1. Feeding intolerance and bilious emesis
      2. Abdominal distension and erythema
      3. Hematochezia

XV. Necrotizing Enterocolitis: Complications
   A. Disseminated intravascular coagulation
   B. Post-surgical complications
      1. Strictures
      2. Short-bowel syndrome

XVI. Necrotizing Enterocolitis: Diagnosis
   A. Abdominal X-ray
      1. Pneumatosis intestinalis (air in bowel wall)
      2. Pneumoperitoneum (bowel rupture)
   B. Blood cultures

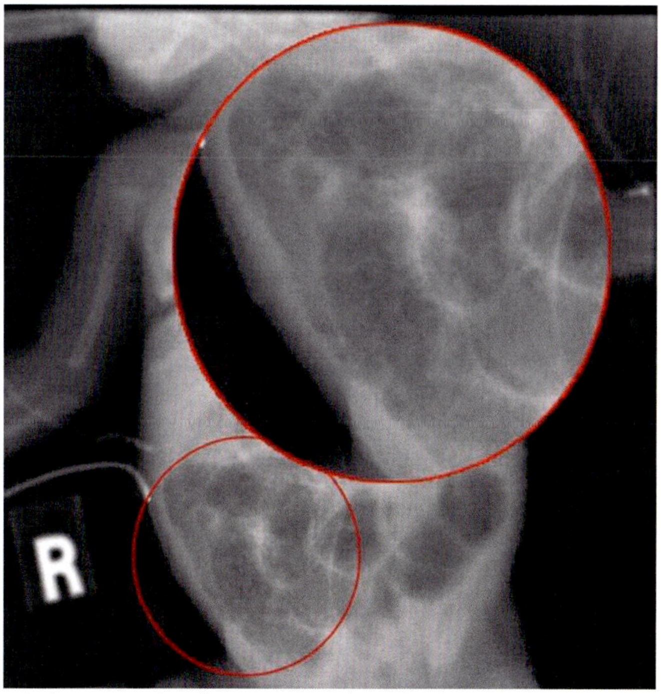

FIGURE 21.9.11 - Abdominal X-ray: Pneumatosis Intestinalis in Necrotizing Enterocolitis

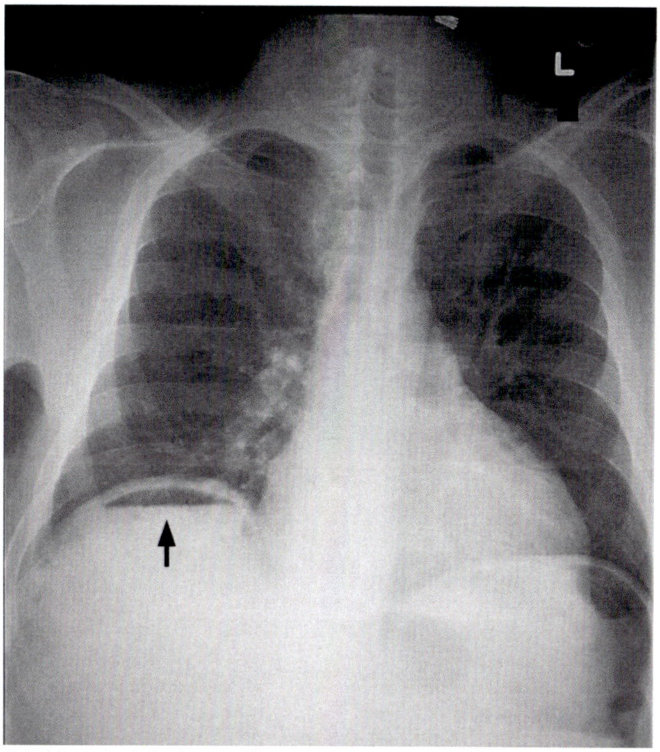

FIGURE 21.9.12 - Chest X-ray: Pneumoperitoneum

XVII. Necrotizing Enterocolitis: Management
   A. Nil per os (NPO) regimen
   B. Nasogastric decompression
   C. IV fluids followed by empiric antibiotics
   D. Indications for surgery
      1. Pneumoperitoneum (bowel perforation)
      2. Clinical deterioration despite optimal medical management (bowel necrosis)

Condition	Etiology	Key Features
Meckel diverticulum	- Most common congenital GI tract anomaly - Remnant of vitelline duct	- Diagnosed by 99mTc-pertechnetate (Meckel) scan - May contain heterotopic gastric and/or pancreatic tissue - Asymptomatic: observation - Symptomatic: surgical excision
Hirschsprung disease	- Absence of Auerbach and Meissner's plexus in sigmoid colon and rectum - Congenital: failure of neural crest cell migration due to loss of function mutation in *RET* gene - Acquired: Chagas disease by *Trypanosoma cruzi*	- Congenital Hirschsprung disease associated with Down syndrome - Positive squirt sign and increased rectal pressure - Diagnosed with rectal suction biopsy - Surgical excision of aganglionic segment
Necrotizing enterocolitis	- Intestinal inflammation and necrosis due to penetration of gas-producing bacteria in GI wall	- Associated with very low birth weight (< 1.5 kg), prematurity, enteral feeding - Pneumatosis intestinalis (air in bowel wall) on X-ray - Treatment: NPO regimen, nasogastric decompression, IV fluids, and empiric antibiotics - Indications for surgery: - Pneumoperitoneum, clinical deterioration despite medical management

TABLE 21.9.2 - Pediatric Gastrointestinal Diseases

REVIEW QUESTIONS

1. A 2-year-old boy is brought to the physician due to bloody stools for the past 2 days. He also has right lower quadrant pain. Right lower quadrant ultrasound shows a protruding mass near the ileocecal valve. ^{99m}Tc-pertechnetate scan reveals increased signal from the terminal ileum. What is the most likely pathophysiology of this patient's current condition?

   - **The most likely pathophysiology of this patient's current condition is incomplete resorption of the proximal vitelline duct during fetal period.**
   - This patient presents with bloody stools and right lower quadrant pain.
   - The right lower quadrant ultrasound shows a protruding mass near the ileocecal valve.
   - 99mTc-pertechnetate scan reveals an increased signal from the terminal ileum.
   - These findings are consistent with the diagnosis of a Meckel diverticulum.
   - Meckel diverticulum is caused by incomplete resorption of the proximal vitelline duct during the fetal period.

2. A 2-year-old girl with Down syndrome presents with chronic constipation and intermittent bilious vomiting. The physician observes an explosive expulsion of feces on digital rectal exam. Rectal tone is increased on rectal manometry. Abdominal X-ray reveals an enlarged descending colon with a narrow sigmoid colon and rectum. Which test can definitively diagnose this patient's condition?

   - **The test that can definitively diagnose this patient's condition is a rectal suction biopsy.**
   - This patient presents with chronic constipation and intermittent bilious vomiting.
   - He has a history of Down syndrome.
   - The physician observes an explosive expulsion of feces on the digital rectal exam.
   - Rectal tone is increased on the rectal manometry.
   - Abdominal X-ray shows an enlarged descending colon with a narrow sigmoid colon and rectum.
   - All these findings suggest the diagnosis of Hirschsprung disease.
   - Hirschsprung disease can be definitively diagnosed with rectal suction biopsy.

3. A 3-week-old boy is brought to the primary care physician because of fussiness and poor feeding for the last 3 days. He was born at 34 weeks of gestation with a birth weight of 1 kg. His vital signs include temperature of 102.2° F (39° C), blood pressure of 60/35 mmHg, heart rate of 175 beats/min, and respiratory rate of 62 breaths/min. The physical exam shows diffuse abdominal tenderness with no rigidity. Abdominal X-ray shows gas in the bowel wall but no air in the peritoneal cavity. He is placed on NPO regimen, and he undergoes nasogastric decompression. Which of the following is the best next step in the management of this patient?

   A. IV fluids
   B. IV antibiotics
   C. Blood culture
   D. Surgery

   - **The correct answer is option A.**
   - This patient presents with nonspecific symptoms of fussiness and poor feeding.
   - He was born at 34 weeks of gestation with a birth weight of 1 kg. Therefore, he is premature with a very low birth weight.
   - His vital signs show fever, hypotension, tachycardia, and tachypnea.
   - Abdominal X-ray shows gas in the bowel wall but no air in the peritoneal cavity.
   - These findings are consistent with the diagnosis of necrotizing enterocolitis.
   - He is placed on NPO regimen, and he undergoes nasogastric decompression.
   - The best next step in the management of this patient is intravenous fluids to increase blood pressure to the normal range.
   - Option B is incorrect because antibiotics are administered after a blood culture is obtained. IV fluids are prioritized to support this patient hemodynamically.
   - Option C is incorrect because blood culture is usually done after IV fluids are initiated.
   - Option D is incorrect because surgery is performed when the patient has pneumoperitoneum or is deteriorating despite medical management. Therefore, one should first try medical management.

Pediatrics | Section 3: Urology - Cryptorchidism, Vesicoureteral Reflux & Posterior Urethral Valves

I. Cryptorchidism
   A. Most common congenital urogenital tract anomaly where one or both testicles fail to descend fully into the scrotum
   B. Risk factors: prematurity, low birth weight, DES exposure in utero, small for gestational age
   C. Clinical features: failure to palpate the testicle in the scrotum, hypoplastic scrotum, ↓ rugation of the scrotum; inguinal fullness
   D. Multiple locations (e.g. abdominal, inguinal)
   E. Diagnosis: mostly clinical
      1. Lab: ↓ testosterone (if bilateral), normal testosterone (if unilateral)
   F. Management
      1. Cryptorchidism usually resolve spontaneously by age 4-6 months
      2. If not, orchidopexy should be performed before age of 1
   G. Complications: infertility/subfertility, testicular cancer, testicular torsion, inguinal hernia

II. Vesicoureteral Reflux: General Information
   A. Retrograde flow of urine from the bladder and into the ureters
   B. Girls > boys (2:1)

III. Vesicoureteral Reflux: Etiology
   A. Primary (more common): short intramural part of the ureter
   B. Secondary: bladder outlet obstruction (e.g. posterior urethral valves, urethral meatal stenosis, neurogenic bladder), congenital ureteral anomalies, iatrogenic (post surgery)

IV. Vesicoureteral Reflux: Clinical Features
   A. Prenatally detected hydronephrosis/oligohydramnios
   B. Asymptomatic
   C. Recurrent UTI: fever, irritability (neonates); urgency, frequency, dysuria (older children); flank/abdominal pain
   D. Complications
      1. Nephropathy (interstitial nephritis), hypertension, kidney failure, renal scarring, urosepsis

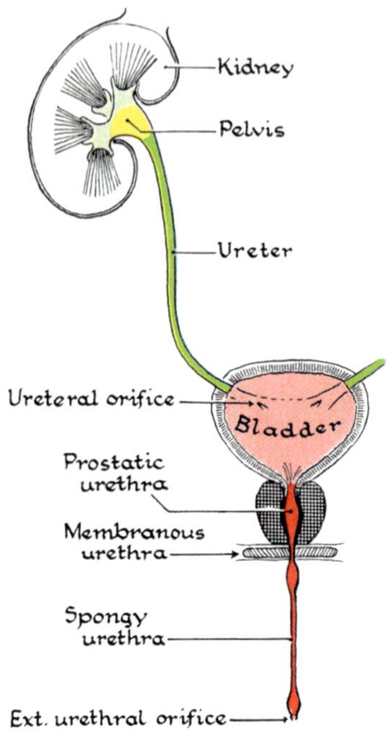

Grant, John Charles Boileau, Public domain, via Wikimedia Commons

FIGURE 21.9.14 - The Urinary System

V. Vesicoureteral Reflux: Diagnosis
   A. Laboratory examination
      1. Urinalysis and urine culture
      2. Renal function tests: to look for evidence of reflux nephropathy
         a) Serial creatinine, urea
      3. CBC: anemia, leukocytosis
   B. Ultrasound
      1. Antenatal ultrasound may show evidence of hydronephrosis
      2. Postnatally in all patients with febrile UTI: hydronephrosis
      3. Follow-up
   C. Contrast voiding cystourethrogram (VCUG): reflux of urine from the bladder into the ureters during micturition
      1. Classifies severity: grades I-V

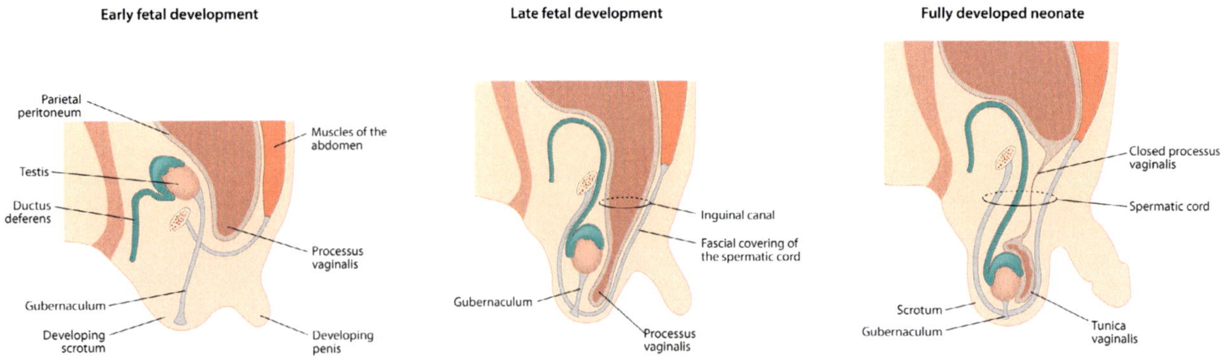

FIGURE 21.9.13 - Pathway of Normal Descent of the Testicle

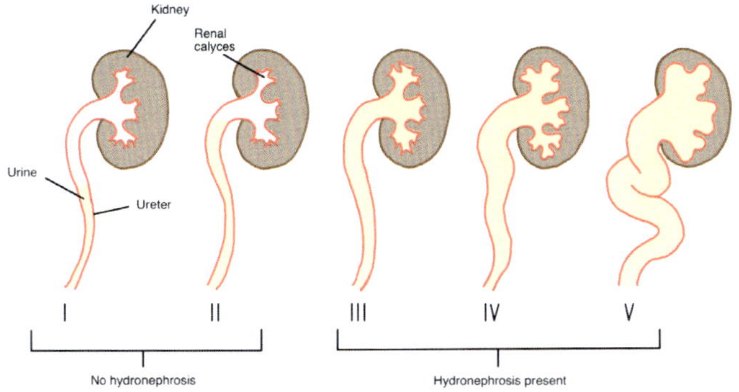

FIGURE 18.1.40 - Grades of Vesicoureteral Reflux

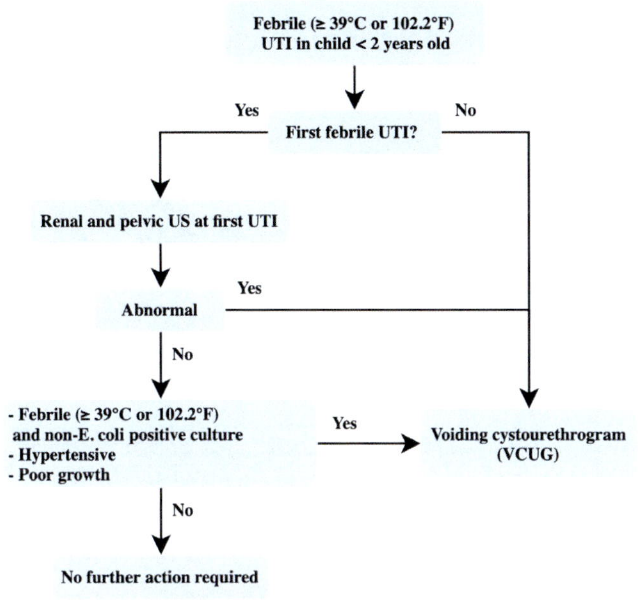

FIGURE 21.9.15 - Management of Febrile UTI in Child < 2 Years of Age

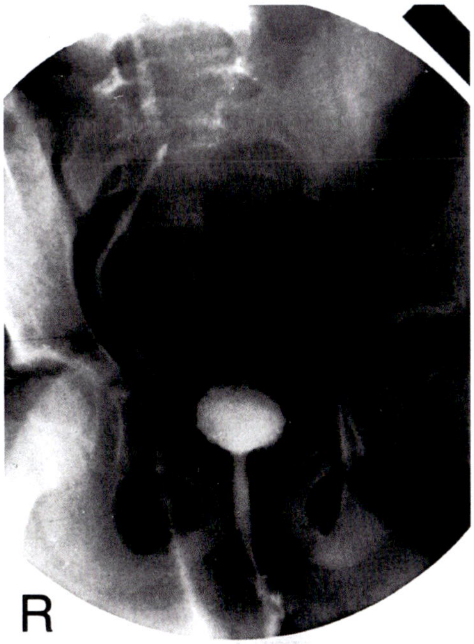

FIGURE 21.9.16 - Voiding Cystourethrogram: Unilateral Vesicoureteral Reflux

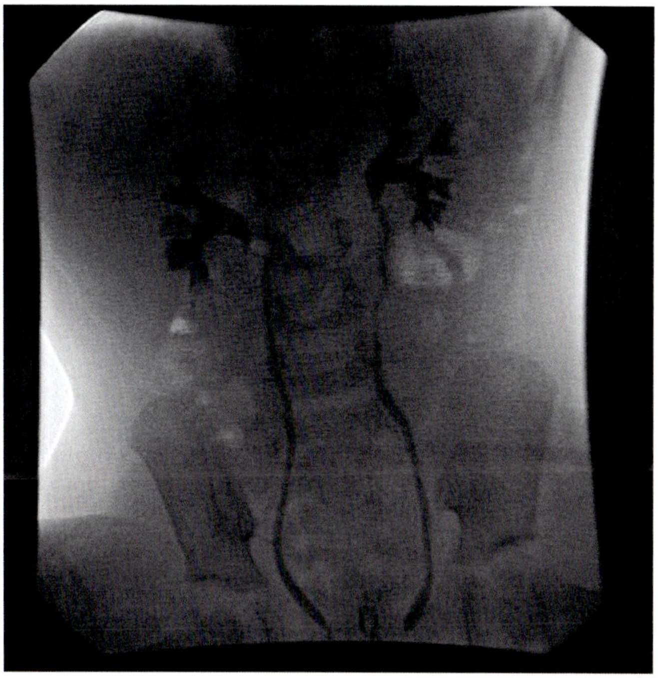

FIGURE 21.9.17 - Voiding Cystourethrogram: Bilateral Vesicoureteral Reflux

VI. Vesicoureteral Reflux: Management
   A. Initial management: treat infection
   B. Patients with low risk of pyelonephritis and renal scarring (children < 5 years with grades 1 - 3)
      1. Long-term prophylactic antibiotics; monitor closely with urinalysis and renal imaging
   C. Patients with high risk (grades 4 - 5, bilateral VUR, refractory disease despite treatment)
      1. Surgery: ureteral transplantation (high success rate)
   D. Renal scintigraphy with dimercaptosuccinic acid: for long-term evaluation of renal scarring

VII. Posterior Urethral Valves
   A. Congenital anomaly in boys where membranous folds obstruct urinary flow in the distal prostatic urethra
   B. This causes the urine to back up into the bladder and ureters → progressive bladder dilation, ureteral dilation → hydronephrosis
   C. Most common cause of urinary bladder obstruction in newborn males

VIII. Posterior Urethral Valves: Clinical Features
   A. Respiratory distress: Potter's sequence (flat facies, pulmonary hypoplasia, and limb deformities)
   B. Abdominal distension (distension of the bladder)
   C. Voiding problems: straining, poor urinary stream
   D. VUR, urinary tract infections, urosepsis, renal failure
   E. Failure to thrive

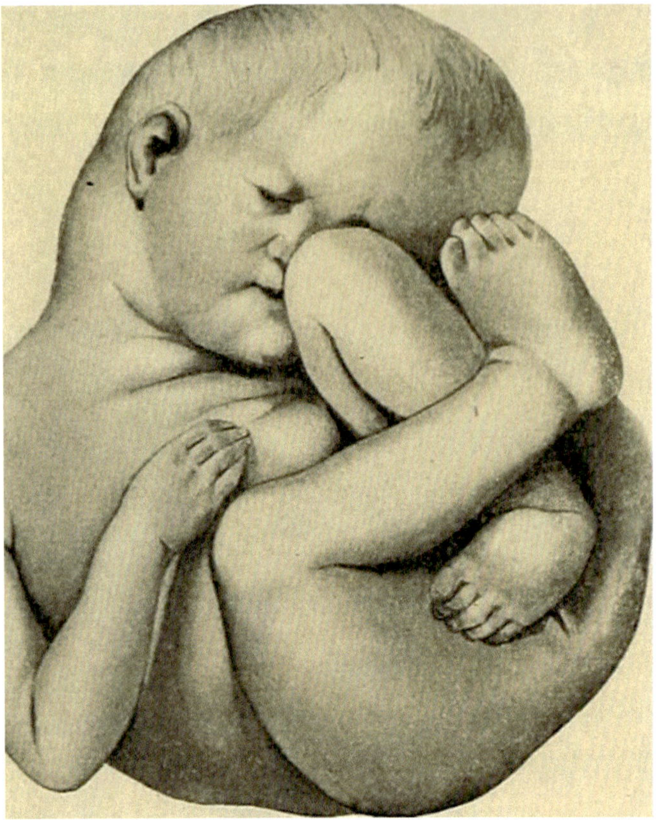

FIGURE 21.9.18 - Potter Sequence

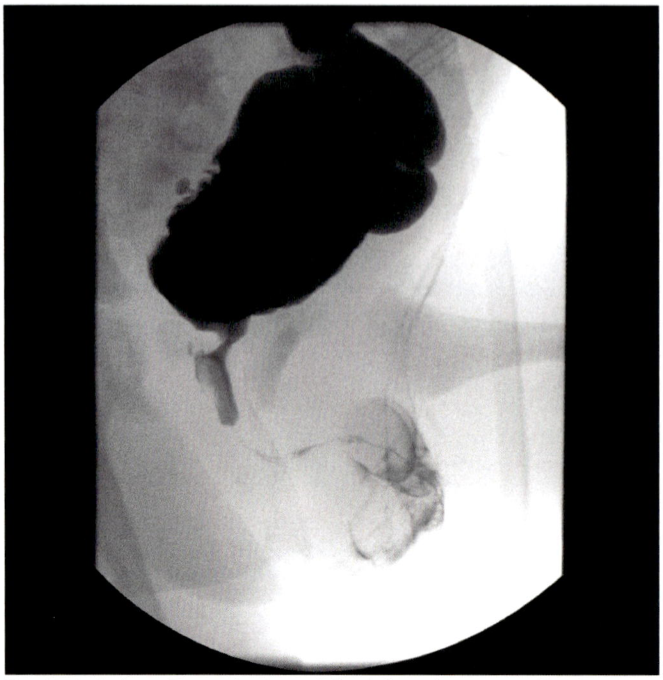

FIGURE 21.9.19 - Posterior Urethral Valve

IX. Posterior Urethral Valves: Diagnosis and Management
  A. Diagnosis
    1. Voiding cystourethrogram (method of choice): dilation of prostatic urethra
    2. Ultrasound: thick, dilated bladder; bilateral hydronephrosis
  B. Management
    1. Valve ablation: 1st line

REVIEW QUESTIONS

1. A 6-month-old boy is brought to the primary care physician for a well-child examination. He is at the 60th percentile for length and 70th percentile for weight. Physical examination shows only one testicle is palpated in the scrotum, but the examination is otherwise normal. What is the recommended treatment for this patient's condition?
    - **The recommended treatment for this patient's condition is orchidopexy.**
    - This 6-month-old boy has only one testicle palpated in the scrotum, which is consistent with cryptorchidism.
    - Since he's 6 months old, orchidopexy is the recommended treatment because spontaneous descent of the testes is very unlikely after this age. Orchidopexy will prevent complications such as infertility and testicular cancer and should be performed before the age of 1 year.

REVIEW QUESTIONS

2. A 15-month-old girl is brought to the primary care physician due to irritability and fever for the past 2 days. Her mother says she cried every time she passed urine for the past 2 days. She was treated for a urinary tract infection 4 months ago, but is otherwise healthy. A renal ultrasound shows hydronephrosis of the right kidney. What is the best next step in management of this patient?

    - **The best next step in management of this patient is a voiding cystourethrography.**
    - This 15-month-old girl is presenting with irritability, fever, and crying while passing urine, which are signs and symptoms of an upper urinary tract infection.
    - She has been treated for a previous UTI , so this is a recurrent infection.
    - Renal ultrasound shows hydronephrosis.
    - All of these features suggest vesicoureteral reflux as the most likely diagnosis.
    - Therefore, a voiding cystourethrography is the best next step. It will measure the reflux of urine from the bladder into the ureters during micturition and will classify the severity of the reflux into grades from I-V.

3. A 10-day-old newborn boy is brought to the primary care physician because of high fever, irritability, and lack of feeding for 2 days. The pregnancy was complicated with oligohydramnios. On physical exam, his abdomen appears distended and his urine stream is weak. What is the method of choice to confirm the diagnosis of this patient?

    - **The method of choice to confirm the diagnosis of this patient is voiding cystourethrogram.**
    - This 10-day-old newborn boy is presenting with high fever, irritability, lack of feeding, and signs of urinary tract infection.
    - Oligohydramnios, distended abdomen, and weak urinary stream are all characteristic of posterior urethral valves.
    - Posterior urethral valves is the most common cause of urinary tract obstruction in newborn males. On ultrasound, a thick, dilated bladder and bilateral hydronephrosis are characteristic.
    - However, the method of choice for diagnosing posterior urethral valves is voiding cystourethrogram, which shows dilation of the prostatic urethra.

4. A newborn boy is being evaluated in the delivery room for weak cry, irregular breathing, and respiratory distress. His pulse oximetry shows an oxygen saturation of 76%. The pregnancy was complicated by oligohydramnios. Physical examination shows facial dysmorphisms and limb deformities. He has low-set ears, flat nose, and a small jaw. Breath sounds are decreased bilaterally. Ultrasound examination shows dilation of the ureters bilaterally as well as dilation of the bladder. Which of the following is the next step to confirm the diagnosis of the patient?

    A. Chest X-ray
    B. Nasogastric tube insertion
    C. Voiding cystourethrogram
    D. Karyotyping

    - **The correct answer is option C.**
    - This newborn male has irregular breathing, is in respiratory distress due to pulmonary hypoplasia, and has limb deformities, and facial abnormalities due to oligohydramnios.
    - This is consistent with Potter's sequence.
    - Ultrasound examination shows dilation of the ureters bilaterally as well as dilation of the bladder characteristic of posterior urethral valves.
    - Therefore, the next step to confirm the diagnosis is ordering voiding cystourethrogram.
    - Option A is incorrect because chest X-ray will reveal pulmonary hypoplasia and will explain the symptoms of respiratory distress. However, it will not reveal the underlying cause.
    - Option B is incorrect because nasogastric tube insertion is helpful to diagnose patients with esophageal atresia, commonly associated with tracheoesophageal fistula. However, tracheoesophageal fistula is associated with polyhydramnios, not oligohydramnios during pregnancy.
    - Option D is incorrect because karyotyping will confirm chromosomal abnormalities which are associated with facial and limb abnormalities, but the combination of these features along with the bladder and bilateral ureteral dilation is highly characteristic of urinary tract obstruction due to posterior urethral valves.

Pediatrics | Section 4: Urology - Penile Conditions

I. Epispadias
   A. Rare embryonic urogenital malformation where the urethra opens on the dorsal penis
   B. Commonly associated with bladder exstrophy
   C. Clinical diagnosis: dorsally located urethral opening, short phallus, dorsal penile curvature, urinary incontinence
   D. Complications: infertility, erectile dysfunction
   E. Management: surgical closure, urethroplasty

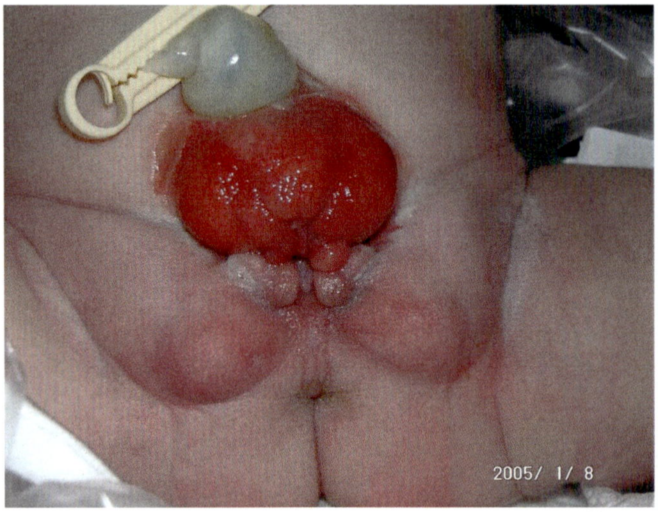

FIGURE 21.9.20 - Bladder Exstrophy

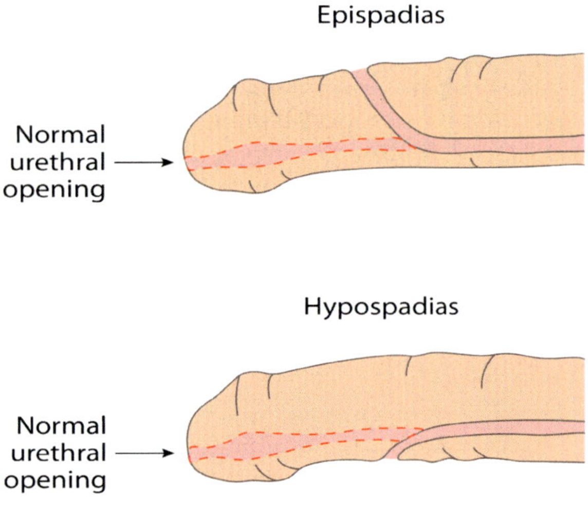

FIGURE 21.9.21 - Epispadias

II. Hypospadias
   A. Common embryonic urogenital malformation where urethra abnormally opens on the ventral penis due to failure of urethral folds to close
   B. Associated with syndromes (e.g. WAGR, Denys-Drash), ↓ androgen sensitivity, genetic disorders of sex development
   C. Clinical diagnosis: dorsal hood, ventrally located urethral opening, ventral penile curvature
   D. Circumcision is contraindicated: skin flap can be used in reconstruction
   E. Management
      1. Reconstruction surgery: urethroplasty, correction of the curvature if present

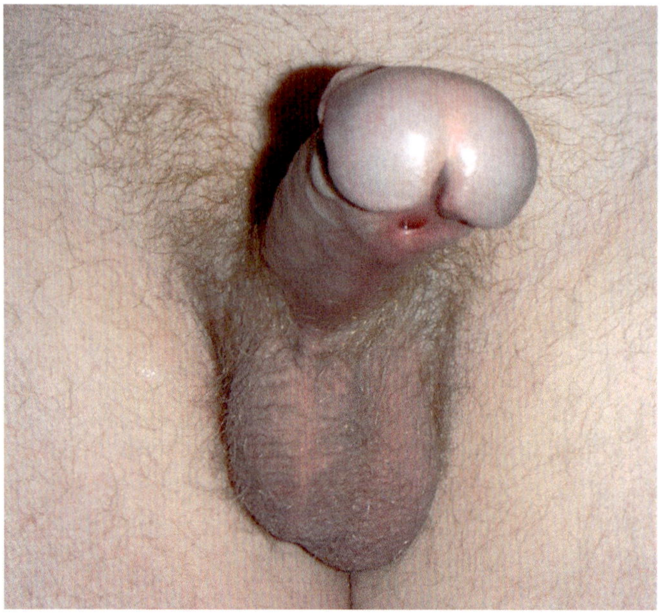

FIGURE 21.9.22 - Hypospadias

III. Phimosis
   A. Inability to completely retract the skin over the glans penis due to tight foreskin
      1. Physiologic: in uncircumcised newborns, resolves at age 6 - 7 years
      2. Pathologic: occurs as a result of inflammation and scarring
   B. Clinical diagnosis: inability to completely retract the foreskin, painful erection, dysuria, ballooning of the foreskin during urination
   C. Complications: tearing and bleeding, paraphimosis
   D. Management: depends on the extent and severity of the phimosis
      1. Daily gentle retraction and stretching
      2. Topical corticosteroid cream
      3. Circumcision (definitive treatment and the treatment of choice)

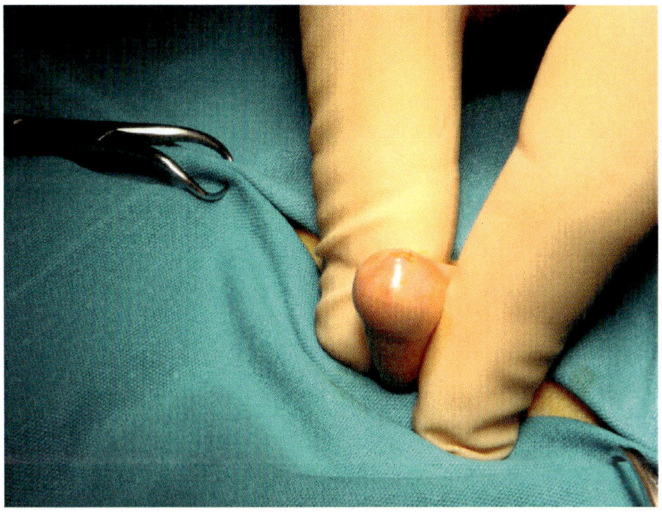

FIGURE 21.9.23 - Phimosis (Before Surgical Treatment)

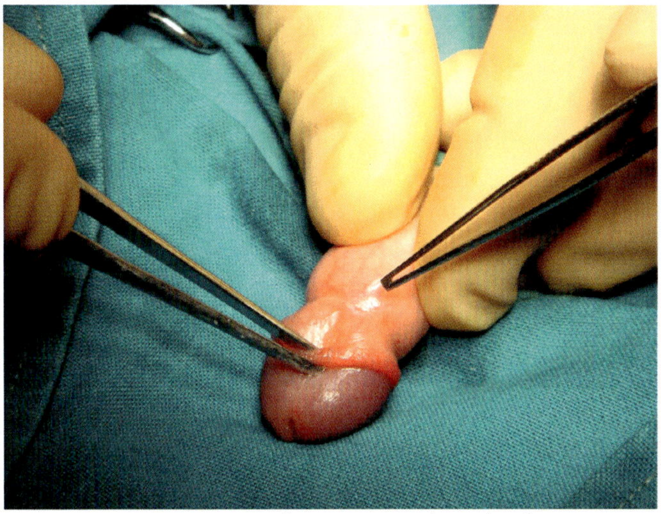

FIGURE 21.9.24 - After Surgical Treatment of Phimosis

IV. Paraphimosis
   A. A condition affecting uncircumcised males where the retracted foreskin cannot be pulled over the glans penis to its original position
   B. Etiology: complication of phimosis, iatrogenic (after retracting the foreskin for cleaning, for placing a urinary catheter)
   C. A medical emergency: foreskin is trapped → strangulation of the glans penis → vascular compromise → edema and possibly necrosis
   D. Clinical diagnosis: foreskin cannot be pulled to its original position, edematous foreskin, painful glans penis
   E. Management
      1. Manual reduction: for mild, uncomplicated cases
      2. Surgical treatment
         a) Incising the constricting band
         b) Circumcision (definitive treatment and the treatment of choice)

REVIEW QUESTIONS

1. A 2-day-old newborn boy presents with a urethral opening on the dorsal aspect of the penis. What other associated genitourinary abnormality is likely present in this patient?
   - **Bladder exstrophy is a congenital deformity that is often associated with epispadias.**
   - This 2-day-old newborn boy is presenting with epispadias suggested by the urethral opening on the dorsal aspect of the penis.

2. A three week old boy is brought to the emergency deparatment by his parents because of swelling of his penis. The patient was delivered vaginally with no complications, and his parents elected not to have him circumcised at the time of birth. Upon closer inspection of the newborn, it is noticed that his glans penis is swollen and the foreskin cannot be pulled back over it. The parents state they noticed it this morning and immediately rushed him to the office. What is the best treatment for this newborn's condition?

   A. Topical Corticosteroids
   B. Gentle Stretching
   C. Circumcision
   D. Urological Surgery

   - **The correct answer is option C.**
   - This three week old male is noticed to have swelling of his penis.
   - He is not circumcised.
   - The glans is swollen and the foreskin is stuck in the retracted position.
   - This is a condition known as paraphimosis, and it presents as an emergency due to possible strangulation of the glans penis.
   - The best and definitive treatment is circumcision.
   - Options A and B are incorrect because topical corticosteroids and gentle stretching are initial treatment options for phimosis, where the foreskin is stuck over the glans penis and unable to retract.
   - Option D is incorrect because circumcision is the definitive treatment for this patient's condition. Urological surgery is unnecessary, and would instead be used in the management of epispadias or hypospadias.

Pediatrics | Section 5: MSK Disorders - Hip Conditions

I. Legg-Calvé-Perthes Disease
   A. Idiopathic avascular necrosis of the femoral head
   B. Affects children (age 4-10 years); peak incidence at age 5-7 years
   C. Boys > girls
   D. Etiology: idiopathic, familial; can be due to hemophilia or repetitive trauma
   E. Clinical features: insidious onset hip pain projecting to the knee, limp, antalgic gait; unilateral or bilateral; ↓ ROM
   F. Physical examination: ↑ pain and limited ROM on internal rotation and abduction; atrophy of thigh muscles
   G. Diagnosis: x-ray may be normal (early stages), fragmentation and sclerosis of the femoral head (late changes); MRI if the x-ray is inconclusive
   H. Differential diagnosis: transient synovitis which occurs after a viral infection; resolves in 1-4 weeks
   I. Management
      1. Conservative with rest, NSAIDs, bracing, avoid weight-bearing exercises
      2. Surgery with femoral osteotomy: age ≥ 6 years, extensive damage where the femoral head is not contained in the acetabulum
   J. Complications include early-onset osteoarthritis
   K. Prognosis: depends on the age of onset and degree of femoral involvement
      1. Early onset (< 6-8 years) is associated with a better prognosis

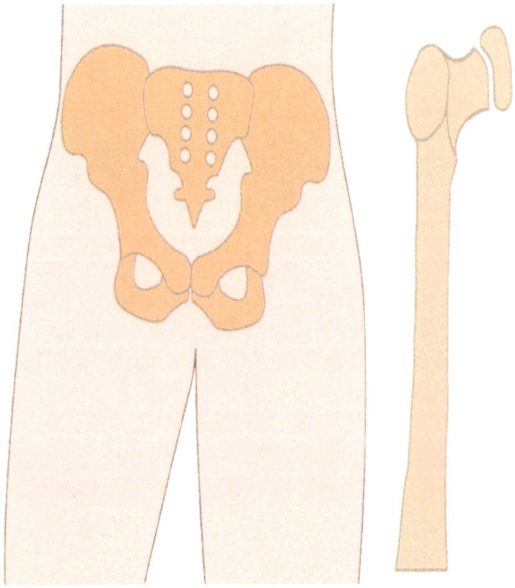

FIGURE 21.9.25 - Subluxation and Displacement of Femoral Head After Necrosis

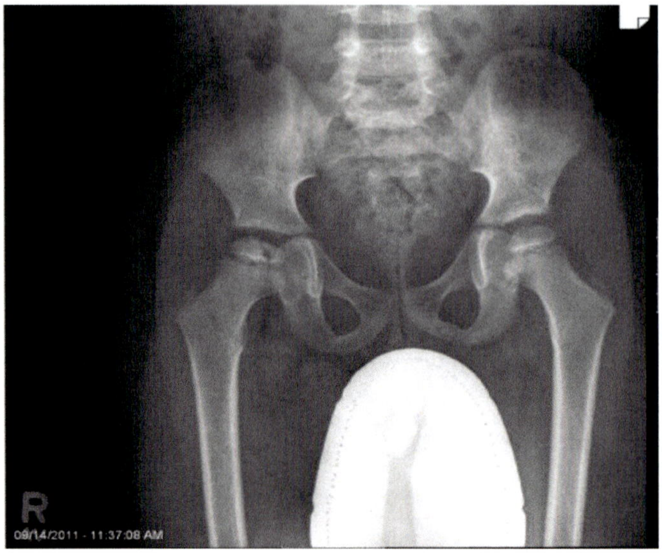

FIGURE 21.9.26 - Pelvic X-Ray Showing Flattening of Both Femoral Heads

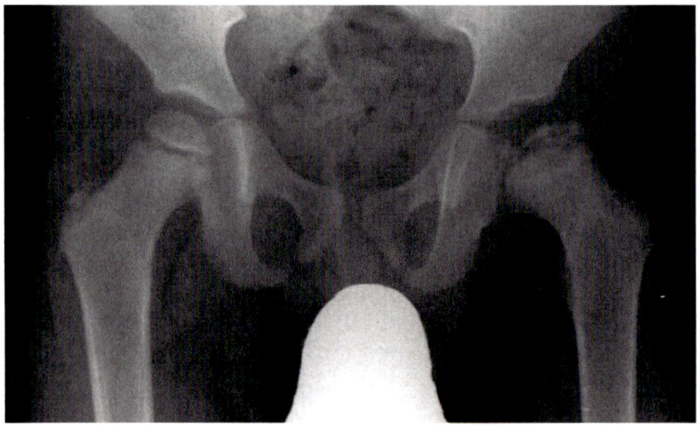

FIGURE 21.9.27 - Pelvic X-Ray Showing Necrosis and Fragmentation of the left Femoral Head

II. Slipped Capital Femoral Epiphysis (SCFE)
   A. A hip disorder characterized by displacement of the femoral head at the proximal growth plate relative to the femoral neck
   B. Affects adolescent males 10-16 years (↑ growth)
   C. Due to weakening of the epiphyseal plate and increased shearing
   D. Risk factors include positive family history, obesity, trauma, endocrine disorders, renal failure, and history of radiation
   E. Clinical features: pain and gait disturbance
      1. Dull, aching hip, groin, or knee pain; increases with physical activity; acute or chronic; limp
   F. Physical exam
      1. ↓ ROM, decreased internal rotation and abduction; limb shortening, inability to bear weight
      2. Patients hold the hip in external rotation

G. Diagnosis
   1. X-ray, ultrasound, MRI
   2. Posterior and inferior displacement of the femoral head and widened joint space; both hips should be assessed
H. Management
   1. Urgent surgical internal fixation
   2. Avoid weight-bearing
I. Follow-up: risk of involvement of the other hip
J. Complications: avascular necrosis of the femoral head, early-onset hip osteoarthritis

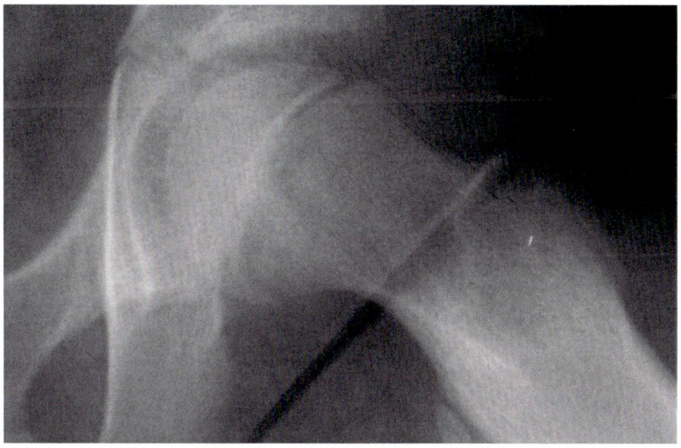

Mikir at English Wikipedia, Public domain, via Wikimedia Commons

FIGURE 21.9.28 - X-Ray of the Hip Joint

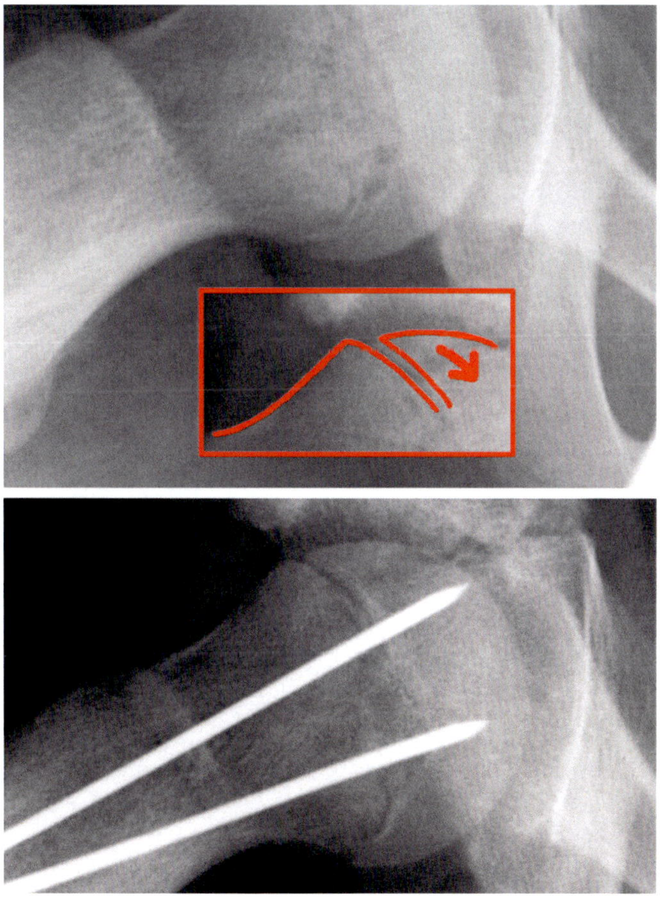

Dr. Jochen Lengerke, Public domain, via Wikimedia Commons

FIGURE 21.9.29 - X-Ray Showing Slipped Capital Femoral Epiphysis, Before and After Surgical Intervention

III. Developmental Dysplasia of Hip
   A. Subluxation or dislocation of the femoral head, and/or dysplasia of the acetabulum
   B. Unknown etiology
   C. Risk factors
      1. Breech positioning
      2. Positive family history
      3. Female sex, first born child
   D. Clinical features
      1. Click or clunk in the hip
         a) When the hip is flexed and abducted while applying anterior force (Ortolani sign)
         b) When the hip is flexed and adducted while applying posterior force (Barlow sign)
         c) Can be detected in patients < 6 months of age
   E. Clinical features
      1. Galeazzi sign, difficulty in hip abduction
      2. Hip pain, trendelenburg gait
      3. Asymmetrical folds of thigh, gluteal and inguinal regions; limb length discrepancy (absent in bilateral conditions)
   F. Diagnosis
      1. Screening physical examination on every well visit <6 months
      2. Age < 4 months: hip ultrasound
      3. Age > 4 months: pelvic x-ray
      4. Imaging helps confirm the diagnosis and assess acetabular development
   G. Treatment
      1. Pavlik harness: < 6 months; splint to hold the hip in flexion and abduction position
      2. Closed reduction with hip spica cast: 6-18 months
      3. Open reduction with hip splice cast: > 18 months; pelvic or femoral osteotomy

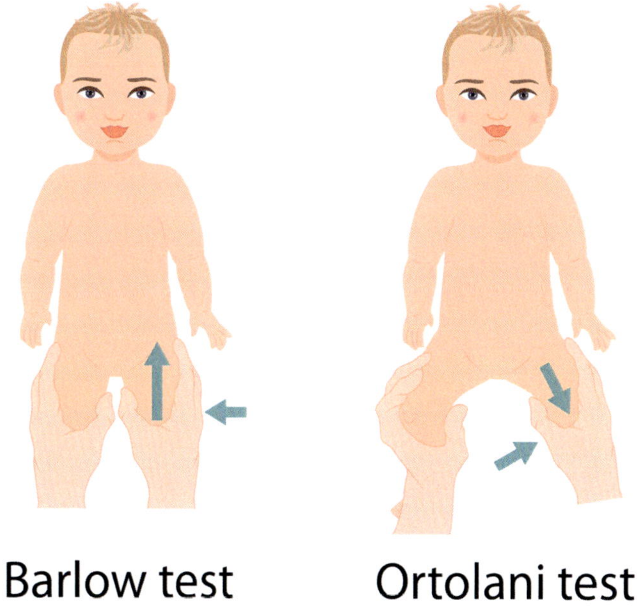

FIGURE 21.9.30 - Barlow & Ortolani Tests

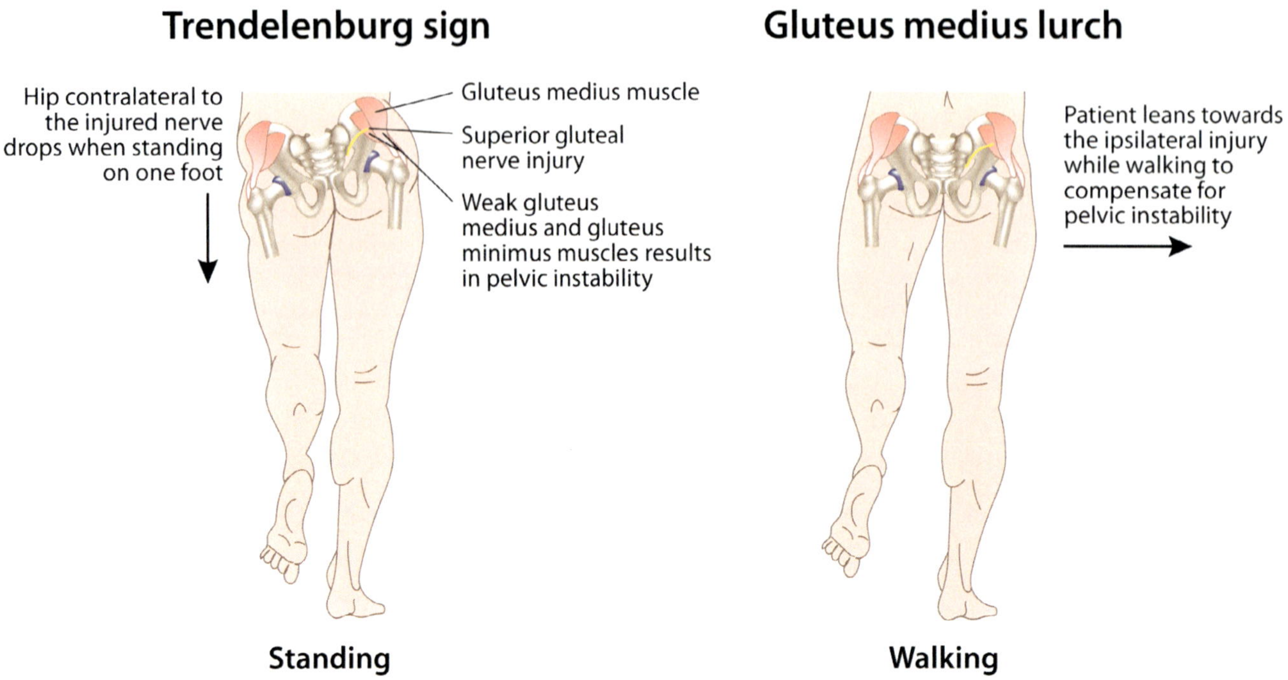

FIGURE 21.9.31 - Trendelenburg Gait

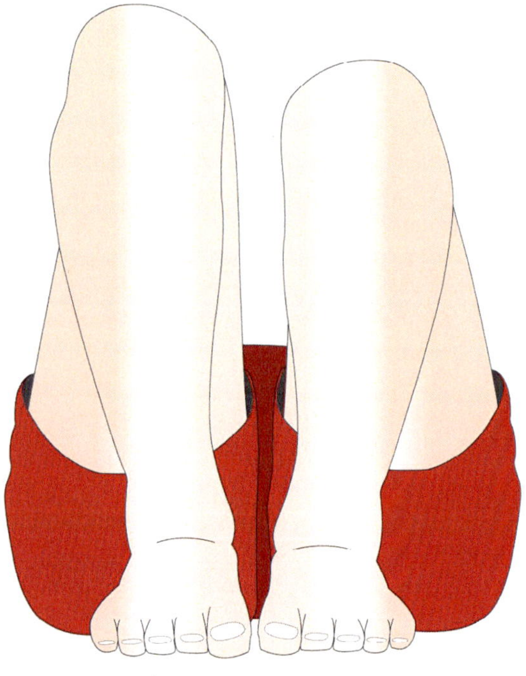

FIGURE 21.9.32 - Galeazzi Sign

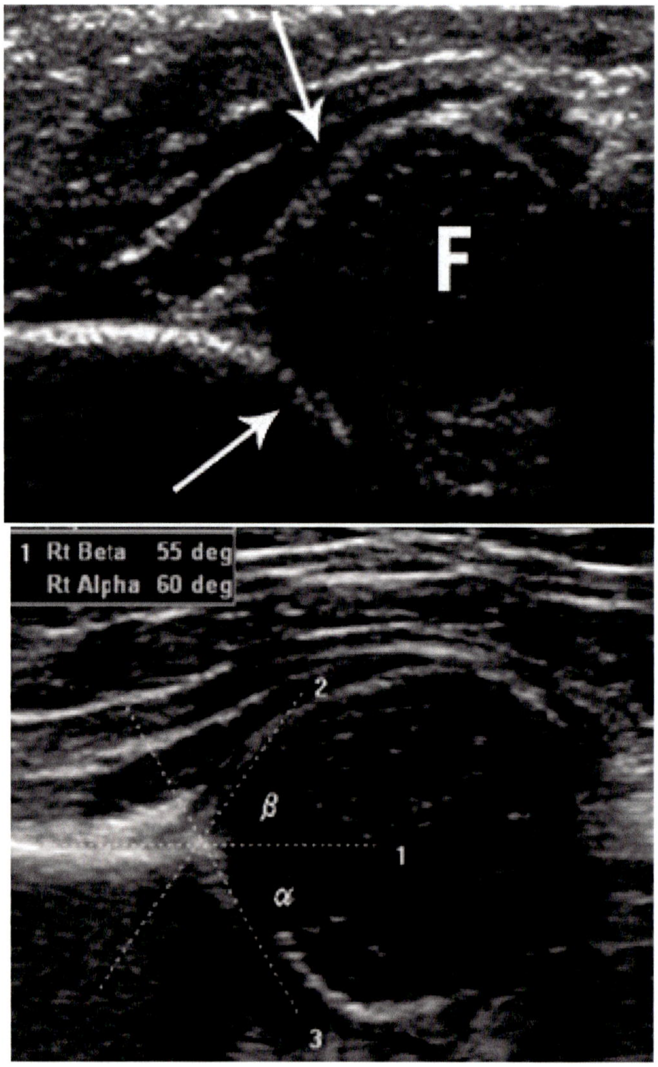

FIGURE 21.9.33 - Normal Hip Ultrasound in an Infant

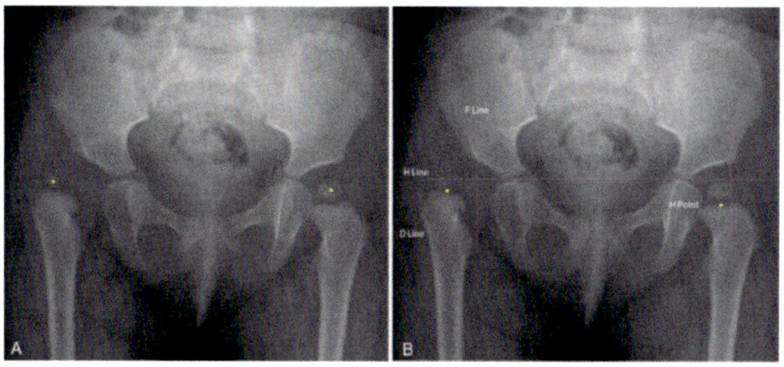

"Retrospective observational study comparing the international hip dysplasia institute classification with the Tonnis classification of developmental dysplasia of the hip" by Mingyuan Miao et al., Medicine is licensed under CC BY 4.0

FIGURE 21.9.34 - Pelvic X-Ray Showing Developmental Dysplasia of the Right Hip

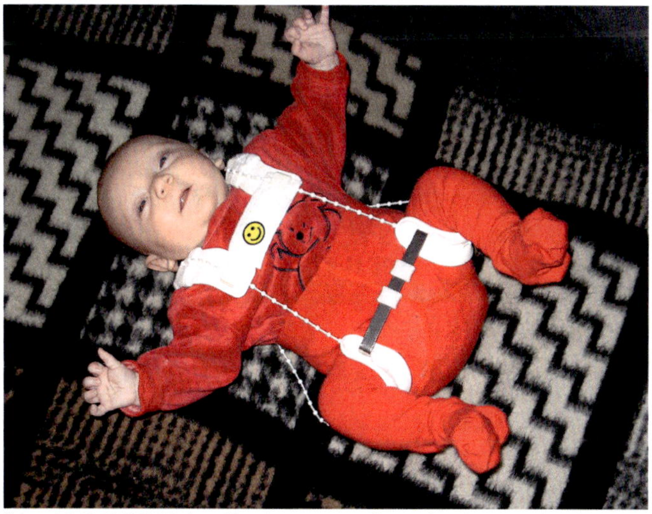

Thiemo Schuff, CC BY-SA 3.0 <https://creativecommons.org/licenses/by-sa/3.0>, via Wikimedia Commons

FIGURE 21.9.35 - Baby Wearing Pavlik Harness

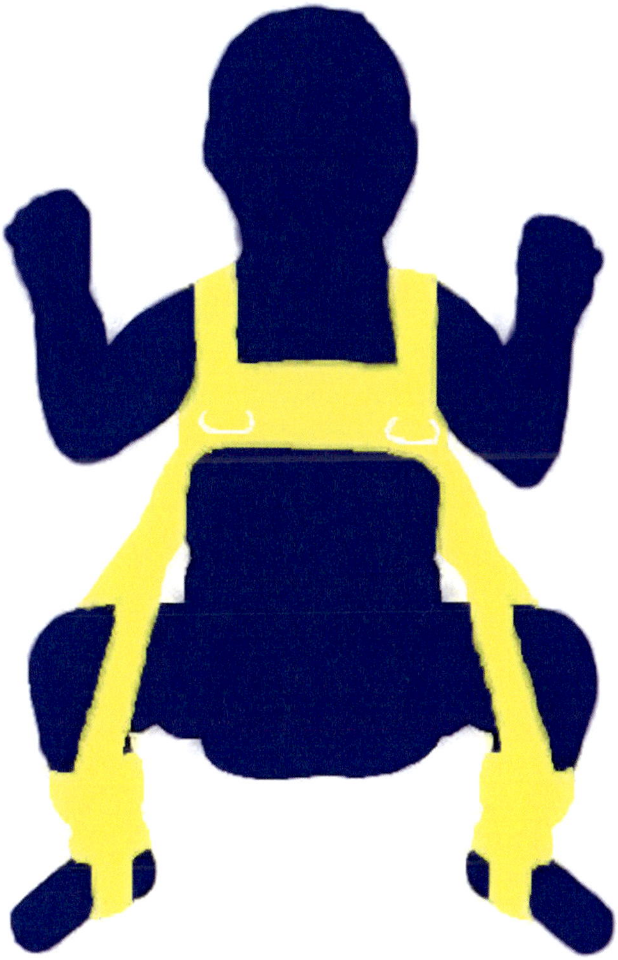

Londenp, CC BY-SA 3.0 <http://creativecommons.org/licenses/by-sa/3.0/>, via Wikimedia Commons

FIGURE 21.9.36 - Diagram of Baby Wearing a Pavlik Harness

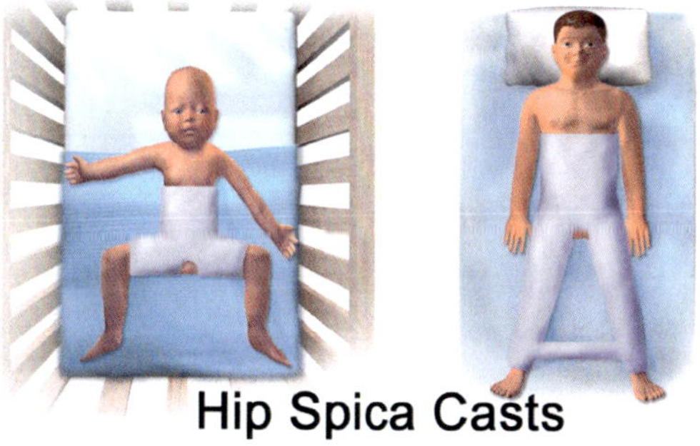

BruceBlaus, CC BY-SA 4.0 <https://creativecommons.org/licenses/by-sa/4.0>, via Wikimedia Commons

FIGURE 21.9.37 - Hip Spica Cast Treatment

REVIEW QUESTIONS

1. A 6-year-old boy is brought to his primary care physician by his parents because of insidious limping and hip pain for the past 4 months. He has recently refused to play with other children in the yard due to hip pain. The physical examination shows pain exacerbation upon internal rotation and abduction of his left hip. Pelvic X-ray shows flattened femoral epiphysis with hyperlucent areas. What is the most likely diagnosis in this patient?
   - **The most likely diagnosis in this patient is Legg-Calvé-Perthes disease.**
   - This boy presents with insidious limping and hip pain for the past 4 months.
   - The physical examination shows pain exacerbation upon internal rotation and abduction of his left hip.
   - His age, gender, and symptoms are all classic for Legg-Calve-Perthes disease.
   - Legg-Calvé-Perthes disease is confirmed by the pelvic X-ray findings of flattened femoral epiphysis with hyperlucent areas.

2. A 2-month-old girl is brought to her primary care physician by her parents because of a "shorter right leg". She was born at 39 weeks of gestation without prenatal or perinatal complications. An audible clunk is elicited by flexing and abducting the hip with applying anterior force or flexing and adducting the hip with applying posterior force. Hip ultrasound shows femoral head dislocated from the acetabular fossa. What is the best initial treatment option for this patient's condition?
   - **The best initial treatment option for the developmental dysplasia of the hip in patients less than 6 months of age is Pavlik harness.**
   - This 2-months-old girl presents with a "shorter right leg".
   - This phenomenon is referred to as leg length discrepancy.
   - An audible clunk is elicited by flexing and abducting the hip with applying anterior force or flexing and adducting the hip with applying posterior force.
   - These findings describe Ortolani and Barlow maneuvers, respectively.
   - Hip ultrasound shows femoral head dislocated from the acetabular fossa.
   - All of these clues are consistent with the diagnosis of developmental dysplasia of the hip.
   - Pavlik harness keeps both hips flexed and abducted so that femoral heads stay in the acetabular fossa.

3. A 14-year-old male is brought to his primary care physician by his mother because of right hip pain. His mother also adds that he has been walking abnormally. The physical exam shows an obese boy sitting in the office in no acute distress. The patient's right hip is noted to be shorter than the left and he is holding the hip in external rotation as he is examined. His vital signs show temperature of 99.7°F (37.6°C), heart rate of 70 beats/min, respiratory rate of 12 breaths/min, and blood pressure of 120/80 mmHg. His BMI is 33 Kg/m2. Based on this patient's most likely diagnosis, which of the following options is a potential complication of his condition?

   A. Rheumatoid arthritis
   B. Avascular necrosis
   C. Osteosarcoma
   D. Osteomyelitis

   - **The correct answer is B.**
   - A 14-year-old male presents due to right hip pain and an abnormal gait.
   - On physical exam, he is noted to be obese which is confirmed by the BMI of 33.
   - Additionally, his right hip is shorter than the left and he is holding it in external rotation.
   - Based on this presentation, the patient most likely has slipped capital femoral epiphysis aka SCFE.
   - Answer choice A is incorrect because early onset hip osteoarthritis is a potential complication of SCFE, but rheumatoid arthritis is not.
   - Answer choice C is incorrect because the risk of osteosarcoma is associated with retinoblastoma, not SCFE.
   - Answer choice D is incorrect because the risk of osteomyelitis is not associated with SCFE, but rather can be seen when an adjacent infection spreads to the bone in a diabetic.

Pediatrics | Section 6: MSK Disorders - Foot Deformities

I. Club Foot
   A. Also known as congenital talipes equinovarus
   B. Widely common congenital deformity
   C. Mostly due to dominance of posterior tibial muscle
   D. Cavus of midfoot: high-arched foot
   E. Adductus of forefoot: toes are turned inwards
   F. Varus of hindfoot: heel is turned inwards
   G. Equinus of hindfoot: abnormal plantar flexion of foot
   H. Diagnosis
      1. Clinical
      2. X-ray: parallelism of talus and calcaneus long axes
   I. Management
      1. Serial stretching, manipulation and casting (Ponseti method)
      2. Surgery: if above method fails; usually performed within 3 - 6 months of age

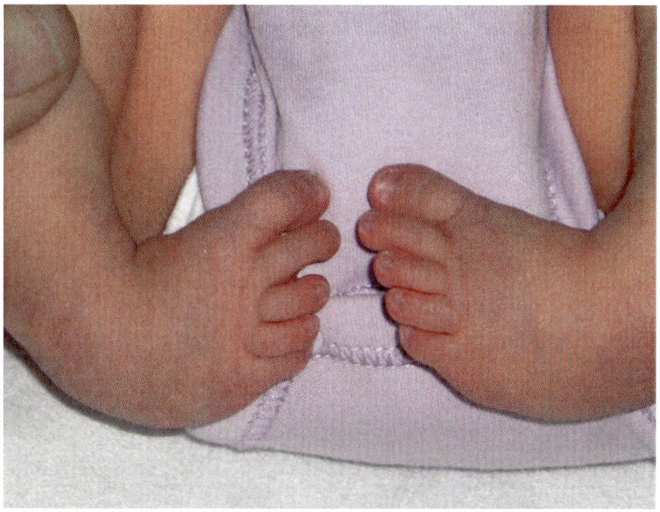

FIGURE 21.9.38 - Club Foot

II. Metatarsus Adductus
   A. Adduction of the forefoot with convex lateral border and concave medial border
   B. Hindfoot is in neutral position
   C. Mostly seen in the first born infants
   D. Can be associated with hip dysplasia
   E. Causes intoeing in children
   F. Diagnosis: clinical; imaging is not required
   G. Management
      1. Mostly spontaneous resolution
      2. Corrective shoes or cast required for special cases

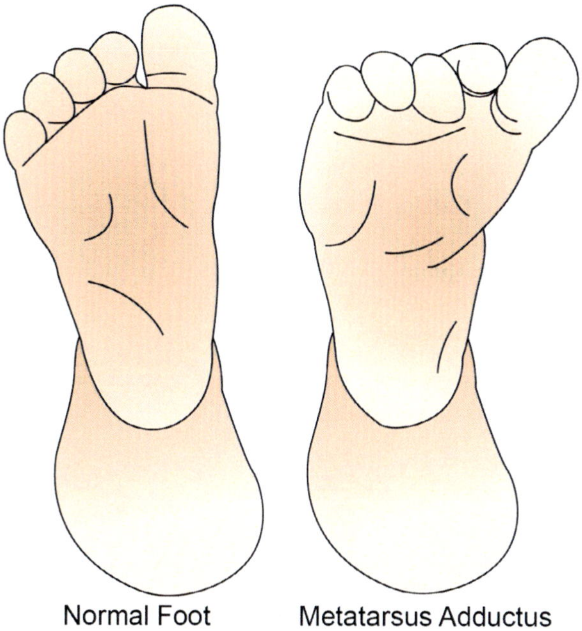

FIGURE 21.9.39 - Metatarsus Adductus

III. Pes Planus
   A. Flat foot; loss of medial longitudinal arch of foot
   B. Etiology
      1. Congenital: isolated or associated with neurological conditions
      2. Functional (e.g. dysfunction of posterior tibial tendon, trauma)
   C. Two types: rigid and flexible
      1. Flexible: intact arch during heel elevation or non weight-bearing
      2. Rigid: absent arch during weight-bearing and heel elevation
   D. Diagnosis
      1. Mainly clinical
      2. Lateral foot X-ray
   E. Management
      1. Serial casting after birth
      2. Surgery in case of failure

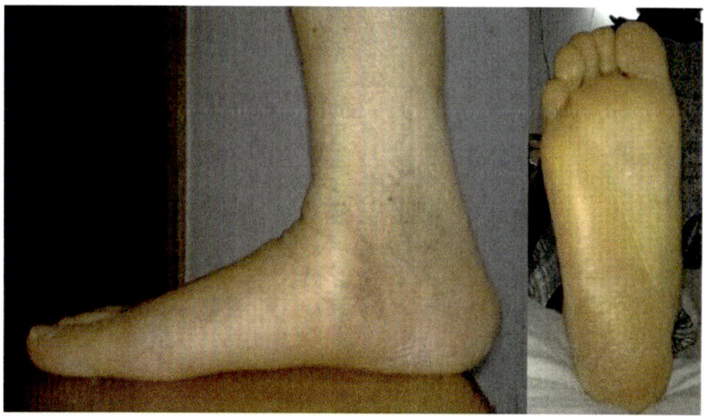

FIGURE 21.9.40 - Pes Planus

IV. Pes Cavus
   A. High-arched foot; high longitudinal plantar arch of foot
   B. Mostly idiopathic; can be associated with neurological and muscular disorders or Charcot-Marie-Tooth disease
   C. Imbalance between strong plantar flexion and weak dorsiflexion
   D. Diagnosis
      1. Mainly clinical
      2. X-ray of foot and ankle joint
   E. Management
      1. Corrective shoes and physiotherapy
      2. Surgery in case of resistant pes cavus

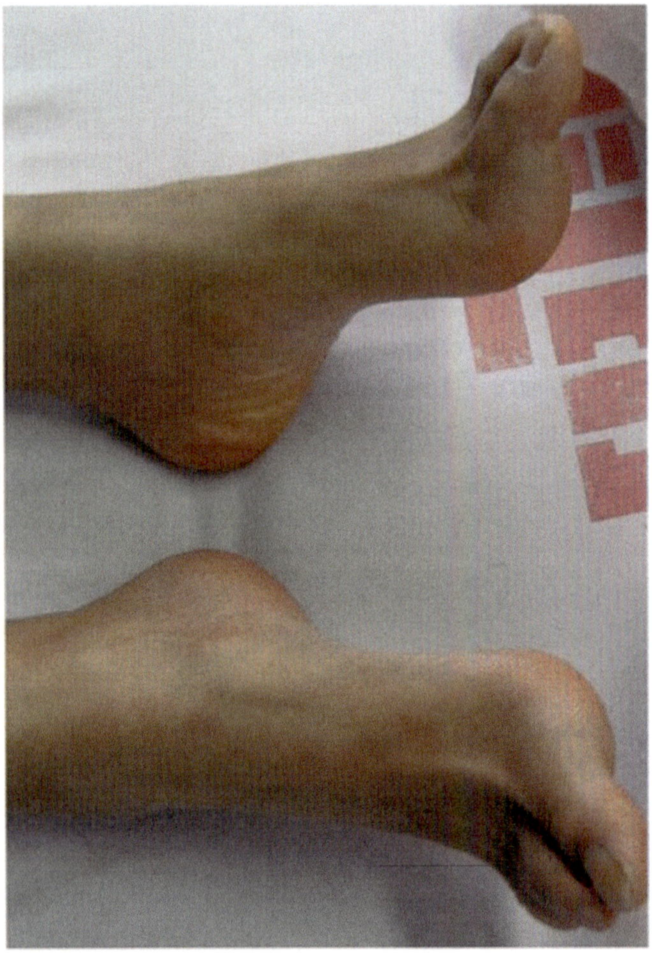

FIGURE 21.9.41 - Pes Cavus

REVIEW QUESTIONS ?

1. A 3-month-old boy is brought to his primary care physician by his parents because of a deformed foot. Physical examination shows adduction of the forefoot with convex lateral border and concave medial border. The hindfoot is in a neutral position. What is the most likely prognosis of this patient's condition?

   - **The most likely prognosis of this patient's condition is spontaneous resolution.**
   - This 3-month-old boy presents with a deformed foot.
   - Physical examination shows adduction of the forefoot with convex lateral border and concave medial border. The hindfoot is in a neutral position.
   - This is a classic description of metatarsus adductus.
   - Metatarsus adductus resolves spontaneously most of the time. Corrective shoes or casts may be needed for resistant cases.

2. A 6-month-old baby girl is brought to her primary care physician because of a deformity in both of her feet. Physical examination shows the posterior tibial muscles of the child is larger compared to the other muscles. X-ray of the child's feet shows, the long axes of the talus and calcaneus bones are parallel. Based on this child's diagnosis which additional feature would be expected on physical examination of the child's feet?

   A. Normal plantar flexion
   B. Toes turned outwards
   C. High arch
   D. Heel turned outwards

   - **The correct answer is option C.**
   - This 6-month-old baby girl presents with a deformity of both feet.
   - Physical examination is notable for dominance of posterior tibial muscles.
   - On X-ray of the feet, talocalcaneal parallelism is noted.
   - Based on these features, this child most likely has a club foot deformity.
   - The mnemonic CAVE can remember the features of club foot. This stands for Cavus of midfoot, which causes a high arch; Adductus of forefoot, where toes are turned inwards; Varus of hindfoot, where the heel turns inwards; and Equinus of hindfoot, which is abnormal plantar flexion.
   - Options A, B, and D are all incorrect because they represent the opposite of what would be expected in a club foot deformity.

Pediatrics | Section 7: MSK Disorders - Orthopedic Injuries

I. Clavicular Fracture
   A. Most common birth trauma
   B. Commonly seen in children and adolescents with fall on the shoulder
   C. Most common fracture site: junction of lateral and middle segments
   D. Clinical features
      1. Sagging of shoulder, short clavicle, skin tenting
      2. Symptoms of neurovascular involvement (e.g. weak pulses in upper extremity, brachial plexus injury)
   E. Diagnosis
      1. Physical examination shows swelling and concomitant injuries
      2. X-ray is best initial test; ultrasound in neonates
      3. CT/MRI if there is neurovascular involvement
   F. Management
      1. Midshaft fracture: conservative treatment with shoulder sling; surgery is reserved for largely displaced fractures
      2. Lateral segment fracture: shoulder sling; consider surgical plating or pinning for unstable fracture
      3. Medial segment fracture: shoulder sling

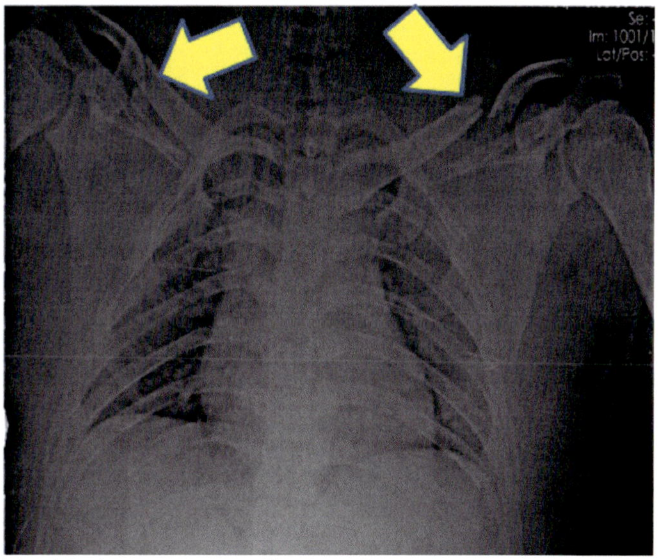

FIGURE 21.9.42 - Chest X-ray: Clavicular Fracture

II. Greenstick Fracture
   a. Partial thickness fracture
   A. Cortex and periosteum of the tension side (convex) are interrupted but these of compression side (concave) remain intact
   B. Angulation might be present
   C. Mostly present in diaphysis of radius, ulna, and fibula
   D. Most commonly due to fall on an outstretched hand
   E. Other risk factors: vitamin D deficiency, malnutrition
   F. Clinical features: pain on palpation, decreased range of motion of affected extremity
   G. Diagnosis: X-ray shows fracture line that doesn't travel throughout the bone
   H. Treatment
      1. Immobilization with cast
      2. Closed reduction is considered if there is excessive angulation

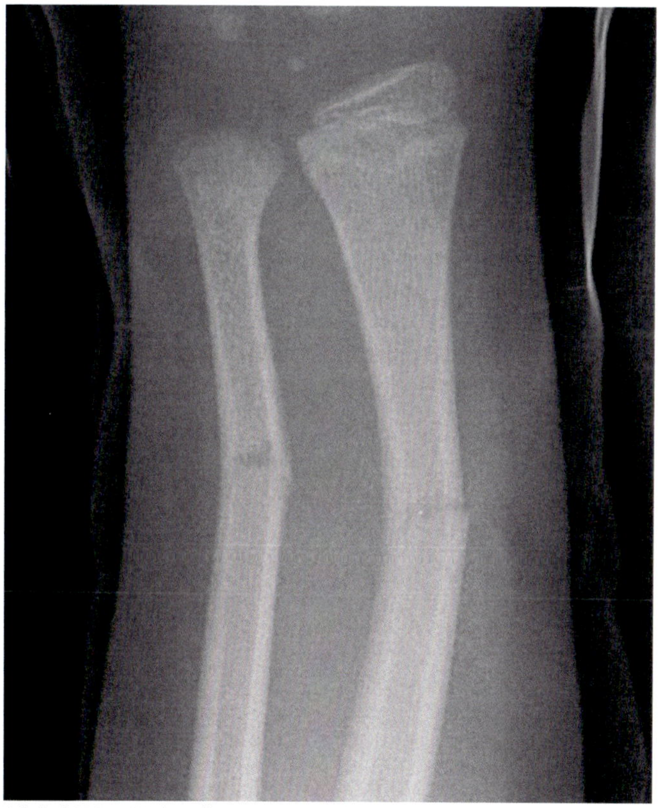

FIGURE 21.9.43 - X-ray of Arm: Greenstick Fracture

III. Torus Fracture
   A. Buckle fracture
   B. Cortex and periosteum are interrupted at the compression side (concave surface), whereas these of tension side are intact
   C. Mostly no angulation
   D. Most common site: distal radius at metadiaphyseal junction
   E. Diagnosis: X-ray
   F. Treatment: immobilization with cast for few weeks

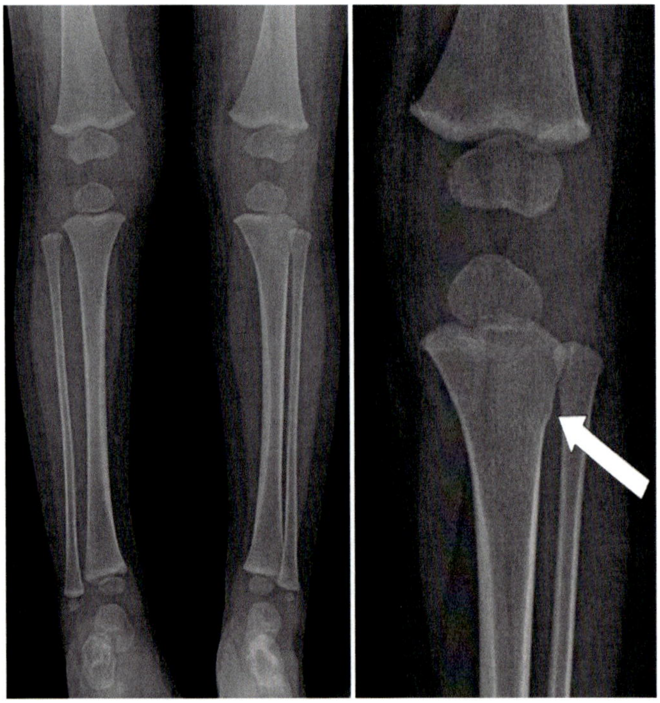

FIGURE 21.9.44 - X-ray of Tibia: Torus Fracture

IV. Nursemaid's Elbow
   A. Radial head subluxation in the presence of immature annular ligament
   B. Axial traction of radius during elbow extension (e.g. child is pulled up quickly or swinged)
   C. Mostly seen in children < 5 years of age
   D. Clinical findings
      1. Arm held flexed and pronated
      2. Pain with movement but no swelling
   E. Diagnosis
      1. Clinical diagnosis; X-ray is not required
   F. Treatment
      1. Closed reduction maneuvers: therapeutic and diagnostic
      2. Hyperpronation of forearm while applying pressure on radial head
      3. Supination of forearm and flexion of elbow while applying pressure on radial head

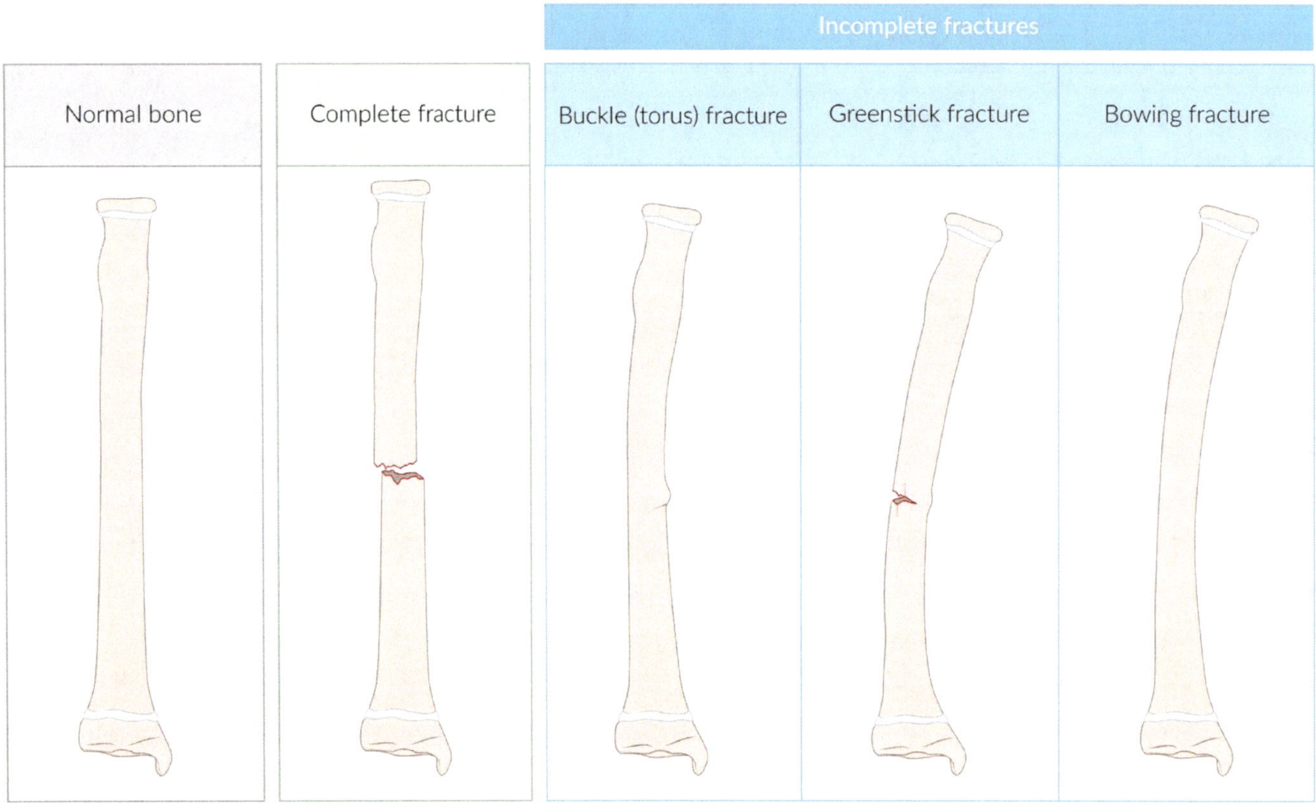

FIGURE 21.9.45 - Torus Fracture vs. Greenstick Fracture

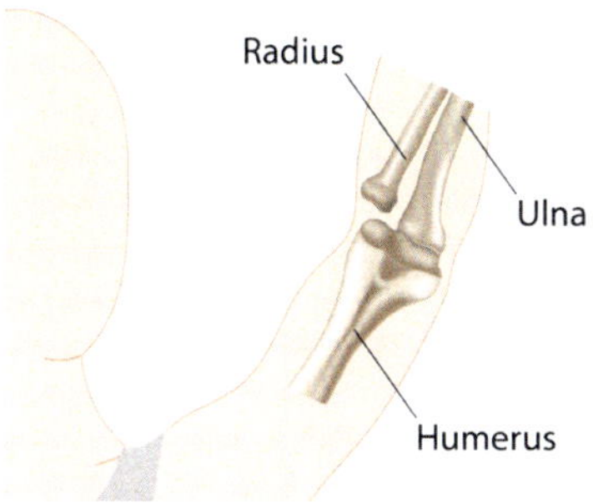

FIGURE 21.9.46 - Nursemaid's Elbow

V. Osgood-Schlatter Disease
   A. Tibial tuberosity apophysitis due to overuse of quadriceps muscle
   B. Mostly seen in adolescents (9 - 14 years)
   C. Excessive running and jumping during the adolescence causes microtrauma to the tibial tuberosity, leading to traction apophysitis
   D. Clinical findings
      1. Anterior knee pain which aggravates with activity and is reproduced with leg extension against resistance
   E. Diagnosis
      1. X-ray: soft tissue swelling, fragmented tubercle, elevated tubercle
   F. Treatment
      1. Conservative management with rest, ice, and NSAIDs
      2. Quadriceps strengthening and stretching exercises

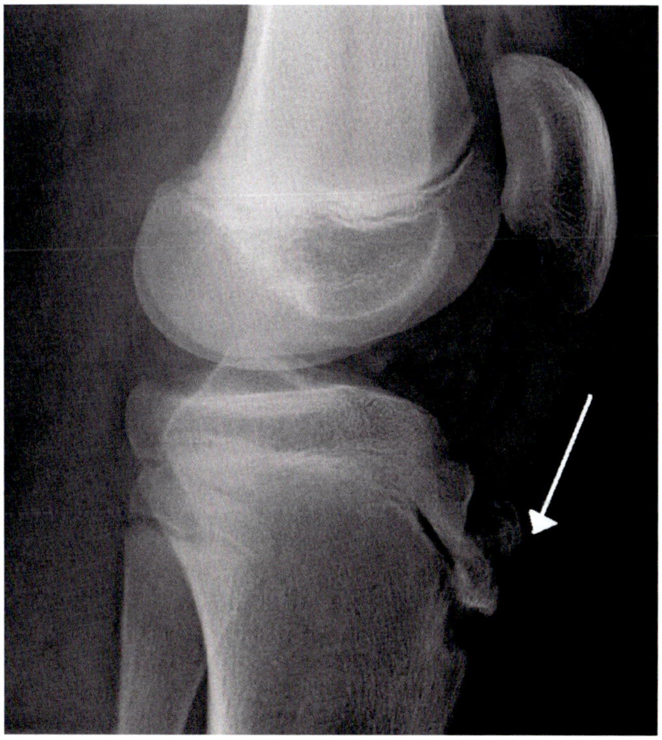

FIGURE 21.9.47 - X-ray of Knee Joint: Osgood-Schlatter Disease

VI. Salter-Harris Fracture
   A. Growth plate fracture
   B. During the time of growth spurts when puberty begins
   C. Most common sites: distal radius and distal humerus
   D. Clinical findings
      1. Joint pain, focal tenderness, swelling, decreased range of motion, inability to bear weight
   E. Diagnosis
      1. X-ray shows widening of the physis; MRI if X-ray is inconclusive
   F. Treatment
      1. Type I and II: closed reduction with cast immobilization; consider surgery if severe
      2. Type III and IV: ORIF (open reduction and internal fixation)
      3. Type V: usually diagnosed late so varies according to age
   G. Complications
      1. Growth arrest due to growth plate involvement
      2. Limb length discrepancies

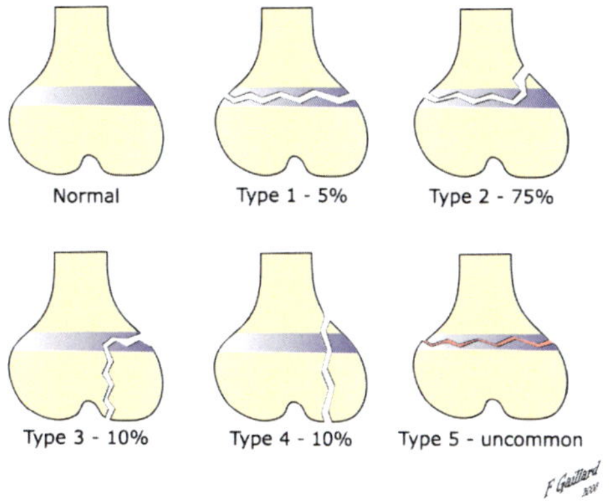

FIGURE 21.9.48 - Types of Salter-Harris Fracture

REVIEW QUESTIONS

1. A 3-year-old girl is brought to the emergency department due to right-sided hand pain after falling on an outstretched hand while she was playing. The physical examination shows distal radial tenderness on the right side. Wrist X-ray in AP view shows a partial thickness fracture at the tension site with an intact compression site. How can this patient's condition be distinguished from torus fracture?

   - **This patient's condition, a greenstick fracture, is characterized by a disrupted tension side and an intact compression side. In contrast, torus fracture is characterized by a disrupted compression side and an intact tension side.**
   - This patient presents with right-sided hand pain after falling on an outstretched hand.
   - The physical examination shows distal radial tenderness.
   - X-ray reveals a partial thickness fracture at the tension site with an intact compression site.
   - This is a classic description of greenstick fracture.

2. A 15-year-old boy is accompanied to the clinic by his father due to a painful right knee. He is a football player and his knee pain has interfered with his practice sessions. The physical examination shows swelling and tenderness below patella without warmth or erythema. Knee X-ray in lateral view shows elevation of right tibial tubercle. In addition to conservative measures, which type of exercise will likely alleviate this patient's symptoms?

   - **Quadriceps stretching and strengthening exercises will likely alleviate this patient's symptoms.**
   - This 15-year-old boy reports a painful right knee.
   - The physical examination shows swelling and tenderness below patella without warmth or erythema.
   - Leg X-ray shows elevation of right tibial tubercle.
   - These clues suggest the diagnosis of Osgood-Schlatter disease.
   - In addition to conversative measures like ice, NSAIDs, and rest, patients with Osgood-Schlatter disease benefit from quadriceps stretching and strengthening exercises.

3. A 6-year-old girl is brought to the emergency department due to left-sided hand pain after falling on an outstretched hand at school. Her vital signs are within normal limits. The physical examination shows a patient in severe distress along with left-sided distal radial tenderness. Wrist X-ray in AP view shows transverse lucency across the radial metaphysis, growth plate, and epiphysis. Which type of Salter-Harris fracture does this patient most likely have?

   A. Type I
   B. Type II
   C. Type III
   D. Type IV
   E. Type V

   - **The correct answer is option D.**
   - This 6-year-old girl presents with left-sided hand pain after falling on an outstretched hand at school.
   - The physical examination shows a patient in severe distress along with left-sided distal radial tenderness.
   - X-ray reveals a transverse lucency across the radial metaphysis, growth plate, and epiphysis. These X-ray findings are classic for type IV Salter-Harris fracture.
   - Type IV fracture is the only one involving all three parts - metaphysis, growth plate, and epiphysis.
   - Option A is incorrect because type I Salter-Harris fracture is characterized by a transverse fracture across the growth plate.
   - Option B is incorrect because type II fracture involves metaphysis and the growth plate.
   - Option C is incorrect because type III fracture involves epiphysis and the growth plate.
   - Option E is incorrect because type V Salter-Harris fracture is characterized by a crush injury of the growth plate.

GYNECOLOGY

Gynecology | Section 1: Benign Breast Diseases: Cysts, Fibrocystic Change & Mastitis

I. Cysts: Definition
   A. A closed fluid-filled sac
   B. Common, usually benign

II. Cysts: Types
   A. Simple cyst
      1. Has thin and regular lining
      2. Completely fluid-filled
   B. Complex cyst
      1. Has thick and irregular lining
      2. May contain solid content or debris

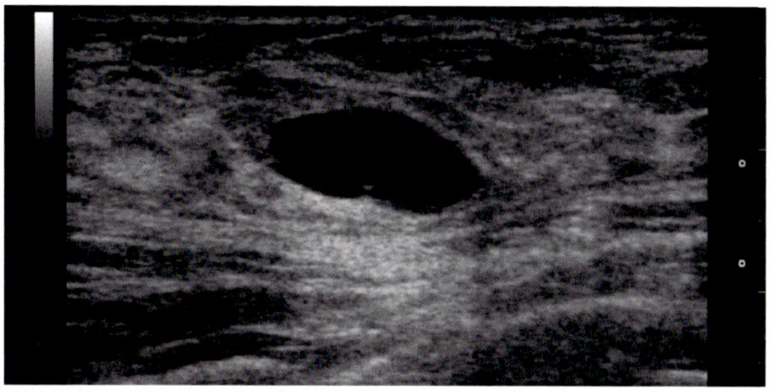

FIGURE 21.10.1 - Ultrasonogram: Simple Breast Cyst

III. Cysts: Clinical Features
   A. Asymptomatic
   B. Round, mobile mass; may be tender

IV. Fibrocystic Change: Definition
   A. Benign breast change characterized by fibrotic and cystic changes
   B. Most common benign lesion of the breast
   C. Unknown etiology
   D. Women age 20 - 50
   E. No increased risk of cancer

V. Fibrocystic Change: Clinical Features
   A. Cyclic, premenstrual, bilateral breast pain; improves after menstruation
   B. Breast nodules: multiple and diffuse; irregular breast consistency
   C. Nipple discharge

VI. Fibrocystic Change: Diagnosis
   A. Clinical diagnosis
   B. History and physical exam
      1. Bumpy, irregular breast
   C. Ultrasound and mammography are first line
      1. Ultrasound: women < 30 years; focal thickening +/- cysts
      2. Mammography: women ≥ 30 years
   D. Fine needle aspiration
      1. Indicated in case cysts are present on imaging, in symptomatic patients, and upon patients' request
      2. Relieves symptoms
   E. Biopsy: if the diagnosis is still not clear

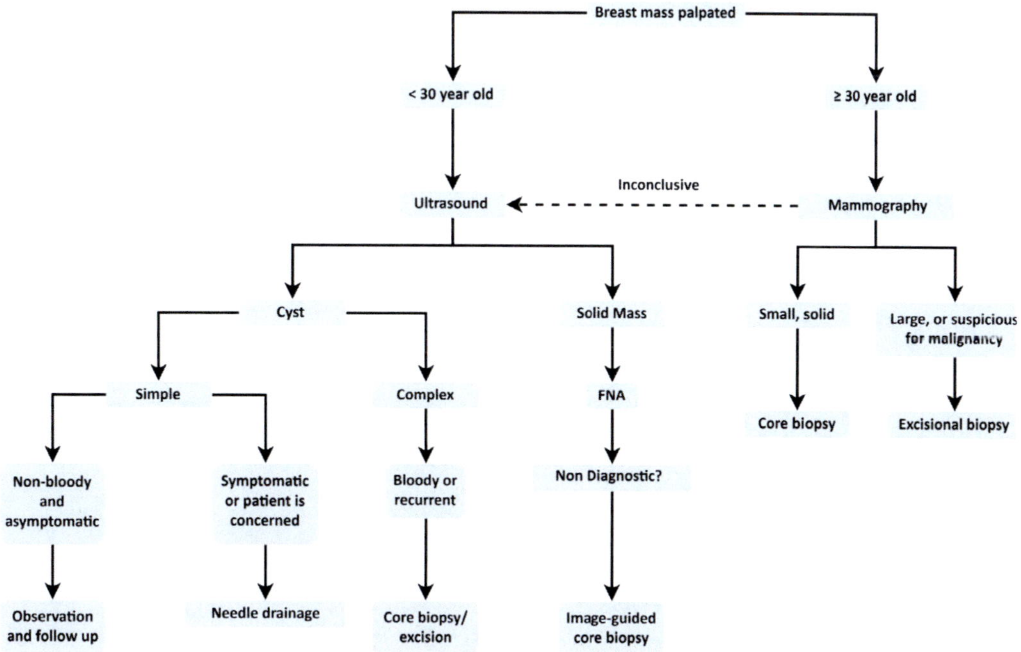

FIGURE 21.10.2 - Evaluation of Palpated Breast Mass

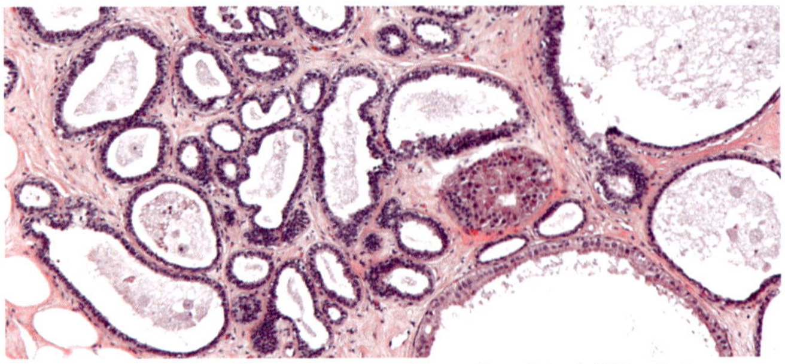

FIGURE 21.10.3 - Light Microscopy: Cystic Ducts and Fibrosis in Fibrocystic Breast Change

VII. Fibrocystic Change: Management
   A. Symptomatic treatment: NSAIDs, OCPs
   B. Cyst drainage (if present): fine needle aspiration
   C. Warm compresses may help
   D. Supportive bra
   E. Follow-up in 4 - 6 weeks

VIII. Mastitis: Definition
   A. Inflammation of the breast

IX. Mastitis: Pathophysiology
   A. Skin breakage and fissures allow entry of skin bacterial flora (most commonly *Staphylococcus aureus*) or from the mouth and nose of a breastfeeding infant → bacteria multiply → inflammation of milk ducts → decreased drainage and breast engorgement

X. Mastitis: Risk Factors
   A. History of mastitis
   B. Factors that impede milk drainage and/or increase breast engorgement (e.g. weaning, tight-fitting bra)

XI. Mastitis: Clinical Features
   A. Inflamed breast: tender, swollen, erythematous breast; usually unilateral
   B. Pain with breastfeeding
   C. Associated symptoms: fever, myalgias, chills, malaise
   D. Complications: breast abscess
   E. Breast abscess occurs as a result of severe or untreated mastitis
   F. Symptoms of breast abscess
      1. Mastitis symptoms (e.g. fever, tender and enlarged breast) in addition to a soft fluctuant breast mass
      2. Purulent nipple discharge

XII. Mastitis: Diagnosis
   A. Mastitis
      1. Clinical diagnosis
      2. Culture if treatment-resistant
   B. Breast abscess
      1. Clinical diagnosis; suspect in patients with mastitis that do not get better with treatment
      2. Ultrasound can also be used

XIII. Mastitis: Management
   A. Pain management (e.g. ibuprofen)
   B. Adequate and frequent breast draining
      1. Direct breastfeeding every 2 - 3 hours
      2. Use both breasts and alternate between them
      3. Breast pumps can be used as an alternative, although less effective
      4. Prevents progression to abscess
   C. Antibiotics
      1. Dicloxacillin or cephalexin (methicillin-sensitive *S. aureus*)
      2. Clindamycin, vancomycin, or TMP-SMX (methicillin-resistant *S. aureus*)
   D. Abscess
      1. Fine needle aspiration and antibiotics: dicloxacillin, cephalexin (first line)
      2. Incision and drainage: non-responsive, large (> 5 cm) abscess

XIV. Mastitis: Differential Diagnosis
   A. Normal breast engorgement
      1. Due to milk accumulation without adequate drainage
      2. During postpartum and early breastfeeding period (or anytime during breastfeeding): ↑ milk production
      3. Clinical diagnosis: tender, warm, enlarged breasts; usually bilaterally; no erythema or fever
      4. Management
         a) Ensure proper nursing techniques
         b) Frequent breastfeeding or pumping
         c) Cool breast compresses
         d) Analgesics (e.g. acetaminophen, NSAIDs)
         e) Symptoms should improve after breast drainage

Condition	Key Features
Cysts	- Asymptomatic; round, mobile mass; may be tender
Fibrocystic changes	- Premenstrual cyclic bilateral breast pain; improves after menstruation - Breast nodules: multiple and diffuse; irregular breast consistency; nipple discharge
Mastitis	- Tender, swollen, erythematous breast; usually unilateral - Pain with breastfeeding, fever, myalgias, chills, malaise

TABLE 21.10.1 - Overview of Benign Breast Diseases

REVIEW QUESTIONS

1. A 28-year-old woman comes to her primary care physician because of a painful left breast mass she noticed one month ago. She appears well and has no fever, or chills. Breast examination shows a tender, well-circumscribed, mobile mass in the upper left quadrant. What is the next best step in management?

    - **The next best step in management is breast ultrasound.**
    - This 28-year-old woman presents with a palpable, tender, well-circumscribed, mobile mass in her left breast.
    - The next step in management depends on her age.
    - Since she is less than 30 years old, an ultrasound examination is indicated. A mammogram would be the answer if she were 30 years or older.

2. A 35-year-old woman comes to her primary care physician because of a painful, swollen right breast for the 3 days. She also reports having fevers and feeling tired over the past 2-days. She gave birth two weeks ago and is currently breastfeeding. Physical examination shows a tender, swollen, erythematous right breast. The left breast appears normal. What is the next best step in management?

    - **The next best step in management is antibiotics, adequate and frequent breast drainage, and NSAIDs.**
    - This breastfeeding woman comes in with a painful, swollen, and erythematous breast.
    - Breast engorgement and mastitis should be on the differential.
    - Because this patient is having a fever and feeling tired and only one breast is affected, mastitis is the most likely diagnosis.
    - In breast engorgement, no fever is present, and both breasts are usually affected.
    - The best next step for mastitis is prescribing an antibiotic such as dicloxacillin or cephalexin and advising the patient to continue breastfeeding from the affected breast to maintain proper breast drainage. NSAIDs can also be prescribed for pain management.

3. A 28-year-old woman comes to her primary care physician because of a breast mass that she palpated yesterday. She is otherwise asymptomatic and prefers non-invasive measures. She does not smoke or drink alcohol and has no history of serious illness. Physical examination shows a non-tender, mobile mass is palpated in the right upper quadrant of the right breast. There are no overlying skin changes. Her temperature is 99° F (37.3° C), pulse is 80/min, and blood pressure is 128/70 mmHg. An ultrasound of the mass shows a well-circumscribed, hypoechoic mass with a thin lining. Which of the following is the next best step in the management of this patient?

    A. Fine needle aspiration
    B. Reassurance and follow-up
    C. Core needle biopsy
    D. Excisional biopsy

    - **The correct answer is option B.**
    - This 28-year-old patient is presenting with a breast mass that she palpated yesterday.
    - Physical examination shows a non-tender, mobile mass is palpated in the right upper quadrant of the right breast.
    - On ultrasound, the mass appears well-circumscribed and hypoechoic with a thin lining consistent with a simple cyst.
    - Patients should be informed that this is a benign condition with no malignant potential, and therefore, the most appropriate management is reassurance and follow-up to monitor patients' symptoms.
    - If the patient is asymptomatic, only reassurance and follow-up are needed.
    - If, on the other hand, the patient remains concerned after counseling or is experiencing pain, fine needle aspiration could be performed.
    - Option A is incorrect because this patient is asymptomatic, is reassured, and wants no further treatment.
    - Option C, core needle biopsy, and option D, excisional biopsy, are incorrect because they are required in patients with masses that raise concern for malignancy. This patient is asymptomatic, with ultrasound findings showing a simple breast cyst.

Gynecology | Section 2: Benign Breast Diseases - Fat Necrosis, Galactocele & Mammary Duct Ectasia

I. Fat Necrosis: Definition
   A. Necrosis of fat tissue of the breast as a result of trauma or surgery
   B. Positive history is not always present
   C. No associated increased risk of carcinoma

II. Fat Necrosis: Clinical Features
   A. Presents as a fixed, irregular mass
   B. Associated skin changes: skin or nipple retraction, ecchymosis, erythema

III. Fat Necrosis: Diagnosis
   A. Ultrasound and mammography: hyperechoic mass; calcifications
   B. Biopsy
      1. Necrotic fat cells
      2. Foam cells and multinucleated giant cells

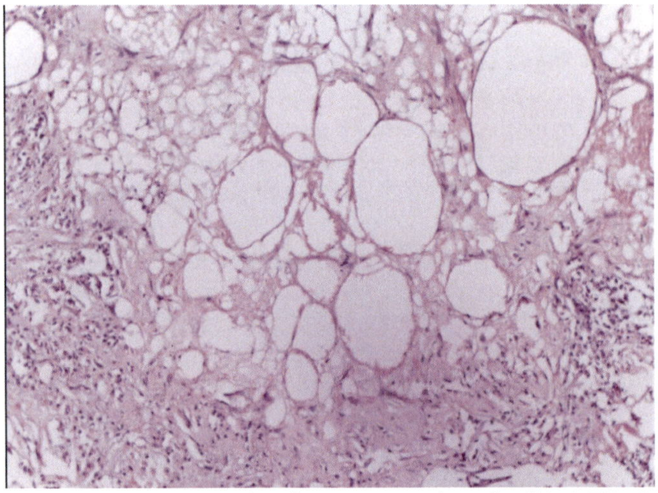

FIGURE 21.10.4 - Light Microscopy: Fat Necrosis of the Breast

IV. Fat Necrosis: Management
   A. Does not require treatment

V. Galactocele: Definition
   A. A cyst composed of accumulated breast milk
   B. During or after lactation
   C. No increased risk of carcinoma

VI. Galactocele: Pathophysiology
   A. Occurs as a result of obstruction of lactiferous ducts which causes stagnant milk accumulation and cyst formation

VII. Galactocele: Clinical Features
   A. Well-circumscribed mass; non-tender
   B. In the subareolar region
   C. If it gets infected will become painful

VIII. Galactocele: Diagnosis
   A. Clinical diagnosis
   B. Fine needle aspiration: milky
   C. Ultrasound: complex lesion

IX. Galactocele: Management
   A. Not needed
   B. Usually resolves spontaneously

X. Mammary Duct Ectasia: Definition
   A. Dilated mammary ducts causing inflammation and leading to clogged ducts
   B. Perimenopausal women (40 - 50 years)

XI. Mammary Duct Ectasia: Clinical Features
   A. Noncyclic breast pain
   B. Greenish-bloody nipple discharge; usually unilateral
   C. Other findings: nipple retraction, subareolar mass

XII. Mammry Duct Ectasia: Diagnosis
   A. Ultrasound or mammogram
   B. Excisional biopsy
      1. Rule out malignancy
      2. Obstruction of ducts and ductal inflammation

XIII. Mammary Duct Ectasia: Management
   A. Usually not required: improves without treatment
   B. Warm compresses and antibiotics: if it progresses to mastitis
   C. Local excision: definitive treatment; for persistent symptoms

Condition	Key Features
Fat necrosis	- Fixed, irregular mass - Nipple retraction, ecchymosis, erythema
Galactocele	- Well-circumscribed non-tender mass in the subareolar region
Mammary duct ectasia	- Noncyclic breast pain - Greenish-bloody nipple discharge

TABLE 21.10.2 - Overview of Benign Breast Diseases

REVIEW QUESTIONS

?

1. A 53-year-old woman comes to her primary care physician because of a mass that she felt in her breast. Physical examination shows a hard, non-tender mass in the upper outer quadrant of the right breast. She does not recall any trauma to the breast. She is a lifetime smoker and drinks alcohol occasionally. Mammography is ordered and shows an irregular breast mass with microcalcifications. Biopsy of the mass shows multinucleated giant cells and foam cells. What is the most likely diagnosis?

- **The most likely diagnosis is fat necrosis of the breast.**
- This 53-year-old woman presents with a mass in her right breast that is hard, nontender and located in the upper outer quadrant.
- Mammography shows an irregular breast mass with microcalcifications, which should raise suspicion for possible malignancy.
- A biopsy is then performed, showing multinucleated giant cells and foam cells, which is characteristic of fat necrosis and requires reassurance to the patient.
- Patients often do not recall trauma to the breast, but that still doesn't rule out the diagnosis.

2. A 27-year-old woman comes to her primary care physician because of mild discomfort in her left breast. She noticed a subareolar mass while taking a shower 2 days ago. The patient gave birth to a healthy neonate 1 week ago. She breastfeeds the baby every 2 - 3 hours. Vital signs include a temperature of 96.8° F (36° C), blood pressure of 110/70 mmHg, heart rate of 86 beats/min, and respiratory rate of 15 breaths/min. Physical examination shows a non-tender subareolar mass with no erythema or induration. An ultrasound shows a complex mass prompting fine needle aspiration. Aspiration yields white fluid. Which of the following is the best next step in the management?

   A. Mammography
   B. Core needle biopsy
   C. Dicloxacillin
   D. Reassurance

- **The correct answer is option D.**
- This 27-year-old woman presents with a subareolar mass that she noticed recently.
- She gave birth to a healthy neonate 1-week ago and breastfeeds the baby every 2 - 3 hours.
- Lactating women are at risk of developing mastitis or galactocele.
- Her temperature is 96.8° F (36° C), making mastitis unlikely.
- Additionally, the mass is non-tender with no erythema or induration. These clues also make mastitis unlikely.
- The fine needle aspiration yields white fluid. This confirms the diagnosis of a galactocele.
- Galactocele is a cyst with accumulated stagnant milk. It usually resolves spontaneously, so the patient needs reassurance.
- Options A and B are incorrect because mammography and core needle biopsy are necessary when there is high suspicion of breast cancer. This patient is young, and the fine needle aspiration yields white fluid, making breast cancer very unlikely.
- Option C is incorrect because dicloxacillin is used to treat acute mastitis. This patient is afebrile, and her subareolar mass is non-tender with no erythema or induration. This practically excludes mastitis.

Gynecology | Section 3: Breast Cancer

I. Breast Cancer: Clinical Features
   A. Depends on the stage
   B. Palpable non-tender lump; most common in upper outer quadrant
   C. Lymphadenopathy
   D. Associated skin changes: nipple inversion, skin dimpling/retraction

II. Breast Cancer: Workup
   A. Additional tests on diagnosed breast cancer
      1. Receptors: estrogen receptor (ER), progesterone receptor (PR), human epidermal growth factor receptor 2 (HER2/neu)
      2. Tumor markers: CEA
   B. Metastasis
      1. Imaging: chest X-ray, CT scan, brain MRI
      2. Lab: ↑ ALP, ↑ calcium

III. Breast Cancer: Management
   A. General approach
      1. Management depends on the TNM stage
      2. Treatment includes surgery, chemotherapy, radiotherapy, targeted therapy, and hormone treatment
   B. Surgery
      1. Breast conserving surgery: only cancerous breast tissue is removed
      2. Mastectomy (e.g. radical, double, total mastectomies)
   C. Radiation: post-surgery for patients at high risk of recurrence
   D. Chemotherapy
   E. Hormone therapy
      1. ER+ and PR+ tumors
      2. Tamoxifen, aromatase inhibitors, and raloxifene
   F. Targeted therapy
      1. Against HER2 receptors
      2. Trastuzumab
   G. Regarding contraception
      1. Hormonal contraception contraindicated; copper IUD is the contraceptive method of choice
   H. Prognostic factors: most important factor is nodal involvement
      1. Good prognostic factors: ER+ and PR+ tumors
      2. Poor prognostic factors: high tumor grade (poorly differentiated), HER2 overexpression

IV. Breast Cancer: Screening
   A. No family history of breast cancer: mammography starting ≥ 50 years
      1. 50 - 74 years: every 2 year
   B. Patients at high risk (e.g. BRCA gene, chest irradiation): start at 40
      1. First-degree relative: begin screening 10 years before the earliest diagnosis in the family

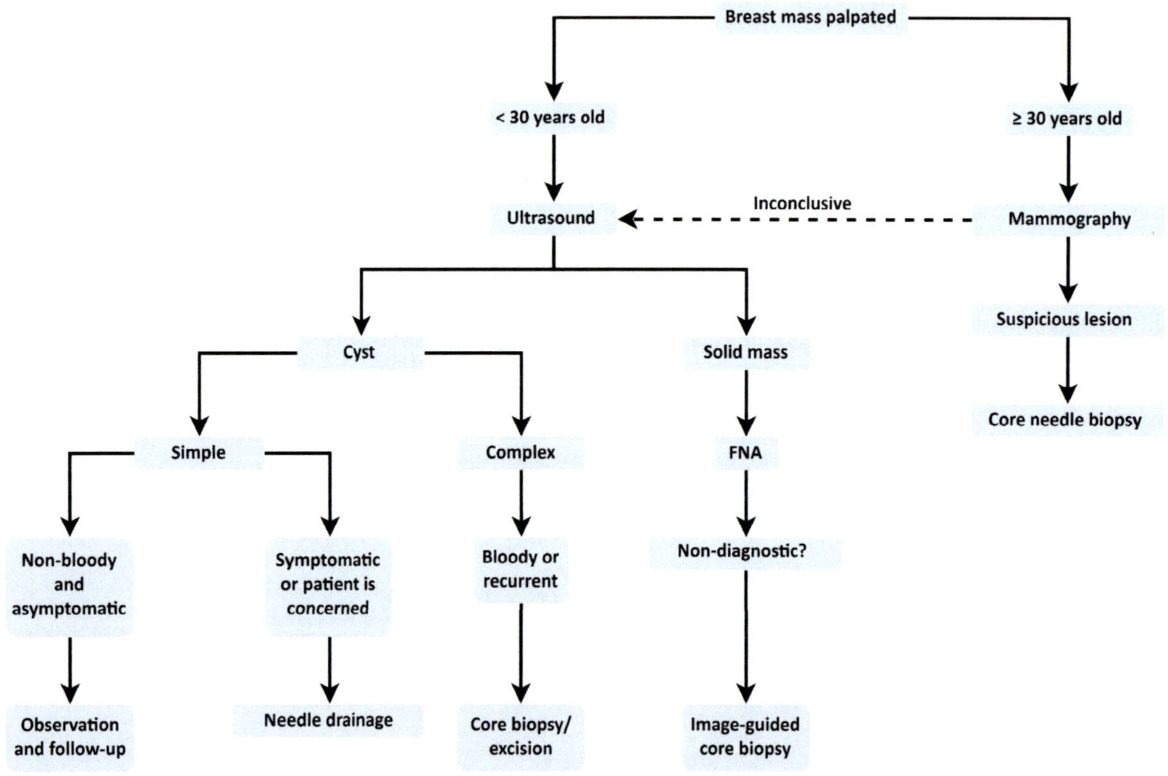

FIGURE 21.10.5 - Evaluation of Palpable Breast Mass

REVIEW QUESTIONS

1. A 54-year-old woman comes to the clinic for a routine screening mammogram. Mammography results show a suspicious 2.5 cm lesion in the right breast. Physical examination of the breast shows a hard, non-tender mass. There are no associated skin or nipple changes, and no lymphadenopathy is present. What is the best next step in the diagnosis?
    - **The best next step in the diagnosis of this patient is an ultrasound-guided core needle biopsy.**
    - This 54-year-old woman has a hard, non-tender mass in her right breast that appears suspicious on mammography.
    - The next best step is to perform an ultrasound-guided core needle biopsy to evaluate the mass histology to determine the diagnosis and determine its receptor profile for further management.
    - In this case, an excisional biopsy would be too invasive. It can be used if the core needle biopsy results are inconclusive.

2. A 2 cm suspicious lesion is detected on routine mammogram screening of a 47-year-old woman. Histology reveals poorly differentiated cells that show HER2 receptor overexpression. Sentinel lymph node biopsy reveals tumor infiltration. What factor has the most effect on the prognosis of this patient?
    - **The factor that has the most effect on the prognosis of this patient is lymph node involvement.**
    - This question presents multiple prognostic factors, including a high tumor grade, HER2 receptor overexpression, and sentinel node biopsy revealing tumor infiltration.
    - Even though a high tumor grade and HER2 receptor overexpression constitute a poor prognosis for this patient, axillary lymph node status is the most important prognostic factor as it makes metastatic spread much more likely.

NEUROLOGY

Neurology | Section 1: Nervous System Tumors - Gliomas, Pilocytic Astrocytoma, GB Multiform

I. Introduction: General Characteristics
   A. Primary brain tumors in adults
   B. 70% occur supratentorial
   C. Adults: glioblastoma multiforme, meningioma, ependymoma
   D. Primary brain tumors in children: second most common cancer
   E. 70% occur infratentorial
   F. Children: pilocytic astrocytoma, medulloblastoma
   G. Schwannomas: sporadically or neurofibromatosis

II. Introduction: Risk Factors
   A. Cigarette smoking
   B. Neurofibromatosis
   C. Turcot syndrome

III. Introduction: Clinical Features
   A. Headache: 20% initially, 60% later
   B. Tend to be worse during the night and often wakes the person up
   C. Visual disturbances
   D. Nausea and vomiting
   E. Seizures: > 30% of cases
   F. Impairment of balance, speech, hearing
   G. Personality or behavior changes

IV. Introduction: Imaging
   A. MRI with gadolinium enhancement
   B. CT scan: if calcium or hemorrhage is present
   C. Functional MRI: lesions in vital areas
   D. Positron emission tomography (PET)

V. Introduction: Treatment
   A. Surgery, irradiation, chemotherapy

VI. Gliomas: Definition
   A. Glial cells
   B. Cerebral hemispheres, brain stem
   C. Benign or malignant
   D. Grade I to IV
   E. Gliomas: Types/Grades
   F. Grade I and II: low grade
      1. Pilocytic astrocytoma (I)
      2. Diffuse astrocytomas (II)
   G. Grade III: diffuse, anaplastic astrocytoma
   H. Grade IV: glioblastoma

VII. Gliomas: Treatment
   A. Approach dependent on stage
   B. Grade I: watch and wait, surgery, radiation
   C. Grade II: surgical removal, radiation
   D. Grade III: chemotherapy, surgery, radiation
   E. Grade IV: surgery, radiation concurrent

VIII. Pilocytic Astrocytoma: General Description
   A. Most common tumor CNS in children
   B. First two decades of life: 8-13 year olds
   C. Midline structures in posterior fossa
   D. Optic nerve (NF1), cerebellum

IX. Pilocytic Astrocytoma: Histology
   A. Rosenthal fibers
   B. Cysts

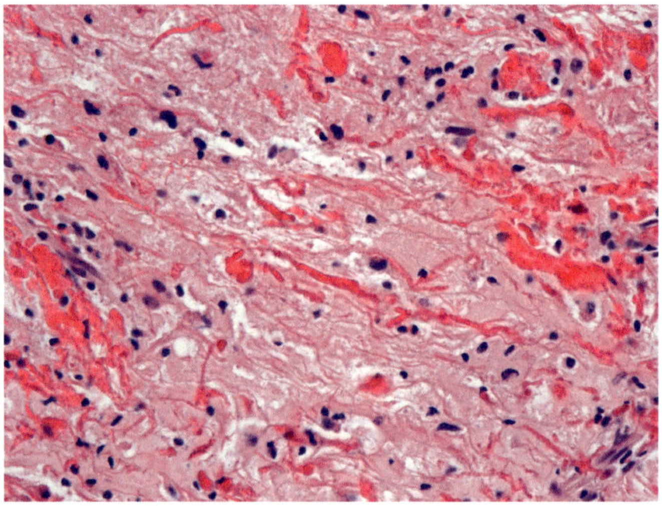

FIGURE 21.11.1 - Light Microscopy of Rosenthal Fibers in Pilocytic Astrocytoma

X. Pilocytic Astrocytoma: Imaging
   A. Cystic mass enhanced by contrast
   B. Mural nodule
   C. Calcifications

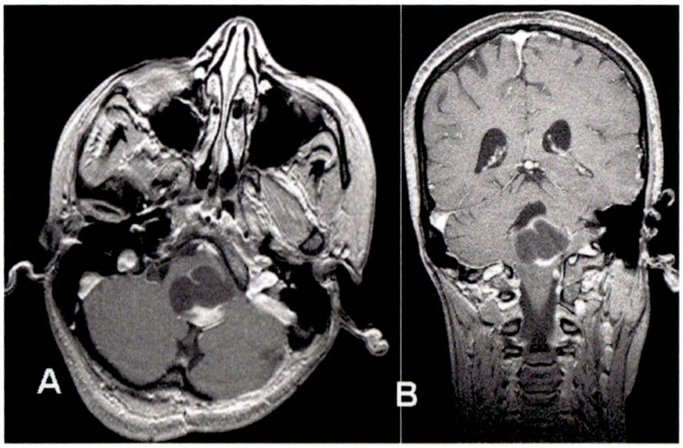

FIGURE 21.11.2 - MRI of the Brain: Pilocytic Astrocytoma

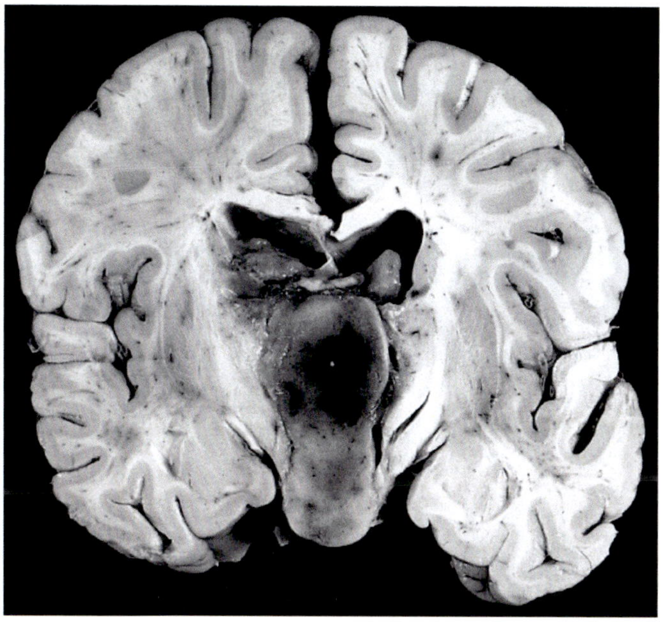

FIGURE 21.11.3 - Pilocytic Astrocytoma

XI. Pilocytic Astrocytoma: Prognosis
   A. 10 year survival is 100%: supratentorial and gross total resection

XII. Glioblastoma Multiforme: General Characteristics
   A. High-grade astrocytoma, stage IV glioma
   B. May arise de novo or from low grade astrocytoma
   C. Supratentorial
   D. IDH and 1p/19q codeletion
   E. Hemorrhagic tumor
      1. Multifocal areas of necrosis and cystic degeneration
      2. Commonly cross the corpus callosum

XIII. Glioblastoma Multiforme: Histology
   A. Marked anaplasia and pleomorphism
   B. Pseudopalisading necrosis
   C. GFAP, vimentin, S100

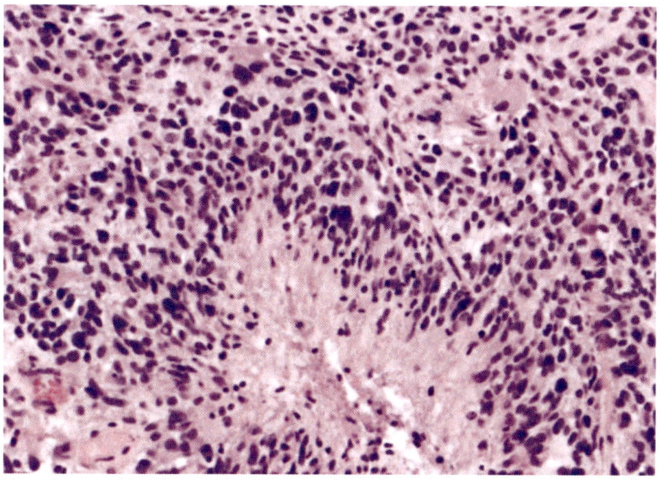

FIGURE 21.11.4 - Light Microscopy showing Pseudopalisading Necrosis in Glioblastoma Multiforme

XIV. Glioblastoma Multiforme: Imaging
   A. Large tumors
   B. Pseudocapsule
   C. Irregular thick margins, low density center
   D. Cross the corpus callosum

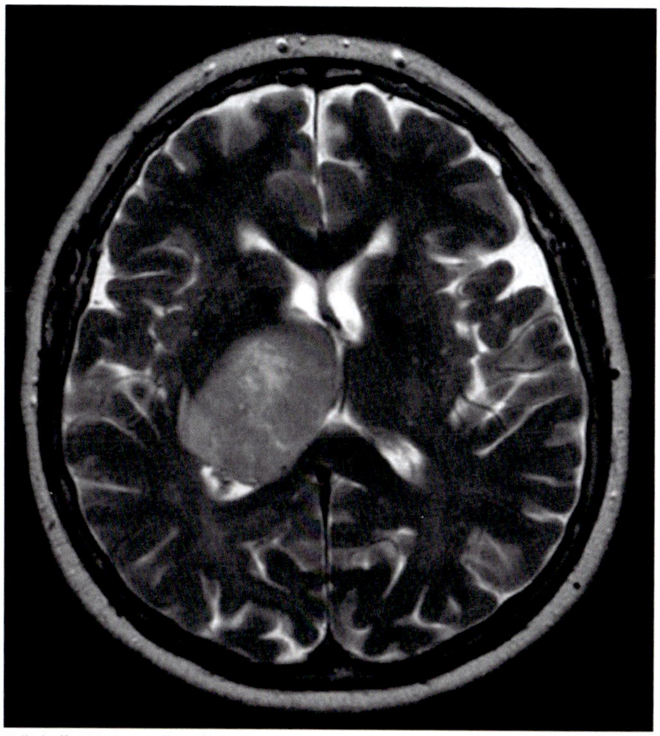

FIGURE 21.11.5 - MRI of the Brain: Glioblastoma Multiforme

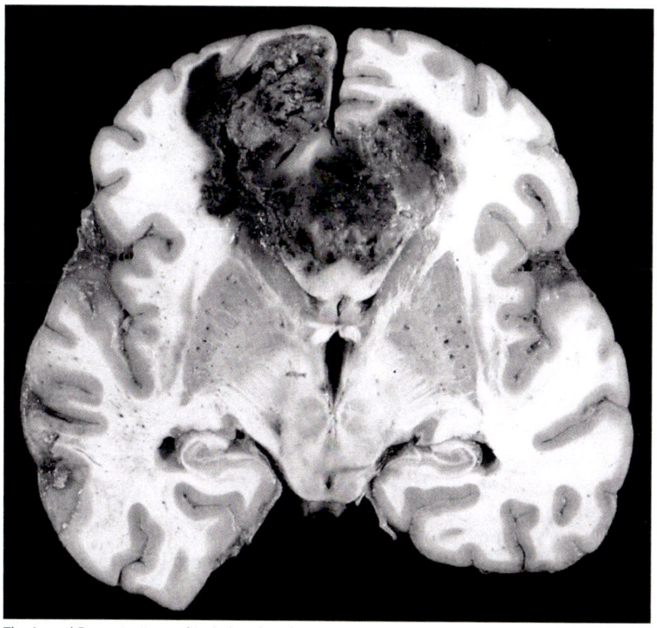

FIGURE 21.11.6 - Glioblastoma Multiforme

XV. Glioblastoma Multiforme: Prognosis
   A. Poor prognosis
   B. Death occurs in less than 1 year

REVIEW QUESTIONS

1. A 34-year-old woman comes to her primary care provider because of recurrent headaches over the last month. She says she has a history of tension migraines that typically occur in the middle of her work day and remit with over-the-counter pain medicines. Over the past month or so, her headaches have persisted despite pain medicines, and she says she occasionally gets woken up by headaches in the mornings. Review of systems is otherwise negative, and the physical examination is unremarkable. What is the next best step in management?
    - **The best next step in management of this patient is an MRI of the brain.**
    - This patient has a history of tension headaches
    - However, there is a new pattern for her headaches. Now, the headaches aren't improving with over the counter pain meds and wake her up from her sleep.
    - The next best step in this situation would be to order a brain MRI due to the pain pattern of her headaches, which could indicate malignancy.
    - There are two notable clues that suggest a brain tumor in this question stem: First her recent headaches no longer improve with pain medications. Second, she gets occasionally woken up by headaches.
    - A brain tumor should always be on the differential when patients report headaches that wake them up.

2. An 11-year-old boy is brought into the emergency department by his mother because of two weeks of worsening headaches and fatigue that have caused him to miss a lot of school. While in the emergency department, the boy vomits and becomes somnolent. An urgent MRI brain is ordered, and it shows a well-circumscribed mass compressing the cerebellum. What is the next best step in management?
    - **The next best step in management is a neurosurgery consultation.**
    - This child has been experiencing worsening headaches and fatigue.
    - MRI of the brain shows well-circumscribed mass compressing the cerebellum, which raises a suspicion of pilocytic astrocytoma.
    - Pilocytic astrocytomas are the most common benign pediatric brain tumors, and they typically originate around the cerebellum. They are considered to be grade I gliomas, which means that surgery can be curative.
    - Hence, the next step in management would be to consult neurosurgery for a potential surgical excision of this boy's brain tumor.

3. A 7-year-old girl is brought to the pediatrician by her dad because of concern for his daughter's vision over the last few weeks . Physical examination shows impaired vision in her right eye, brown spots in her iris bilaterally, and several hyperpigmented macules in her left axillary region. MRI of the brain and orbits is ordered, and shows a mass adjacent to the girl's right optic nerve. A biopsy of the mass reveals "stretched-out eosinophilic inclusions." What is the most likely diagnosis?
    - **The most likely diagnosis is optic glioma - neurofibromatosis type I.**
    - The girl has been experiencing impaired vision.
    - MRI of the brain and orbits shows a mass adjacent to the right optic nerve.
    - The biopsy of the mass shows "stretched-out eosinophilic inclusions," which is a common description of rosenthal fibers.
    - Therefore, this girl is most likely suffering from an optic glioma.
    - However, she also has several other findings on physical examination that are worth considering when deciding on the overarching diagnosis.
    - Specifically, the brown spots in her iris bilaterally are a description of Lisch nodules, and the several hyperpigmented macules in her left axillary region are a description of axillary freckling. Both Lisch nodules and axillary freckling are seen in patients with neurofibromatosis type I.
    - Hence, the most likely diagnosis in this case is a right-sided optic glioma in the setting of neurofibromatosis type I.

4. A clinician receives the biopsy results of her patient with a suspected glioma. The biopsy report describes marked anaplasia with pseudopalisading necrosis. The report also mentions that the tumor sample stained positive for GFAP. What is the grade of this patient's glioma?
    - **The patient's glioma is grade IV.**
    - Both grade I and grade IV gliomas can stain positive for GFAP, which makes this finding unhelpful in distinguishing them.
    - The histological finding of pseudopalisading necrosis, however, is a feature unique to glioblastoma multiforme.
    - Therefore, the most likely grade of this patient's glioma is a grade IV glioma or glioblastoma multiforme.

REVIEW QUESTIONS

5. A 55-year-old man comes to his primary care provider because of headaches for the past month. He says his headaches last for hours, do not resolve with pain medications, and often wake him up at night. Upon review of systems, he says he also lost about 10 lbs over the past two months. He is compliant with his medications. He is a chronic smoker, and denies alcohol use. Family history is unremarkable. His vital signs are within normal limits, along with the physical examination and full neurologic examination. A brain MRI reveals a heterogenous, poorly-demarcated mass that spans from the left parietal lobe to the right frontal lobe. What will the biopsy of the mass most likely show?

   A. Neoplastic cells with eosinophilic hair-like inclusions
   B. Marked anaplasia and pleomorphism with pseudopalisading necrosis
   C. Evenly distributed, uniform and rounded nuclei
   D. Monomorphic cells and perivascular pseudorosettes
   E. Interlacing bundles of elongated cells with palisading nuclei

- **The correct answer is option B.**
- This is a case of an older gentleman with worsening headaches.
- There are three clues that he may have brain cancer: First, his headaches wake him up at night. Second, he lost 10 lbs over the past two months. And third, he has a long-standing history of smoking.
- A brain MRI reveals a heterogenous, poorly-demarcated mass that spans from the left parietal lobe to the right frontal lobe. This description is consistent with glioblastoma multiforme. Additionally, glioblastoma multiforme should always be on the differential when suspecting a brain tumor in an older patient with a long-standing history of smoking because smoking is one of the key risk factors for development of brain tumors.
- Option A is incorrect because it describes rosenthal fibers, which are seen on biopsy of pilocytic astrocytomas. Pilocytic astrocytomas are grade I gliomas typically seen in children.
- Option C is incorrect because it describes the "fried-egg" appearance of cells seen in histology of oligodendroglioma. Oligodendrogliomas can be seen in adults, although they are more often well-circumscribed and homogenous on brain MRI and tend to be found in the frontal lobe.
- Option D is incorrect because it includes the buzz phrase "perivascular pseudorosettes" which are seen in cases of ependymomas. Ependymomas are more common in children and are usually seen around the 4th ventricle on brain MRI.
- Option E is incorrect because it describes the findings seen in Antoni A schwannomas. Schwannomas are most often located in the cerebellopontine angle on brain MRI.

Neurology | Section 2: Nervous System Tumors - Oligodendroglioma & Ependymoma

I. Oligodendroglioma: Definition
   A. Grade II glioma, derived from oligodendrocytes
   B. IDH mutation, codeletion (1p:19q)
   C. Middle age patients: more common in males
   D. Frontal lobe with frequent calcification

II. Oligodendroglioma: Histology
   A. Infiltrating mass
   B. Fried egg cell appearance
   C. Chicken wire pattern

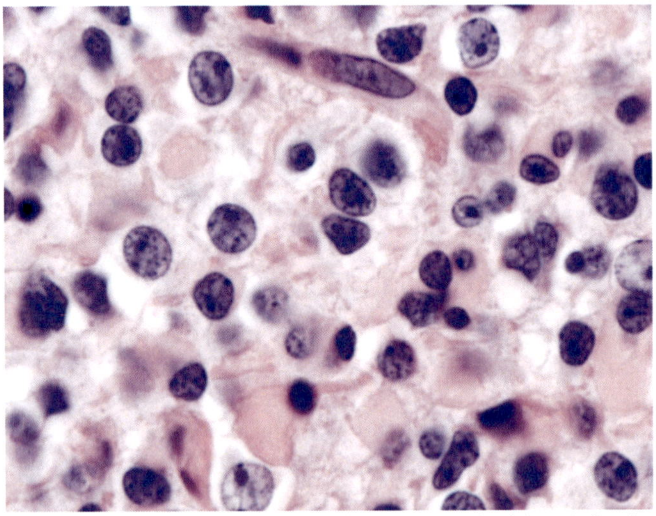

FIGURE 21.11.7 - Light Microscopy Showing Fried-Egg Appearance in Oligodendroglioma

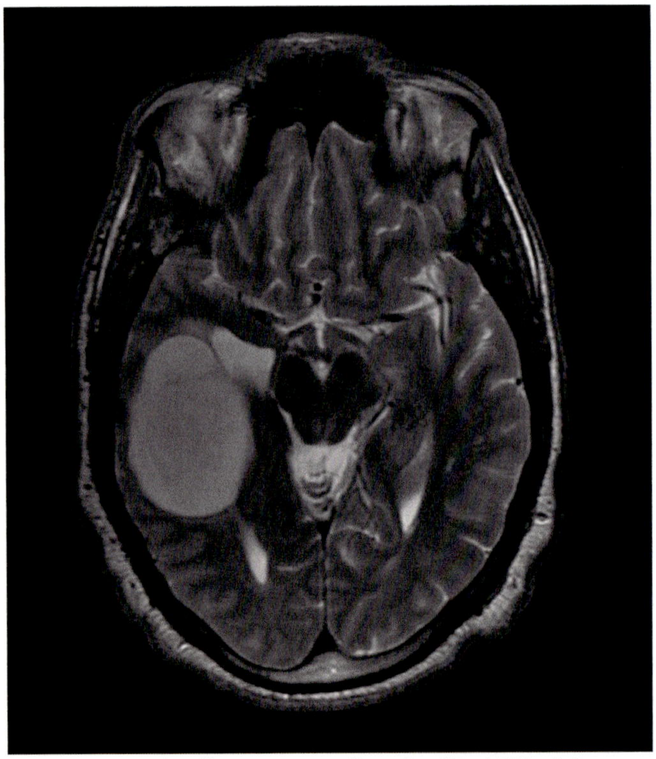

FIGURE 21.11.8 - MRI Displaying Oligodendroglioma

III. Ependymoma: General Characteristics
   A. Benign tumor derived from ependymal cells
   B. Infratentorial ependymomas: children
   C. Spinal tumors: adults
   D. Supratentorial ependymomas: both children and adults
   E. GFAP

IV. Ependymoma: Histology
   A. Monomorphic cells
   B. Perivascular pseudorosettes
   C. Calcifications, hyalinized vessels

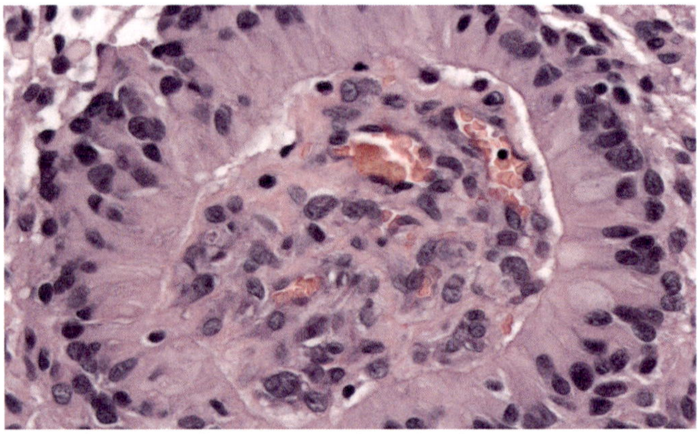

FIGURE 21.11.9 - Light Microscopy: Perivascular Pseudorosettes in Ependymoma

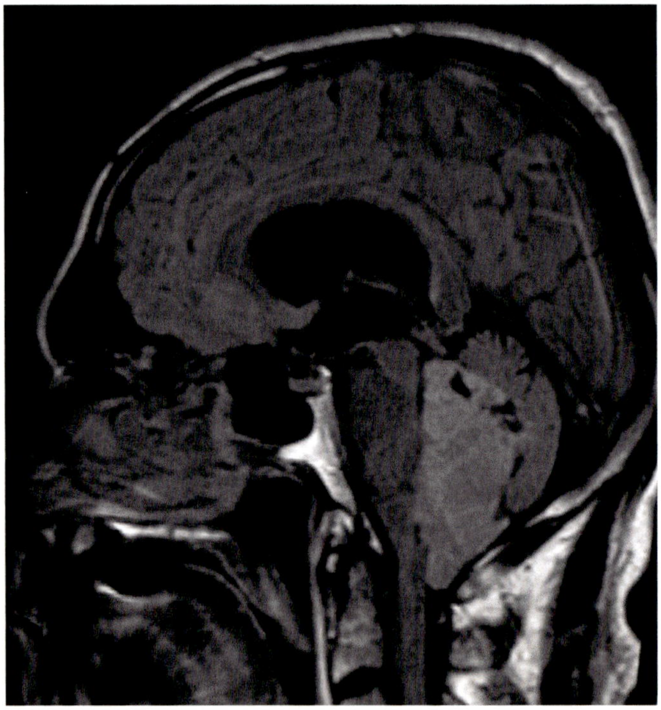

FIGURE 21.11.10 - MRI of the Brain: Ependymoma

V. Ependymoma: Prognosis
   A. Good prognosis

REVIEW QUESTIONS

1. What symptoms would you expect in a patient with an oligodendroglioma in the left frontal lobe?
   - **Symptoms expected in a patient with an oligodendroglioma in the left frontal lobe include personality changes and difficulties in speech.**
   - One of the most unique sets of symptoms that manifest as a result of masses in the frontal lobe are sudden and dramatic personality changes. Patients may become uncharacteristically irritable, impulsive, or aggressive. Some may lose their social awareness or even exhibit social disinhibition in the form of behaviors in public that are not deemed appropriate.
   - Broca's area is located in the left frontal lobe in the majority of people, and it is responsible for articulation and production of speech. Hence, people with masses in the left frontal lobe may report difficulties with speech.

2. What is a common risk factor for development of ependymomas in the pediatric population?
   - **In the pediatric population, a common risk factor for development of ependymomas is neurofibromatosis type 2.**
   - This is in contrast to pilocytic astrocytomas and optic gliomas, which are traditionally associated with neurofibromatosis type 1.

Neurology | Section 3: Nervous System Tumors - Meningioma, Sella & Suprasellar Tumor & Secondary Brain Tumor

I. Meningioma: Definition
   A. Arachnoid cells
   B. Most common benign CNS tumor in adults

II. Meningioma: Clinical Features
   A. Female predominance: estrogen, progesterone receptors
   B. Neurofibromatosis type 2
   C. History of radiation
   D. Seizures
   E. Hearing loss
   F. Anosmia

III. Meningioma: Diagnosis
   A. Swirling masses of meningothelial cells encompass psammoma bodies (calcified bodies)

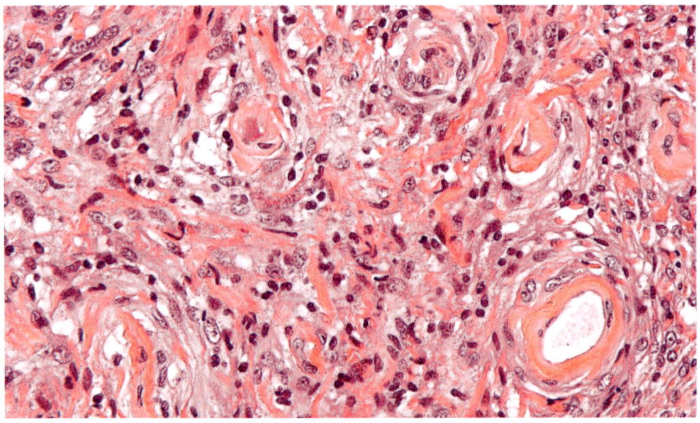

FIGURE 21.11.11 - Light Microscopy: Psammoma Body in Meningioma

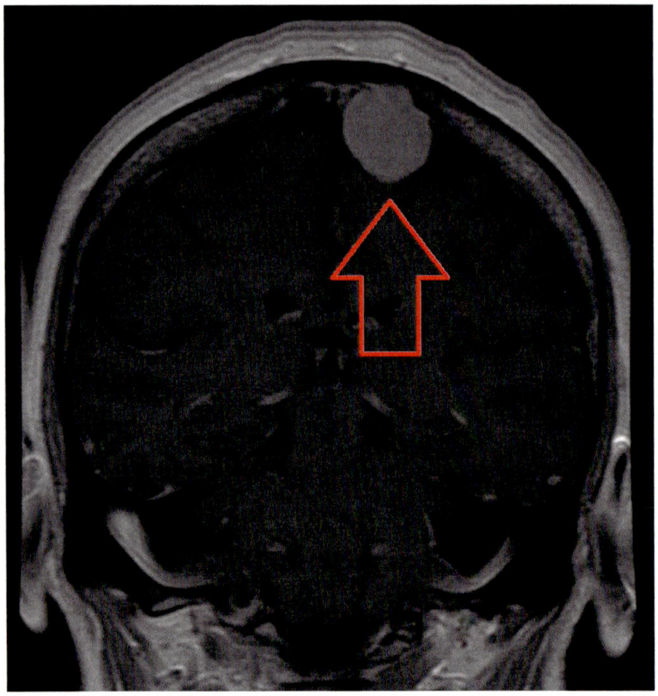

FIGURE 21.11.12 - MRI of the Brain: Meningioma

IV. Sellar and Suprasellar Tumors: Definition
   A. Pituitary adenomas: sellar
   B. Benign tumors anterior pituitary
   C. Suprasellar tumors: extend to neighboring structures (sphenoid sinus, cerebellopontine angle, pineal region)
   D. Craniopharyngiomas: sellar or suprasellar
   E. Remnants of Rathke's pouch

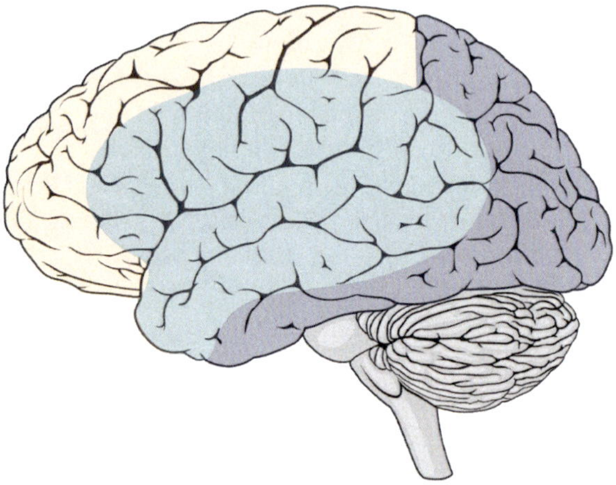

FIGURE 21.11.13 - The Pituitary Gland

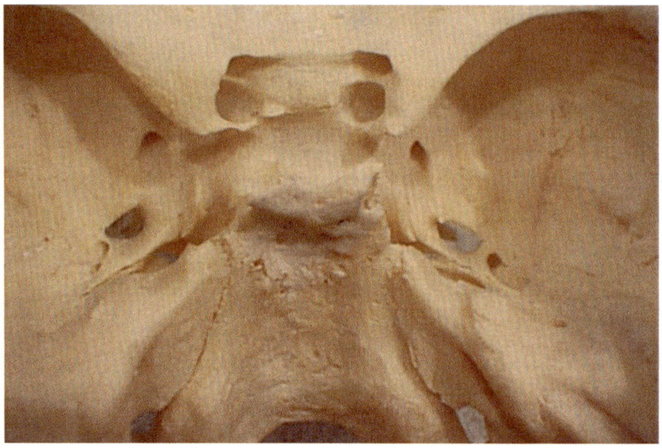

FIGURE 21.11.14 - The Sella Turcica

V. Sellar and Suprasellar Tumors: Clinical Features
   A. Pituitary adenomas: functional or non-functional
      1. Nonfunctional: mass effect
      2. Headaches, hypopituitarism
      3. Prolactinomas, growth hormone, ACTH, TSH, LH, FSH
   B. Craniopharyngiomas
      1. Present in bimodal age distribution:
         a) Children: 5-14 years old
         b) Adults: 50-74 years old
      2. Calcifications commonly seen
      3. Benign but tend to recur after resection
      4. Mass effect
      5. Supratentorial mass compressing optic chiasm

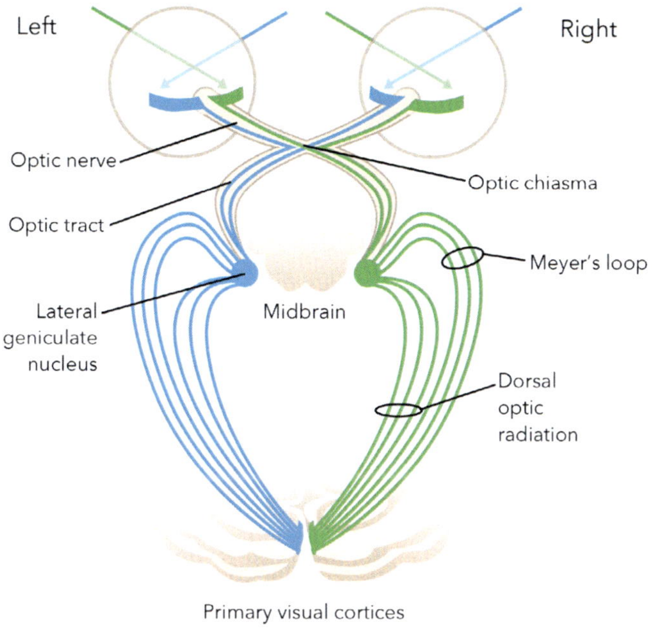

FIGURE 21.11.15 - The Optic Pathway

VI. Sellar and Suprasellar Tumors: Diagnosis
    A. Abundant cytoplasm
    B. Cytoplasmic appearance usually correlates with content of hormone containing secretory cells
    C. Craniopharyngiomas
        1. Sheets of compact cells
        2. Yellow fluid rich in cholesterol crystals

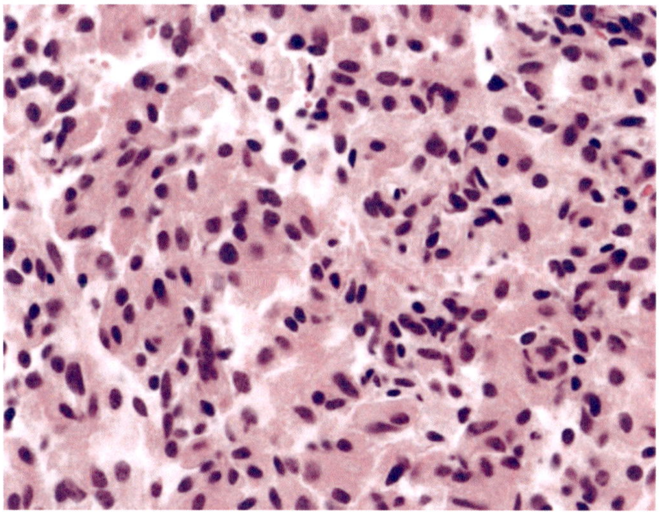

FIGURE 21.11.16 - Light Microscopy: Cells of Pituitary Adenoma

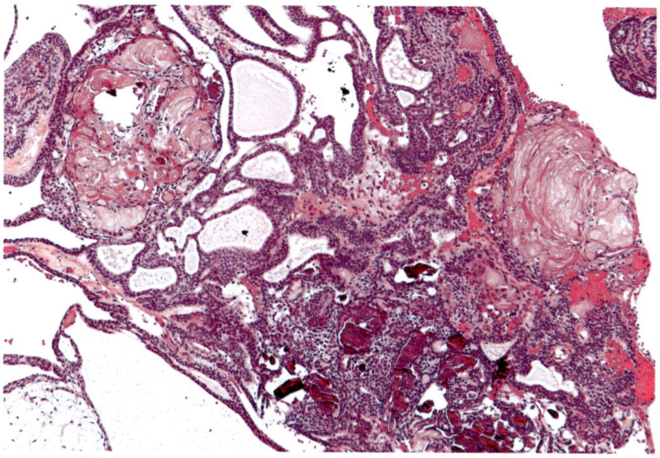

FIGURE 21.11.17 - Light Microscopy: Craniopharyngioma

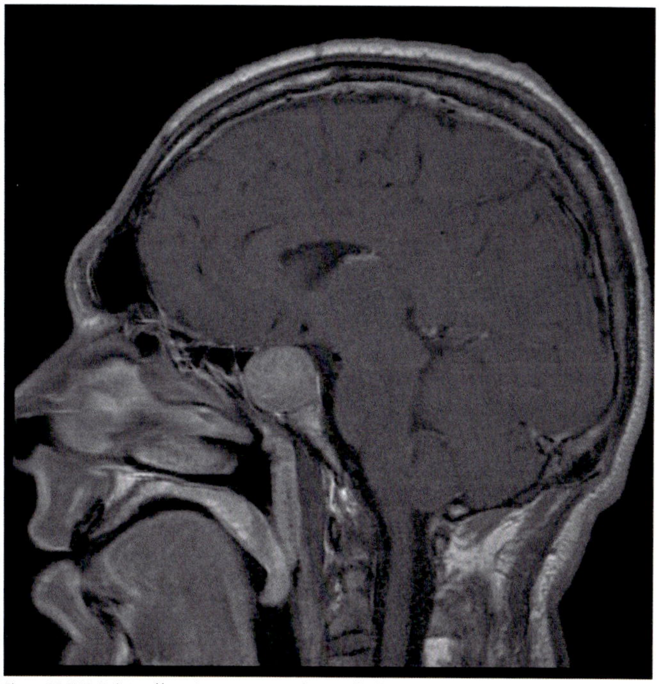

FIGURE 21.11.18 - MRI of the Brain: Pituitary Adenoma

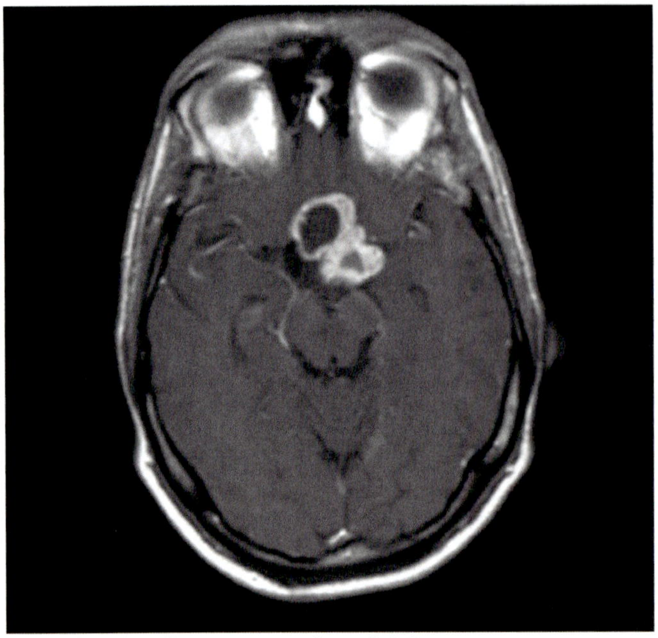

FIGURE 21.11.19 - MRI of the Brain: Craniopharyngioma

VII. Metastatic Brain Tumors: Definition
  A. More common than any primary neoplasm
  B. Multiple, well circumscribed lesions: at gray-white junction
  C. Originate from primary sites: lung, breast, melanoma, kidney, GI
  D. Existing malignancy, stage/grade
  E. More common in adults

VIII. Metastatic Brain Tumors: Clinical Features
  A. Increased intracranial pressure
  B. Headache
    1. Worsens when lying down
    2. Localized or diffuse
    3. "Head in a vise"
    4. Dull, piercing, throbbing
  C. Vomiting, seizures, alteration in consciousness

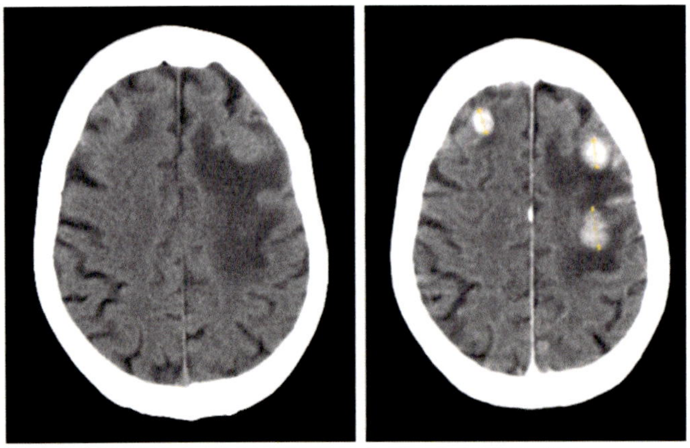

FIGURE 21.11.20 - CT Scan of the Head: Metastatic Brain Tumors

IX. Metastatic Brain Tumors: Treatment
  A. Non-chemotherapeutic drugs
  B. Chemotherapy avoided: absent blood-brain barrier diffusion capacity
  C. Surgery, radiation

REVIEW QUESTIONS

1. Aside from meningioma, which other cancers may exhibit psammoma bodies on histologic examination?
    - **Other cancers that may exhibit psammoma bodies on histologic examination are mesothelioma, papillary thyroid carcinoma, serous papillary endometrial carcinoma, and serous papillary ovarian carcinoma.**

2. What signs and symptoms would be expected in a male patient with a prolactinoma?
    - **Signs and symptoms in a male patient with prolactinoma are erectile dysfunction, decreased libido, and occasionally gynecomastia.**
    - Normally, prolactin inhibits GnRH and sex hormone secretion. It also promotes breast growth. Therefore, elevated levels of prolactin can cause erectile dysfunction, decreased libido, and occasionally gynecomastia.

3. What features of a headache should prompt suspicion for an underlying brain tumor?
    - **Features of a headache that should prompt suspicion for an underlying brain tumor are headaches upon awakening or headaches that no longer respond to treatment.**
    - Headaches caused by brain tumors are often so severe that they wake patients up at night or are worse in the morning, due to the increased intracranial pressure and mass effect.
    - In patients with a history of headaches, if a headache suddenly becomes different and no longer responds to treatments that were known to work in the past, a clinician should consider the possibility of a brain tumor.

REVIEW QUESTIONS

4. A 66-year-old woman with a history of tension headaches comes to her primary care provider because of worsening headaches occurring for the last 5 days. She says her current headaches have been worse than usual, do not resolve to pain medications, and have been waking her up from sleep. Her past medical history is notable for hypertension and hyperlipidemia. Patient has been smoking one pack of cigarettes daily for the past 40 years. Vital signs are notable only for elevated blood pressure. Physical examination, including a full neurologic examination, was unremarkable. Review of records indicates a lung mass was found on a prior screening which the patient never followed-up on. A MRI of the brain is ordered. Which of the following findings will likely be seen on imaging?

    A. A midline mass in the fourth ventricle
    B. A sharply demarcated homogenous mass with a cystic wall and a mural nodule
    C. A homogenous parasagittal mass with a dural tail
    D. A hyperdense mass in the sellar region
    E. Multiple cannonball lesions at the gray-white junction

- **The correct answer is option E.**
- The patient is at high risk of having brain cancer.
- She reports a history of worsening headaches that no longer remit with pain medications and wake her up from sleep. This should immediately prompt suspicion of a brain tumor.
- She reports a 40-pack year smoking history and her records are notable for a lung mass that she never followed-up on. This should raise suspicion for an undiagnosed lung cancer.
- Putting the two clues together, this patient likely has brain metastases from her underlying lung cancer.
- Therefore, the correct option will be one that describes what brain metastases typically look like on brain MRI, and that is option E.
- Option A is incorrect because a midline mass in the fourth ventricle is more suggestive of a medulloblastoma. In general, medulloblastomas are more commonly seen in children rather than adults.
- Option B is incorrect because a sharply demarcated homogenous mass with a cystic wall and a mural nodule is more suggestive of a hemangioblastoma. Hemangioblastomas can be associated with Von Hippel-Lindau syndrome.
- Option C is incorrect because a homogenous parasagittal mass with a dural tail is a classic description of a meningioma. Meningiomas are the most common benign brain tumors in adults and tend to occur more frequently in women than men. Given the likely history of lung cancer in this patient, a meningioma is less likely than brain metastases.
- Option D is incorrect because a hyperdense mass in the sellar region is a finding consistent with suprasellar tumors, such as a pituitary adenoma or a craniopharyngioma. Either of these brain tumors is less likely in the context of this patient's presumed lung cancer.

EMERGENCY MEDICINE

Emergency Medicine | Section 1: Abdominal Trauma

I. Blunt Abdominal Trauma: Definition
   A. Physical trauma
      1. Physical attack
      2. High-velocity impact
      3. Damage to internal organs

II. Blunt Abdominal Trauma: Pathophysiology
   A. Shearing (e.g. distal aortic rupture, hepatic tear)
   B. Crushing (most commonly affecting spleen, liver, kidney)
   C. Compression (e.g. bursting or rupture of vessels)
   D. Hollow organ rupture (e.g. stomach, intestines, gallbladder) → infection
   E. Solid-organ injury (e.g. liver, spleen, pancreas) → hypovolemia

III. Blunt Abdominal Trauma: Etiologies
   A. Vehicle accident (e.g. seat belt injury)
   B. Falls
   C. Industrial and recreational accidents
   D. Iatrogenic (e.g. cardiac resuscitation, Heimlich maneuver)
   E. Sports injury

IV. Blunt Abdominal Trauma: Clinical Features
   A. Nausea, vomiting
   B. Abdominal pain, tenderness
   C. Diminished or absent bowel sounds
   D. Abdominal distention and rigidity
   E. Pneumoperitoneum
   F. Physical exam findings (e.g. abrasions, contusions, lacerations, bone fractures)

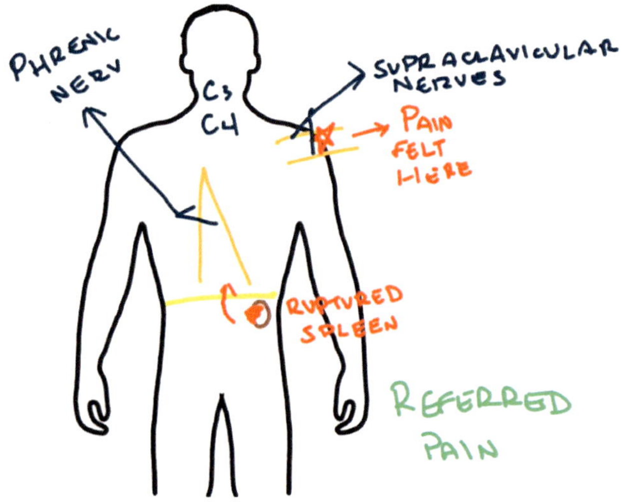

FIGURE 21.12.1 - Kehr Sign in Splenic Rupture

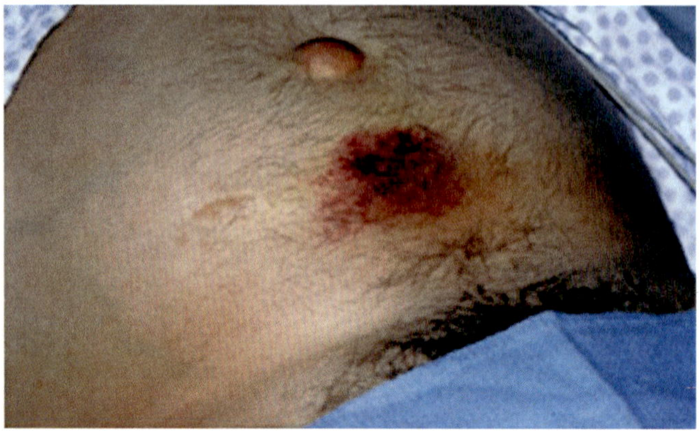

FIGURE 21.12.2 - Cullen Sign Suggesting Intraperitoneal Hemorrhage

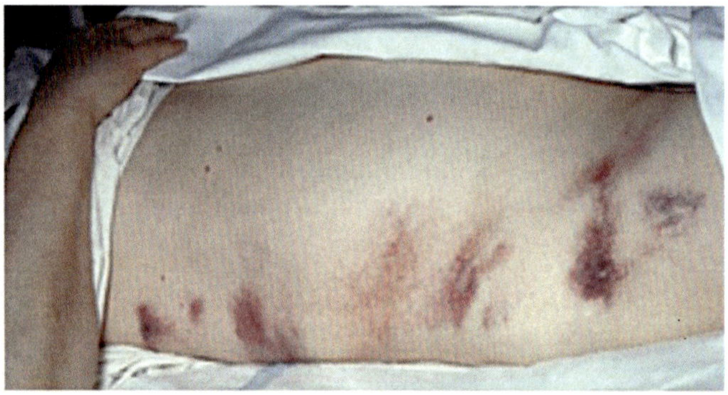

FIGURE 21.12.3 - Grey Turner Sign Suggesting Retroperitoneal Hemorrhage

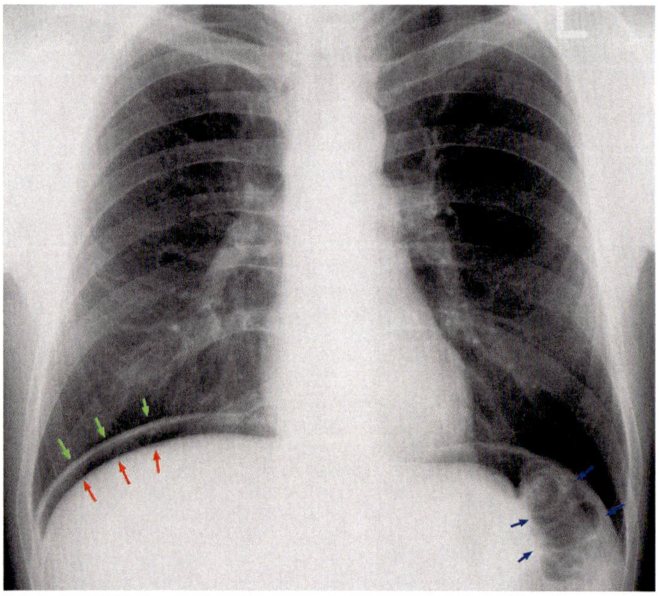

FIGURE 21.12.4 - Chest X-ray Showing Pneumoperitoneum

V. Blunt Abdominal Trauma: Diagnosis
   A. History and physical exam
   B. Imaging studies
      1. FAST ultrasound if hemodynamically unstable; investigates perihepatic and splenic spaces, pericardium, pelvis
      2. Radiography/CT scan if hemodynamically stable
      3. Diagnostic peritoneal lavage
      4. Laboratory workup: CBC, CMP, blood type and screen, and ABG

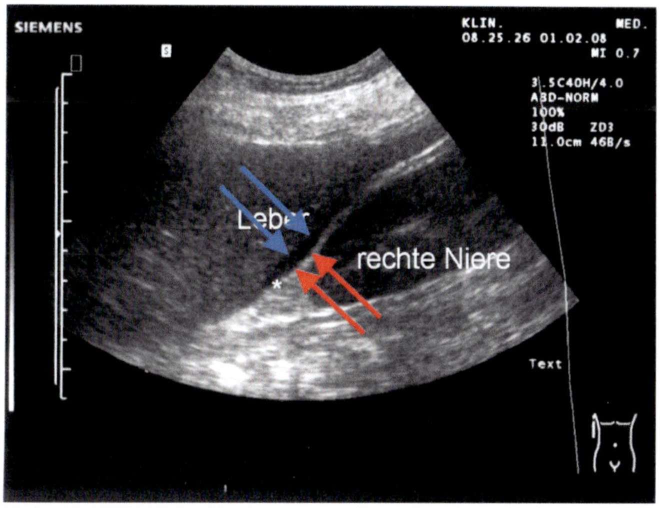

FIGURE 21.12.5 - FAST Image Showing Fluid in Morisson's Pouch (Space between Red and Blue Arrows)

VI. Blunt Abdominal Trauma: Management
   A. Primary survey (e.g. ABCDE system)
   B. Unstable patient → laparoscopy or laparotomy
   C. Stable patient with a normal primary survey → observation
   D. Stable patient with abdominal tenderness → abdominal/pelvic CT
   E. Secondary survey (e.g. history and physical exam)
   F. Diagnostic evaluation
   G. Most common cause of death in abdominal trauma → shock
   H. External bleeding → apply direct pressure
   I. Internal bleeding → IV fluids, blood transfusion, surgery
   J. Sepsis, peritonitis (hollow organ rupture) → antibiotic therapy, update tetanus status
   K. Assess patient first, then fetal status (e.g. airway, breathing, circulation, fetal HR)
   L. If unstable, give oxygen, IV access with fluid resuscitation, uterus displacement to the left if > 20 weeks
   M. CBC, type and screen, Kleihauer-Betke test if Rh-negative
   N. Fetal heart rate monitoring if viable, doppler auscultation if pre-viable
   O. Tocodynamometer

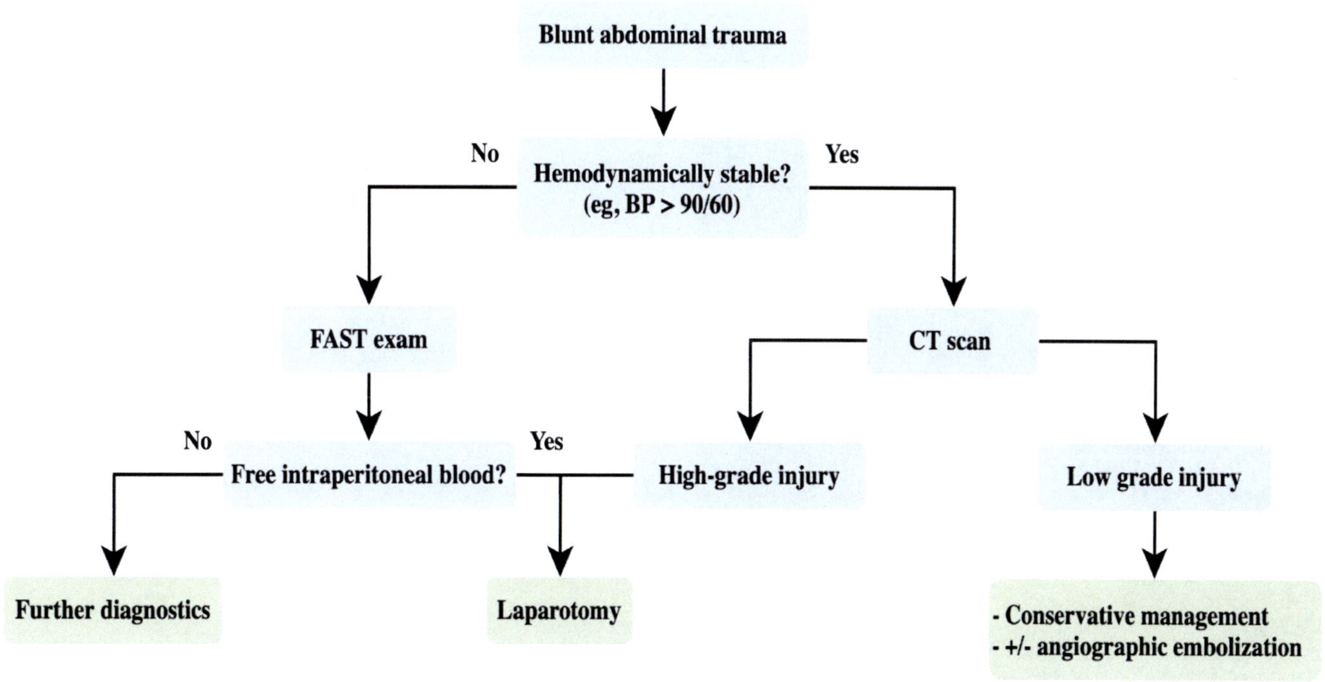

FIGURE 21.12.6 - Algorithm for Management of Blunt Abdominal Trauma

VII. Penetrating Abdominal Trauma: Definition/Etiology
   A. Gunshot wounds
      1. Small bowel, colon, liver, vessels
   B. Stab wounds
      1. Liver, small bowel, diaphragm, colon

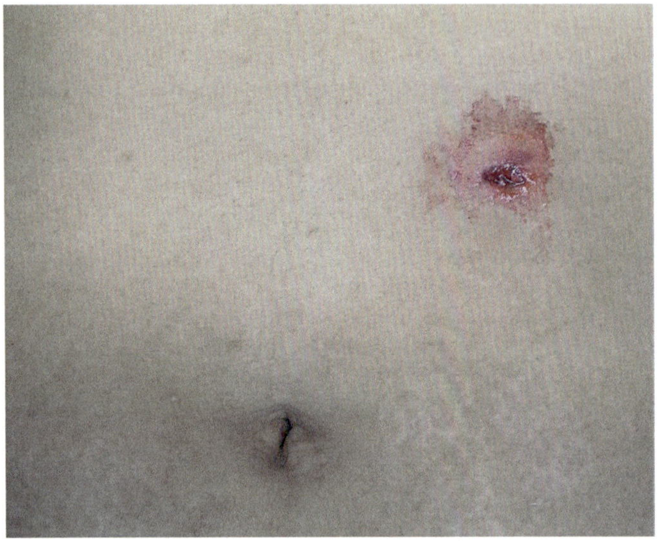

FIGURE 21.12.7 - Gunshot Wound

VIII. Penetrating Abdominal Trauma: Clinical Features
   A. Abdominal pain
   B. Evisceration
   C. Bleeding or perforation
      1. May present with abdominal distension, altered levels of consciousness, peritoneal signs
   D. Shock
      1. Hypotension, tachycardia, changes in respiratory rate

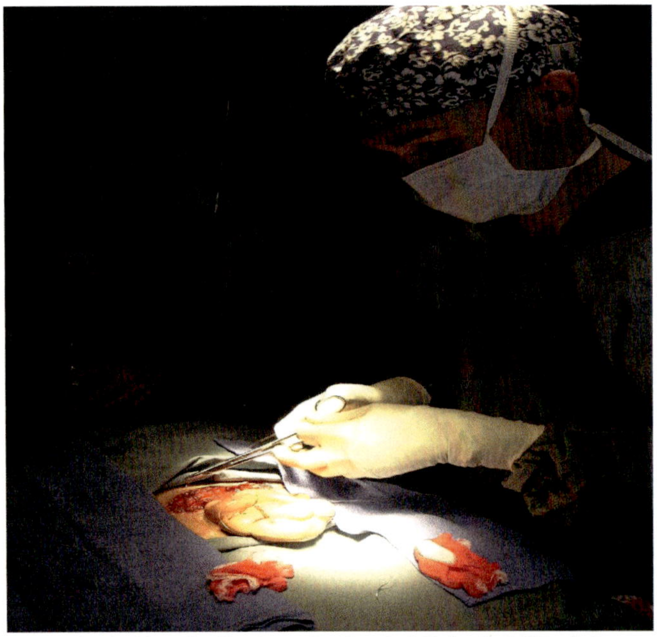

FIGURE 21.12.8 - Evisceration After Penetrating Abdominal Trauma

IX. Penetrating Abdominal Trauma: Diagnosis
   A. Clinical history and physical exam
   B. CBC, blood type, ABG
   C. BUN, creatinine, blood glucose, electrolytes, urinalysis
   D. Imaging, invasive procedures
      1. Stable: X-ray, CT
      2. Unstable: FAST, DPL (if FAST negative), diagnostic laparoscopy

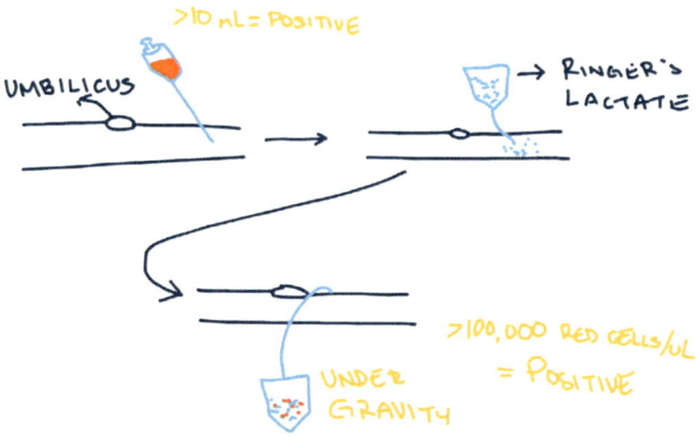

FIGURE 21.12.9 - Diagnostic Peritoneal Lavage

X. Penetrating Abdominal Trauma: Management
   A. ABCDE system
   B. IV fluids and blood transfusions as needed
   C. If unstable: laparotomy, antimicrobials, analgesics
   D. Urinary catheterization
   E. Nasogastric tube placement

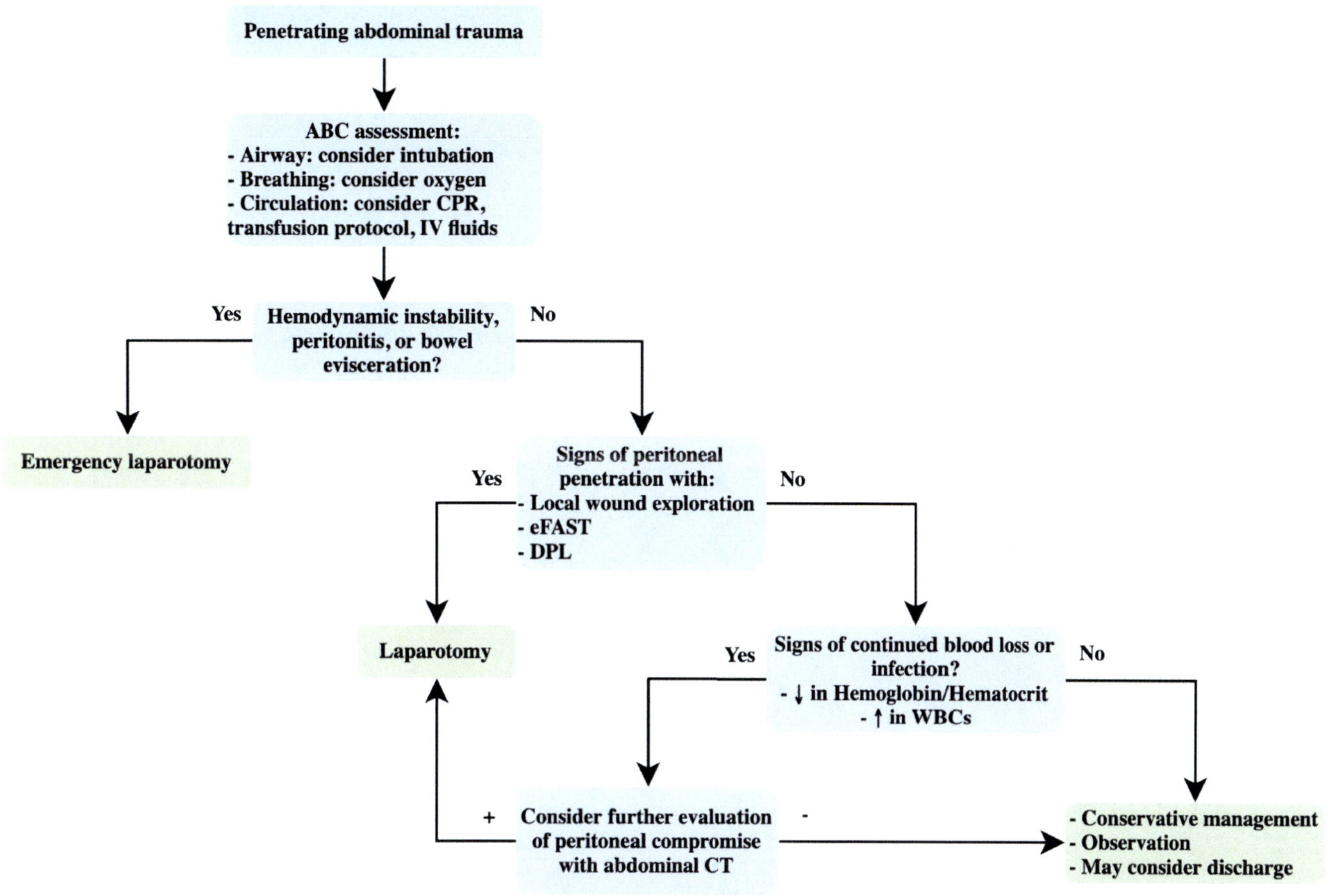

FIGURE 21.12.10 - Algorithm for Management of Penetrating Abdominal Trauma

Tests	Key Features
DPL	- Quick, early diagnosis - Invasive - Misses retroperitoneal and diaphragmatic injuries
FAST	- Quick, early diagnosis - Repeatable - Noninvasive - Can not assess for diaphragm and pancreatic injuries - Operator-dependent
CT scan	- Most specific - Sensitive - High cost and takes time - Needs transportation

TABLE 21.12.1 - Diagnostic Tests Used in Trauma Patients

REVIEW QUESTIONS

1. A 25-year-old gravid woman at 30 weeks gestation comes to the emergency department after a MVC, what is the best approach to this patient?

   - **The best approach is an immediate consultation with obstetrics or transfer to a facility with those capabilities. Continuous fetal monitoring with a tocodynamometer should also be utilized. If the patient is stable and needs a CT scan then it can be done for pregnant trauma patients and is not associated with fetal anomalies. Nitrazine testing should be done to evaluate for rupture of membranes. A Kleihauer-betke test should be performed if the mother is O-negative in order to determine the amount of immunoglobulin that needs to be given to the mother if there has been exposure to the fetal blood.**
   - It can be nerve-racking to have a pregnant trauma patient, but the basic principles of work up here are the same because what is good for the mother is what is good for the baby.
   - As part of the circulatory evaluation, consideration must be given to the uterus compressing the vena cava which may be worsening the cardiac output.
   - While maintaining C-spine precautions the uterus should be manually displaced to the left side.
   - In making the decision of stable vs. unstable, keep in mind the vital sign changes associated with pregnancy.
   - Pregnant patients have increased intravascular volume which allows them to lose a greater amount of blood volume before their heart rate or blood pressure will change- so the fetus may be in distress, due to the decreased perfusion to the placenta, despite the mother having normal vitals signs.
   - During the abdominal exam evaluation for placental abruption or uterine rupture are critical, and these may or may not have vaginal bleeding associated with them.
   - Immediate consultation with obstetrics is required or transfer to a facility with those capabilities.

2. In what scenarios would a diagnostic peritoneal lavage be indicated? In which scenario is DPL an absolute contraindication?

   - **A diagnostic peritoneal lavage would be indicated for a penetrating abdominal trauma, if there is fascial penetration then a DPL is indicated. For blunt abdominal trauma if the patient is hemodynamically unstable and the FAST exam is not available, negative, or equivocal, then DPL is also indicated.**
   - **Previous abdominal surgery is the only absolute contraindication due to the increased risk of damaging an organ or interference from adhesions. Relative contraindications include coagulopathies, advanced cirrhosis, and morbid obesity.**
   - Historically, diagnostic peritoneal lavage was used to a greater extent than it is today because it has high accuracy for evaluating intraperitoneal hemorrhage and rupture of a hollow viscus.
   - Now, it is less common due to the FAST exam and availability of CT scans.
   - For penetrating trauma, if there is hemodynamic instability then the patient will go for a laparotomy.
   - If the patient is hemodynamically stable and does not have peritoneal signs then the wound should be explored; if there is fascial penetration then a DPL is indicated.

REVIEW QUESTIONS

3. A 15-year-old man is brought via ambulance to the emergency department because of a gunshot wound to his abdomen that occurred 20 minutes ago. After initial resuscitative measures, the bullet was removed from the edge of the exit wound. What characteristics indicate the patient requires emergent laparotomy?

- **Key features that indicate the patient needs a laparotomy would include signs of evisceration, peritoneal signs, rectal bleeding, or bloody aspirate from a nasogastric tube.**
- If all of those are negative, but the patient continues to be hemodynamically unstable, then he will also qualify for exploratory laparotomy.

4. A 14-year-old man is brought via ambulance to the emergency department after doing belly flops into the local lake with friends 30 minutes ago. The patient became unresponsive after jumping down and landing on a rock directly under his abdomen. Vitals signs are notable for tachycardia and significant hypotension. On arrival he had a GCS of 8. After initial resuscitative measures, the patient remains hypotensive. A FAST exam is performed. Which findings on the FAST exam would indicate a need for emergent laparotomy?

A. Anechoic stripe in Morrison's pouch
B. Anechoic collection in the pericardial sac
C. No echogenic changes
D. Ovoid anechoic lesion with few septa and no wall thickening of the liver
E. Echogenic foci in the gallbladder

- **The correct answer is option A.**
- This patient has had major abdominal trauma and continues to be unstable despite resuscitative measures.
- The finding on a FAST exam that would indicate the need for a laparotomy in an unstable patient is any evidence of free fluid.
- Fluid is going to appear black, or anechoic, on ultrasound.
- Morrison's pouch refers to the space between the liver and kidney where intra-abdominal fluid will collect, so an anechoic stripe in Morrison's pouch indicates there is free fluid in the abdomen and this patient needs to go for a laparotomy.
- Option B is incorrect because an anechoic collection in the pericardial sac is consistent with the pericardial effusion or cardiac tamponade.
- Cardiac tamponade necessitates pericardiocentesis, not a laparotomy.
- Option C is incorrect because it is describing a normal fast exam.
- Option D is incorrect because an ovoid anechoic lesion with few septa and no wall thickening describes a liver cyst, which generally does not require treatment.
- Option E is incorrect because echogenic foci in the gallbladder are the sonographic description of gallstones, which is not an indication for laparotomy.

Emergency Medicine | Section 2: Chest Trauma: Aortic Injury & Cardiac Contusion

I. Aortic Injury: General Characteristics
   A. Rapid deceleration from blunt trauma produces shearing forces
   B. Most common site of the injury: aortic isthmus

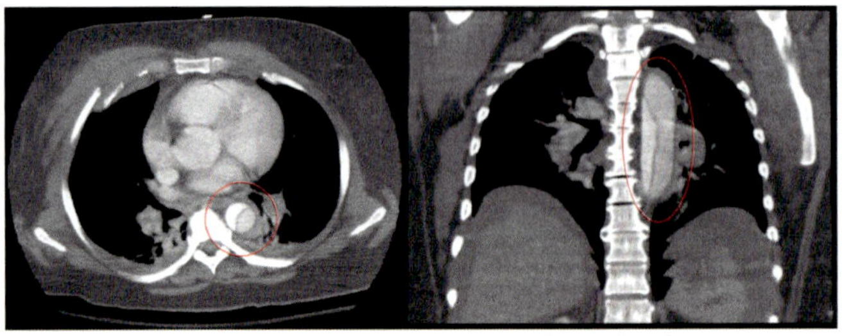

FIGURE 21.12.11 - CT of Chest with IV Contrast: Type B Aortic Dissection

II. Aortic Injury: Etiology
   A. Motor vehicle accidents
   B. Falls from heights

III. Aortic Injury: Clinical Features
   A. Chest pain, dyspnea
   B. Interscapular pain, dysphagia
   C. Physical exam findings
      1. Absent femoral pulses
      2. Interscapular murmur
      3. Hypertension (upper body)
      4. Left subclavian hematoma

IV. Aortic Injury: Diagnosis
   A. Chest CT (stable patients): intimal flap, hematoma, or aneurysm
   B. Chest X-ray: enlarged mediastinum, tracheal displacement, or hemothorax
   C. TEE (unstable patients): mediastinal hematomas, pseudoaneurysms, lacerations
   D. Aortography: location and type of the injury

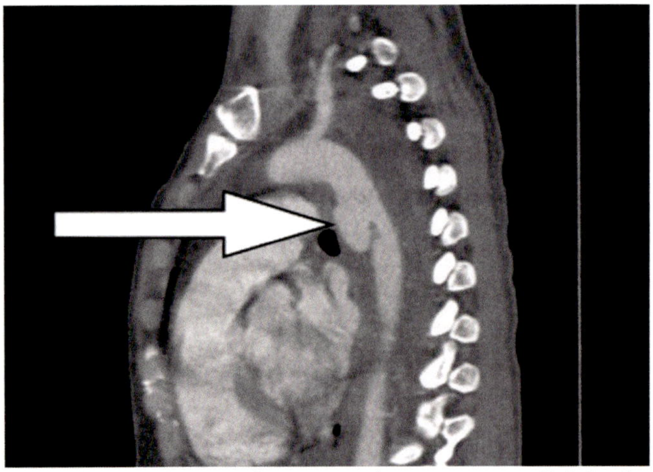

FIGURE 21.12.12 - CT of Chest: Saccular Aneurysm of Aorta

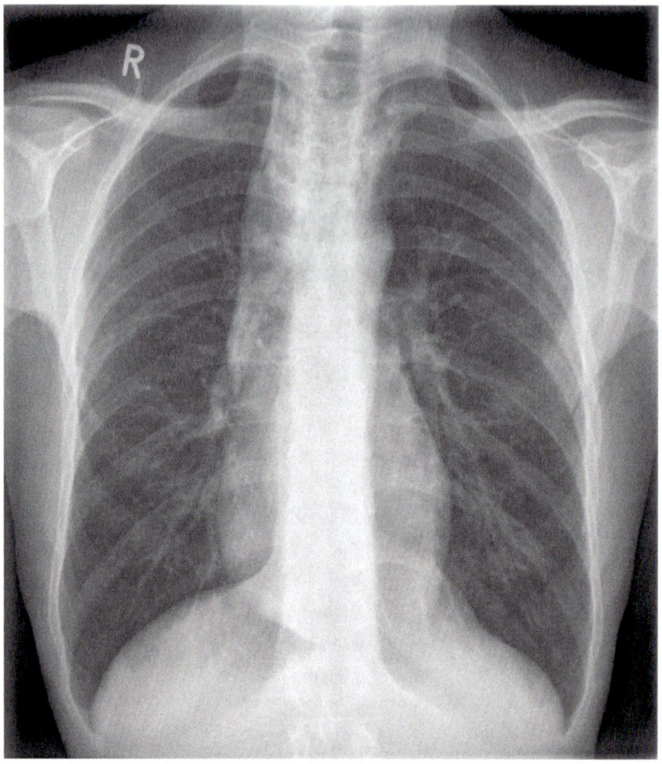

FIGURE 21.12.13 - Chest X-ray: Mediastinal Widening

V. Aortic Injury: Management
   A. Small intimal tear or small aortic hematoma
      1. Conservative management (e.g. blood pressure monitoring)
   B. Larger injuries or complete tears
      1. Open surgical repair
      2. Endovascular stent therapy

VI. Cardiac Contusion: General Characteristics
   A. Bruising of the myocardium due to decelerating force, direct or indirect pressure to the chest wall
   B. Can lead to LV dysfunction and cardiogenic shock
   C. Blow to the chest wall most commonly impacts the right ventricle

VII. Cardiac Contusion: Etiology
   A. Chest compressions
   B. Motor vehicle accidents
   C. Fall from height

VIII. Cardiac Contusion: Clinical Features
   A. Pain above ribs
   B. Bruising over the chest and upper abdomen
   C. Nausea, vomiting
   D. Dyspnea
   E. Arrhythmias
   F. Tachycardia

IX. Cardiac Contusion: Diagnosis
   A. 12-lead ECG: arrhythmias or ST changes

X. Troponins: Myocardial Injury
   A. TTE, TEE: ejection fraction, wall motion, and valvular function

XI. Chest X-ray or CT: Injuries of Chest Wall
   A. Cardiac Contusion: Management
   B. Oxygen
   C. Chest tube placement
   D. Pericardiocentesis if signs of tamponade
   E. Follow ACLS protocol for life-threatening rhythm abnormalities
   F. Cardiac telemetry
   G. Surgical repair

REVIEW QUESTIONS

1. A 27-year-old man is brought into the emergency department via ambulance after a motor vehicle accident 20-minutes ago. On arrival at the emergency department he complained of crushing chest pain. Rated 10/10 in severity, located substernally and radiated to the back. Vitals signs are unremarkable. What would be the best imaging modality to order if the patient?

   - **The best imaging modality to order is a CT chest. If this patient were brought in unconscious, the best imaging modality would be a transesophageal echocardiography.**
   - Stable patient → CT of chest; unstable patient → TEE.
   - One of the risk factors for aortic injury is rapid deceleration injury such as in a car accident.
   - Additionally, the common symptoms of aortic dissection include chest pain and interscapular pain.

2. A patient with a history of recent myocardial infarction requiring numerous chest compressions returns to the emergency department and is later diagnosed with a cardiac contusion. What is the effect on cardiac function?

   - **Cardiac contusion causes myocardial injury leading to cardiac dysfunction.**
   - This patient recently required numerous chest compressions which causes acute myocardial injury secondary to blunt force trauma.
   - Cardiac contusion → myocardial injury → ↓ LV function → ↓ CO

REVIEW QUESTIONS

3. A 25-year-old man who works as a professional athlete is brought to the emergency department via ambulance because of severe chest pain after being involved in a motor vehicle accident 30 minutes ago. Rapid deceleration led him to hit his chest against the steering wheel. Past medical history and family history are non-contributory. Vital signs include a temperature of 36° C (96.8° F), blood pressure of 80/60 mmHg, heart rate of 125 beats/min, and respiratory rate of 21 breaths/min. Physical examination shows a large bruise across his chest. ECG shows non-specific ST-T wave changes. Initial Troponin I is 1 ng/mL with 2-hour repeat of 0.8 ng/mL (< 0.04 ng/mL). CXR is unremarkable. Which of the following is the most likely diagnosis in this patient?

   A. STEMI
   B. Stable angina
   C. Unstable angina
   D. Myocardial contusion

   - **The correct answer is option D.**
   - This young athlete presents with severe chest pain after being involved in a motor vehicle accident 30 minutes ago.
   - Rapid deceleration led him to hit his chest against the steering wheel.
   - Vital signs are significant for hypotension with a blood pressure of 80/60 mmHg, tachycardia with a heart rate of 125 beats/min, and tachypnea evidenced by respiratory rate of 21 breaths/min.
   - Physical exam shows a large precordial bruise.
   - ECG shows non-specific ST-T wave changes.
   - Troponin I is 1 ng/mL with a 2-hour repeat of 0.8 ng/mL.
   - All these findings within the context of chest trauma in a young patient suggest the diagnosis of myocardial contusion.
   - Myocardial injury due to contusion can induce ECG changes and increased troponin levels.
   - Option A is incorrect because ST-elevation myocardial infarction, also known as STEMI, is characterized by ST elevation on ECG. This patient, in contrast, has non-specific ST-T wave changes.
   - Option B is incorrect because there is no troponin rise with stable angina.
   - Option C is incorrect because unstable angina does not lead to increased troponin levels.

Emergency Medicine | Section 3: Chest Trauma: Pulmonary Contusion & Diaphragmatic Rupture

I. Pulmonary Contusion: General Characteristics
   A. Injury to the lung parenchyma, most commonly from blunt trauma, leading to lung consolidation and collapse secondary to edema and blood accumulation in the alveoli
   B. Hypoxic pulmonary vasoconstriction
      1. Attempt to prevent V/Q mismatch

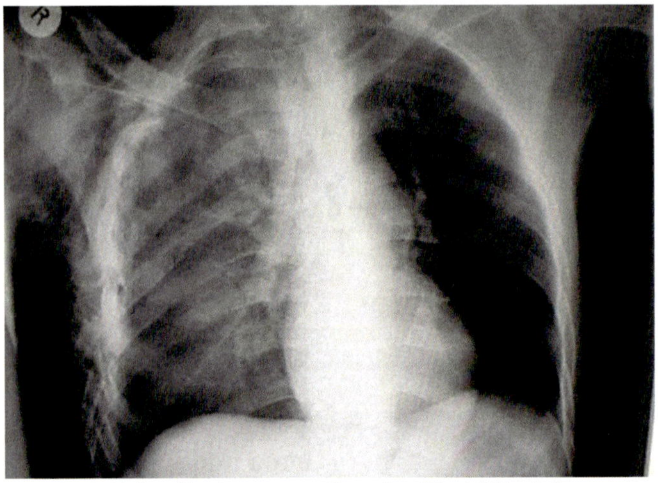

FIGURE 21.12.14 - Chest X-ray: Pulmonary Contusion

II. Pulmonary Contusion: Etiology
   a. Blunt trauma (e.g. rapid deceleration, sports injury, falls)
   b. Penetrating trauma
   c. Localized lesions (e.g. fractured ribs)
   d. Lung tissue shearing

III. Pulmonary Contusion: Clinical Features
   A. Dyspnea, hemoptysis, wheezing
   B. Hypotension, tachycardia, tachypnea
   C. Decreased breath sounds
   D. May be asymptomatic initially and can develop signs slowly

IV. Pulmonary Contusion: Diagnosis
   A. Chest X-ray
      1. Pulmonary changes may take 24 - 48 hours to be visible
      2. Will show irregular opacifications or diffuse opacifications (white out)
   B. CT scan
      1. May show better resolution of the injury

V. Pulmonary Contusion: Management
   A. Oxygen therapy
   B. CPAP, BiPAP
   C. Intubation, mechanical ventilation
   D. Pain control
   E. Chest physiotherapy
   F. Optimal positioning

VI. Diaphragmatic Rupture: General Characteristics
   A. Usually secondary to blunt or penetrating trauma
   B. Anterior compression
   C. Lateral compression
      1. Posterolateral diaphragm is weakest point
   D. Most diaphragmatic injuries occur on the left side as the right side is protected by liver

VII. Diaphragmatic Rupture: Etiology
   A. Penetrating injury (e.g. gunshots, stab wounds)
   B. Blunt trauma (e.g. motorcycle and car accidents)

VIII. Diaphragmatic Rupture: Clinical Features
   A. Dyspnea, chest pain, abdominal pain
   B. Nausea, vomiting
   C. Physical exam findings
      1. Displacement of abdominal organ into the thorax
      2. Bowel sounds on cardiac, lung auscultation
      3. Decreased breath sounds
      4. Scaphoid abdomen

IX. Diaphragmatic Rupture: Diagnosis
   A. FAST: large tears through the diaphragm, eviscerated organs
   B. Chest X-ray: elevated diaphragm, gastric or colonic bubble in the left chest, coiled NGT, rib fracture, pneumoperitoneum
   C. If the chest X-ray is non-diagnostic or abnormal → CT scan

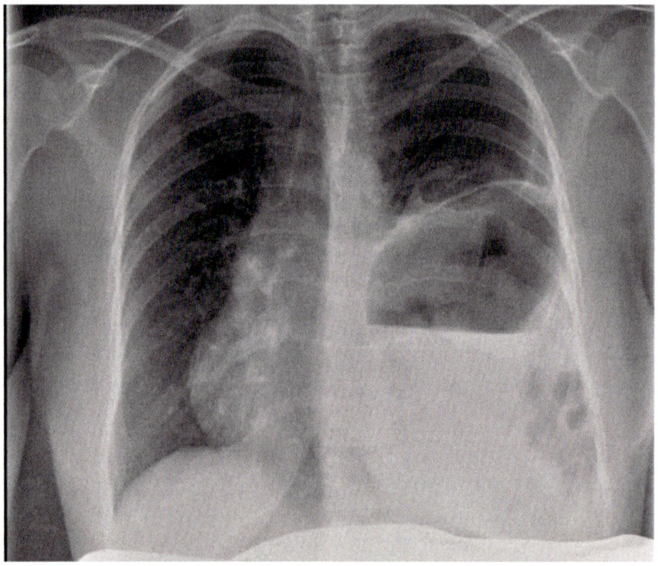

FIGURE 21.12.15 - Chest X-ray: Diaphragmatic Rupture

X. Diaphragmatic Rupture: Management
   A. IV fluids if hypotensive
   B. Pain control
   C. Exploratory laparoscopy, laparotomy

REVIEW QUESTIONS

1. How can a chest X-ray be used to differentiate between pulmonary contusion and a pneumothorax?
    - **In the setting of a pulmonary contusion, a chest X-ray would show diffuse opacification (white off) because edema and/or blood accumulate in the alveolar spaces. While a pneumothorax, would show loss of lung markings secondary to lung collapse.**
    - Contusion → consolidation; pneumothorax → loss of lung markings, collapsed visceral pleura.

2. A 35-year-old man is brought via ambulance to the emergency department because of a motorcycle accident 30 minutes ago. Physical examination is notable for bowel sounds when auscultating the heart. What additional findings would you expect in this patient on examination of the lungs?
    - **Additional findings on lung examination would likely be decreased breath sounds as the lungs have less room in the thorax as abdominal contents are now in the thorax.**
    - Based on the recent motorcycle accident paired with the finding of bowel sounds in the chest region, a ruptured diaphragm is suspected.
    - A ruptured diaphragm means there is no longer an acting barrier separating the abdominal viscera from the thorax, this allows contents to be displaced superiorly.
    - Abdominal viscera in thorax → ↓ breath sounds + scaphoid abdomen.

3. A 28-year-old man is brought to the emergency department because of severe chest and abdominal pain after being involved in a motorcycle accident 1 hour ago. His past medical history is non-contributory. Vital signs include temperature of 98.6° F (37° C), blood pressure of 100/70 mmHg, heart rate of 92 beats/min, and respiratory rate of 25 breaths/min. Physical examination shows a scaphoid abdomen along with bowel sounds on lung auscultation. ECG is unremarkable and cardiac troponin I is normal. Intravenous normal saline is initiated, and a FAST exam has been performed. Which of the following is the next best step in the diagnosis of this patient?

    A. Chest X-ray
    B. Chest CT scan
    C. PET scan
    D. PET-CT scan

    - **The correct answer is option A.**
    - This young man presents with severe chest and abdominal pain after being involved in a motorcycle accident 1 hour ago.
    - Vital signs are significant for tachypnea with the respiratory rate of 25 breaths/min.
    - Physical examination is notable a scaphoid abdomen along with bowel sounds on lung auscultation.
    - These findings are classic for a diaphragmatic rupture.
    - Intravenous normal saline is initiated to support the patient's hemodynamic status, and FAST exam has been performed.
    - The best next step in the diagnosis of the diaphragmatic rupture is a chest X-ray.
    - Chest X-ray typically shows an elevated diaphragm and a gastric or colonic bubble in the left hemithorax. It may also show pneumoperitoneum or rib fracture.
    - Option B is incorrect because chest CT scan is only performed in patients with suspected diaphragmatic rupture and the chest X-ray is non-diagnostic or abnormal.
    - Options C and D are incorrect because PET scan and PET-CT scan are not indicated in a patient with diaphragmatic rupture.

Emergency Medicine | Section 4: Chest Trauma: Flail Chest & Penetrating Chest Injury

I. Flail Chest: General Characteristics
   - A. At least 2 fractures per rib in at least adjacent ribs
   - B. Paradoxical chest movement
     1. Flail chest segment is sucked in with inspiration
     2. Flail chest segment is ballooned out outwards with expiration

II. Flail Chest: Etiology
   - A. Motor vehicle collisions (most common)
   - B. Falls (e.g. elderly)
   - C. Chest compression

III. Flail Chest: Clinical Features
   - A. Dyspnea
   - B. Pleuritic chest pain
   - C. Tachypnea
   - D. Physical exam findings
     1. Paradoxical chest wall movement

IV. Flail Chest: Diagnosis
   - A. Physical exam
   - B. Chest X-ray
   - C. CT
   - D. Arterial blood gas

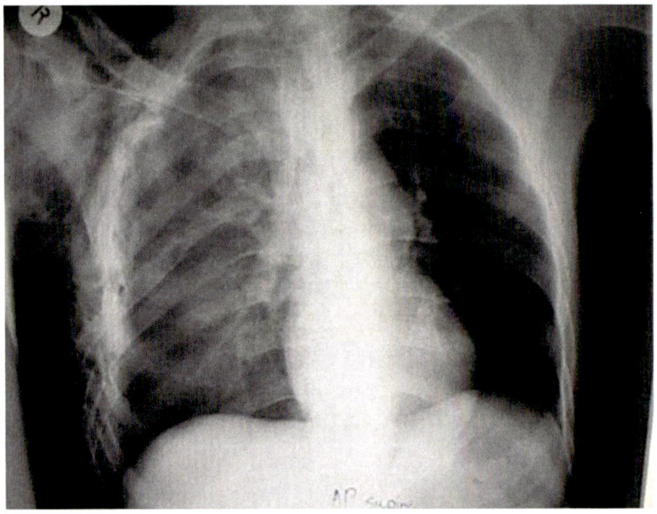

FIGURE 21.12.16 - Chest X-ray: Multiple Rib Fractures

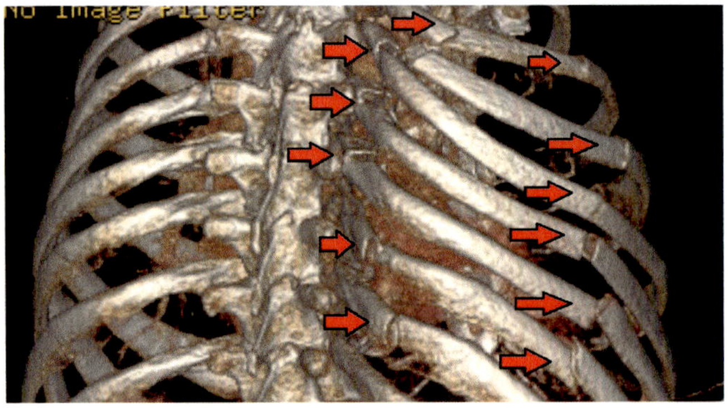

FIGURE 21.12.17 - Flail Chest

V. Flail Chest: Management
   - A. Pain control
   - B. Positive pressure ventilation
   - C. Tube thoracostomy if pneumothorax occurs
   - D. Surgical internal fixation
   - E. Intubation
   - F. Physiotherapy

VI. Penetrating Chest Injury: General Characteristics
   - A. Open chest wound
   - B. Hemothorax (blood accumulation in the pleural space)
   - C. Pneumothorax (air entry into the chest)
   - D. Cardiac tamponade (blood accumulation in the pericardial sac)
   - E. Pneumomediastinum (air escapes from the lung or abdomen into mediastinum)

VII. Penetrating Chest Injury: Clinical Features
   - A. Hemothorax: shock, tracheal deviation, dullness to percussion
   - B. Pneumothorax: respiratory distress, decreased breath sounds, JVD, tracheal deviation, tachycardia, narrow pulse pressure, tympanic sounds on percussion
   - C. Cardiac tamponade: Beck triad (JVD, hypotension, distant heart sounds), electrical alternans
   - D. Pneumomediastinum: pleuritic chest pain, Hamman sign

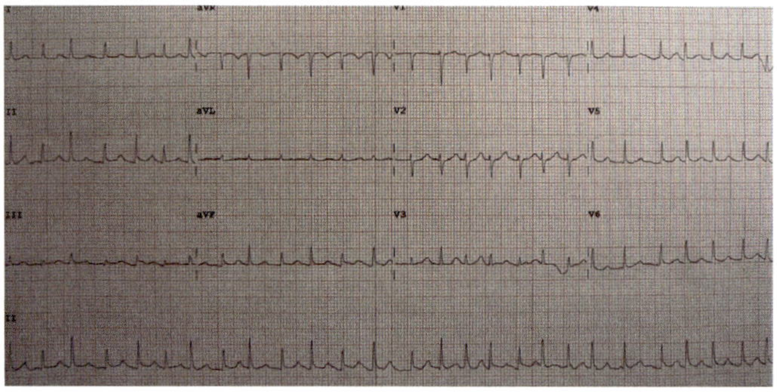

FIGURE 21.12.18 - ECG: Electrical Alternans

VIII. Penetrating Chest Injury: Diagnosis
   - A. ABC trauma evaluation for stability
   - B. ABG, CBC
   - C. FAST
   - D. Chest X-ray, CT
   - E. Echocardiogram

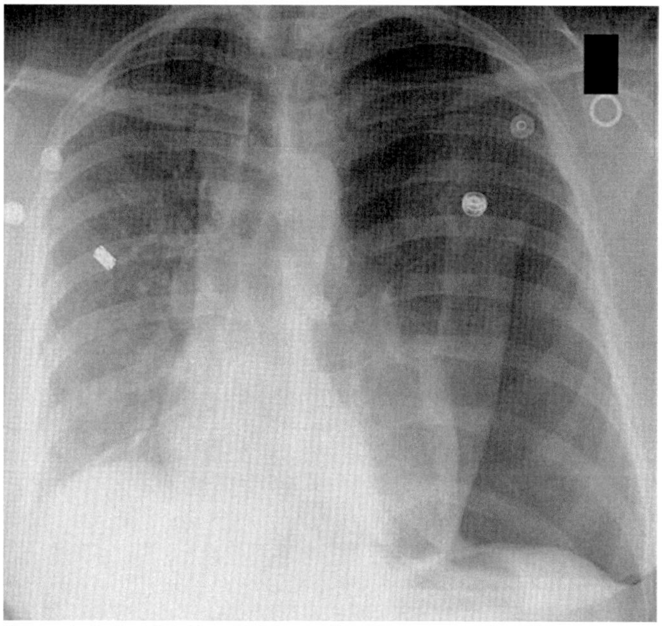

FIGURE 21.12.19 - Chest X-ray: Tension Pneumothorax

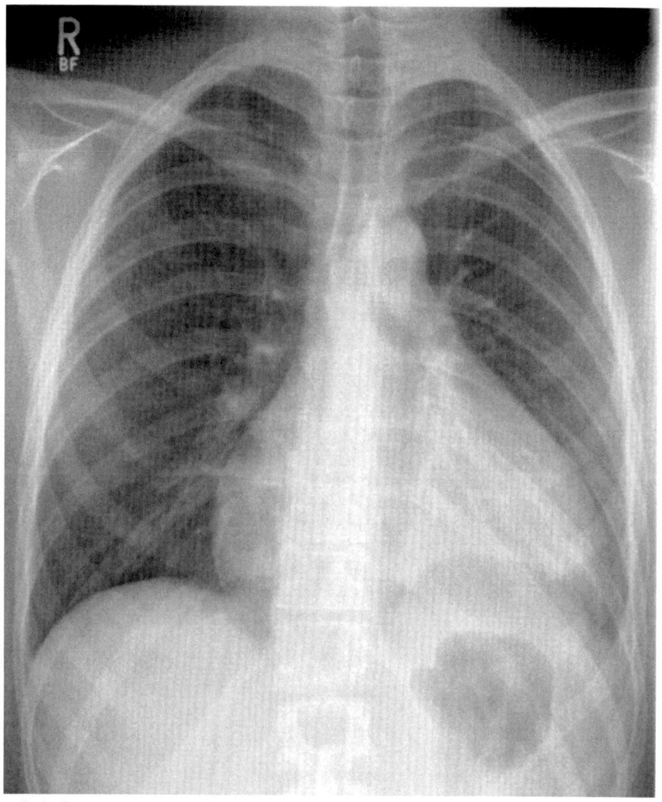

FIGURE 21.12.20 - Chest X-ray: Cardiomegaly

IX. Penetrating Chest Injury: Management
    A. Needle thoracostomy, tube thoracostomy
    B. Pericardiocentesis
    C. IV fluids
    D. Stable
        1. Echocardiogram
        2. Observation
    E. Sternotomy, thoracotomy

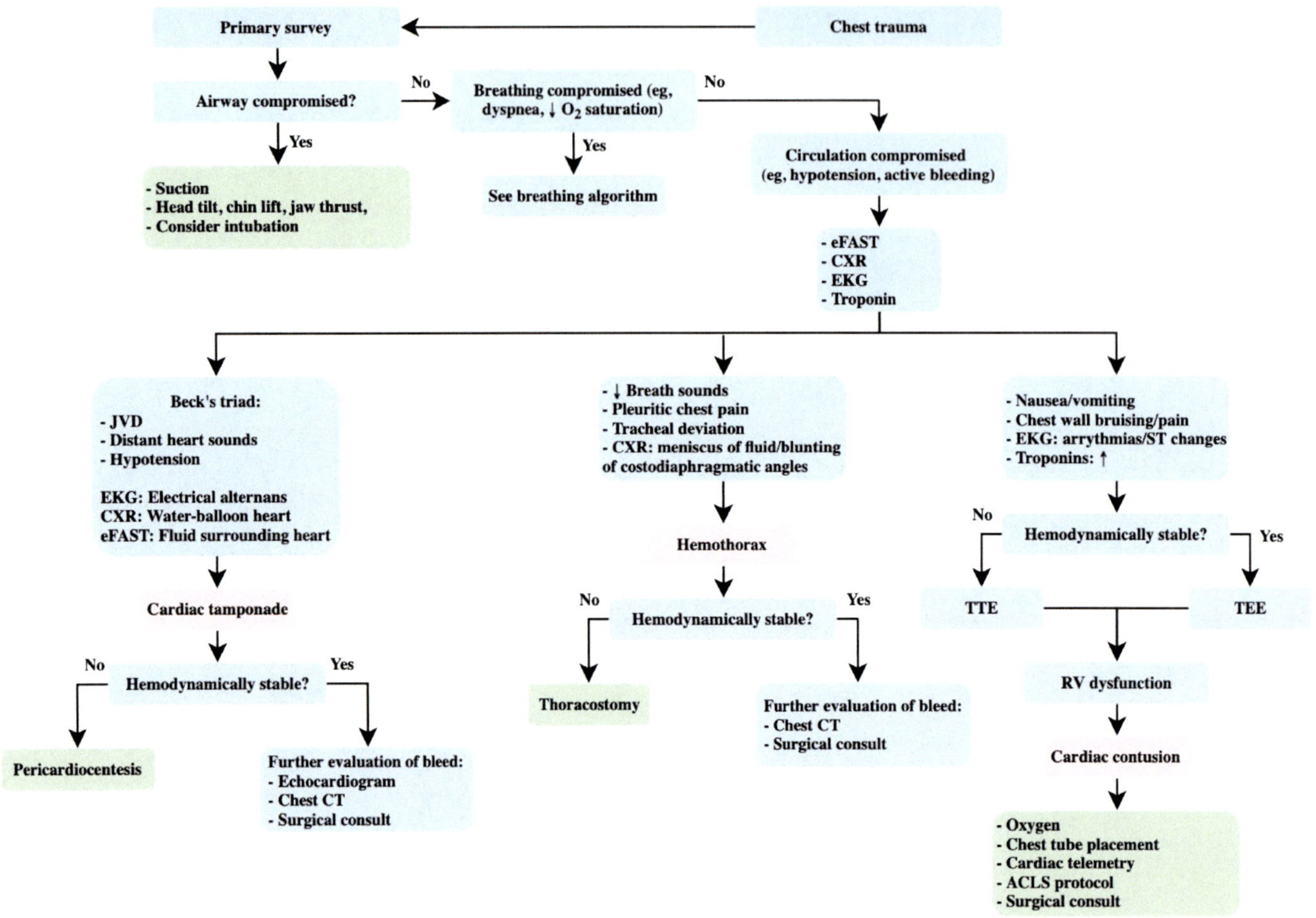

FIGURE 21.12.21 - Diagnosis and Management of Chest Trauma

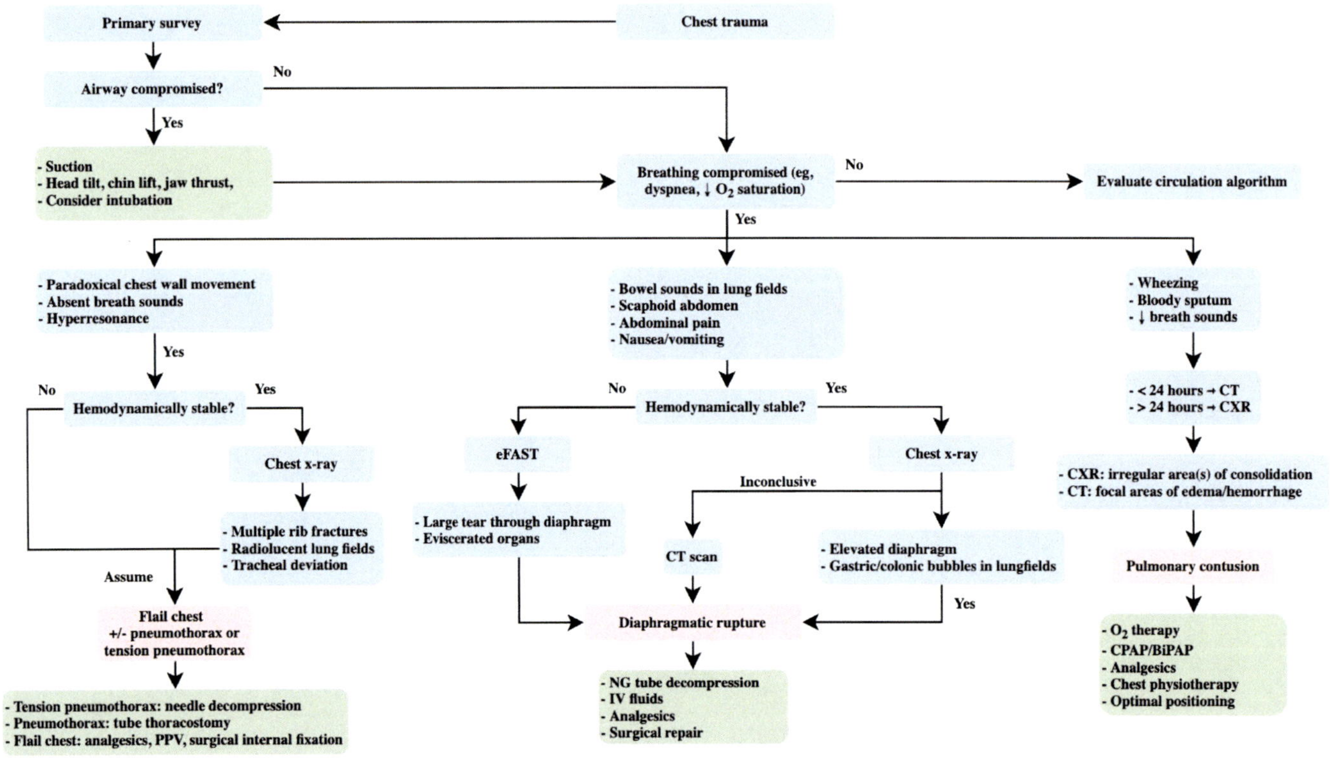

FIGURE 21.12.22 - Diagnosis and Management of Chest Trauma with Difficulty Breathing

REVIEW QUESTIONS

1. A 25-year-old man is brought to the emergency department via ambulance following a motor vehicle accident that occurred 30 minutes ago. On arrival he had chest pain and significant shortness of breath. Initial chest X-ray shows fractures in ribs 4 - 6 on the patient's right side with two fractures per rib. What is the characteristic physical exam finding likely to be seen in this patient?
   - **The characteristic physical exam finding likely to be seen in this patient is paradoxical chest movement (flail chest): when the patient inhales, the chest wall is pulled inwards; when the patient exhales, the chest wall is pushed outwards.**
   - This patient presents to the emergency department following a motor vehicle accident and is complaining of chest pain and dyspnea.
   - Chest X-ray shows fractures in ribs 4-6 on the patient's right side with two fractures per rib, which is consistent with flail chest.
   - The characteristic physical exam finding in flail chest is paradoxical chest movements meaning the chest wall will move opposite that of a healthy patient during respiration.
   - When the patient inhales, the chest is pulled inwards instead of outwards. Additionally, when the patient exhales, the chest wall will be pushed outwards instead of inwards.

2. During a play rehearsal an actor is accidentally 'stabbed' in the right upper chest with what was assumed to be a fake spear. On chest X-ray, there is an absence of peripheral lung markings on the right side and the trachea is shifted to the left. Based on the type of injury and chest X-ray findings, what would be expected on auscultation and percussion of this patient?
   - **Based on the type of injury and chest X-ray findings, decreased breath sounds on auscultation and tympanic sounds on percussion would be expected.**
   - This patient has a penetrating chest injury which has allowed air inside of the pleural cavity, thus making the intrapleural pressure equal to the atmospheric pressure and collapsing the right lung. This is the definition of a pneumothorax.
   - The chest X-ray findings of absent peripheral lung markings help to distinguish this injury from a hemothorax, which is typically associated with opacification of the thorax on the affected side secondary to blood accumulation.
   - On auscultation of a pneumothorax, since the right lung is collapsed, decreased or absent breath sounds on the right side is expected. On percussion, since the right lung is deflated and there is a significant amount of air in the chest, louder tympanic sound is expected.
   - This is in contrast to a hemothorax, where one would expect to hear decreased breath sounds and dull sounds on percussion.

REVIEW QUESTIONS

3. A 48-year-old man is brought to the emergency department via ambulance because of a stab wound to the left side of his chest. He was attacked roughly 30-minutes ago. The patient is A&Ox3, but is moaning in pain. Vital signs include temperature of 98.6° F (37° C), blood pressure of 80/50 mmHg, heart rate of 150 beats per minute, and respiratory rate of 25 breaths per minute. SaO_2 on room air is 97%. Physical examination shows jugular venous distension and distant heart sounds. ECG shows low-voltage QRS complexes with alternating amplitudes. What is the next best step in the management of this patient?

    A. Pericardiocentesis
    B. IV normal saline
    C. Chest tube placement
    D. Intubation

- **The correct answer is option A.**
- This patient presents with a stab wound to the left side of the anterior chest wall.
- He is A&Ox3, but is moaning in pain.
- The patient is hemodynamically unstable, evidenced by the blood pressure of 80/50 mmHg, heart rate of 150 beats per minute, and respiratory rate of 25 breaths per minute.
- Physical examination shows jugular venous distension and distant heart sounds.
- Therefore, this patient has Beck's triad, which includes hypotension, jugular venous distension, and muffled heart sounds. Beck's triad is characteristic of cardiac tamponade.
- ECG shows low-voltage QRS complexes with alternating amplitudes. This sign is known as electrical alternans and is pathognomonic for the cardiac tamponade.
- The best next step in the management of an unstable patient with cardiac tamponade is emergent pericardiocentesis. It relieves the external pressure on the heart chambers and restores the end-organ perfusion.
- Option B is incorrect because although intravenous normal saline is promptly administered in the emergency department to maintain the end-organ perfusion, this patient is unstable and requires immediate stabilization with pericardiocentesis. Additionally, the patient's low blood pressure is a result of fluid in the pericardial sac compressing the heart, decreasing cardiac output. Normal saline will not impact the cardiac output, and will therefore not impact the blood pressure in this patient. The only option to improve their cardiac output is to remove the fluid to improve pumping function of the heart.
- Option C is incorrect because chest tube placement is used to treat pneumothorax, hydrothorax, hemothorax, and chylothorax. It is not useful in the management of cardiac tamponade.
- Option D, intubation, is incorrect because this patient has a secured airway evidenced by the normal oxygen saturation value of 97%.

Emergency Medicine | Section 5: Acute Appendicitis

I. Acute Appendicitis: Definition
   A. Obstruction of the appendiceal lumen leading to inflammation of the appendix
   B. Surgical emergency
   C. Early teens to middle-aged adults

II. Acute Appendicitis: Etiology
   A. Obstruction due to:
      1. Hyperplasia of lymphoid tissue (children)
      2. Fecalith (adults)
      3. Foreign body
      4. Parasites

III. Acute Appendicitis: Pathophysiology
   A. Obstruction leads to:
      1. Accumulation of bacteria due to stasis
      2. Distended appendix and intraluminal pressure exceeds the venous pressure causing vascular congestion
      3. Vascular supply compromised
      4. With ischemia, wall weakens and perforation occurs

IV. Acute Appendicitis: Clinical Presentation
   A. Non-specific symptoms: anorexia, nausea, vomiting and fever
   B. Diarrhea or constipation
   C. Diffuse and dull periumbilical pain
   D. Localized sharp right lower quadrant pain (McBurney's point)
   E. Physical examination
      1. Pain at McBurney's point
      2. Rovsing sign
      3. Psoas sign
      4. Obturator sign
   F. Pseudoappendicitis
      1. Presents like appendicitis but with bloody diarrhea
      2. Classically due to *Yersinia enterocolitica*
      3. Typically self-limited, but can be fatal in immunocompromised patients
      4. Treat with doxycycline if immunocompromised

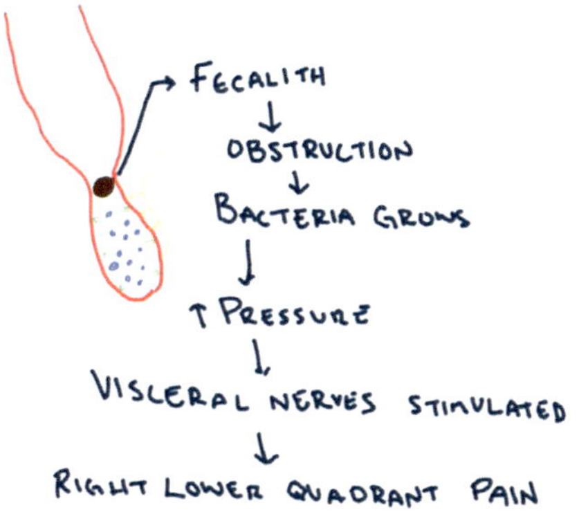

FIGURE 21.12.23 - Pathophysiology of Acute Appendicitis

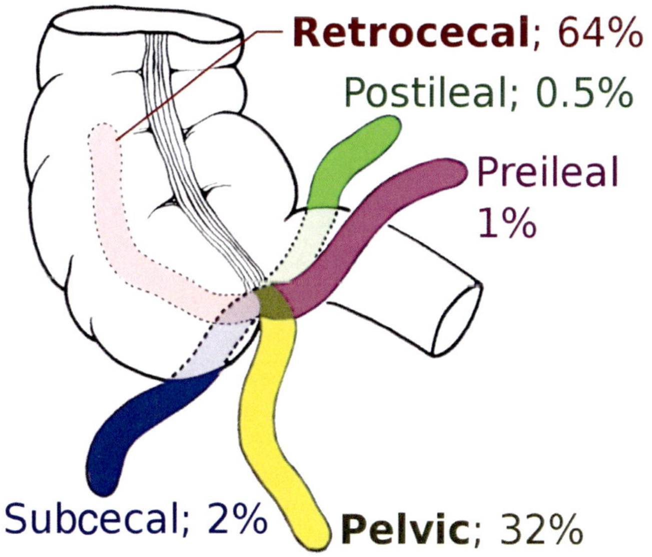

FIGURE 21.12.24 - Locations of Appendix

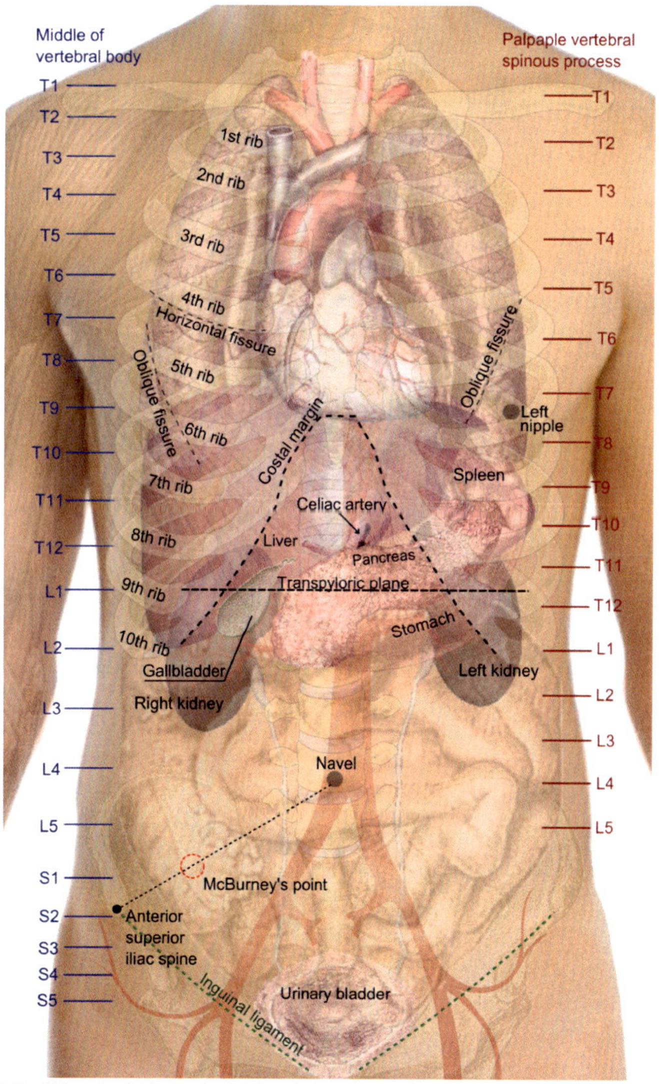

FIGURE 21.12.25 - McBurney's Point

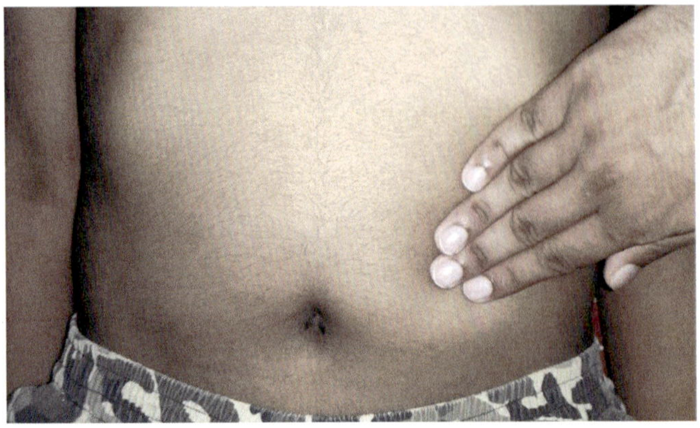

FIGURE 21.12.26 - Palpation of Left Lower Quadrant of Abdomen to Screen for Rovsing Sign

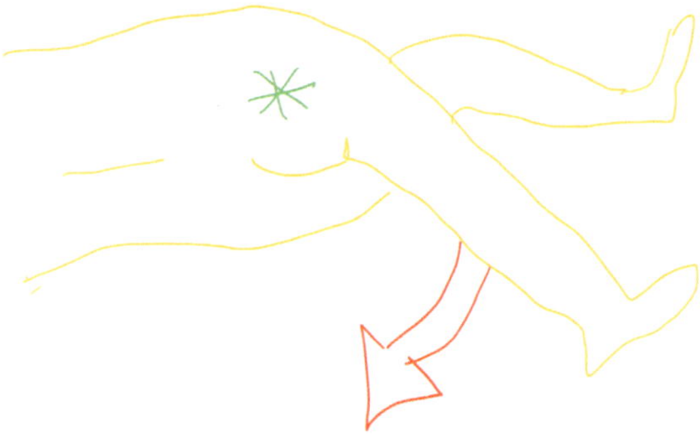

FIGURE 21.12.27 - Psoas Sign

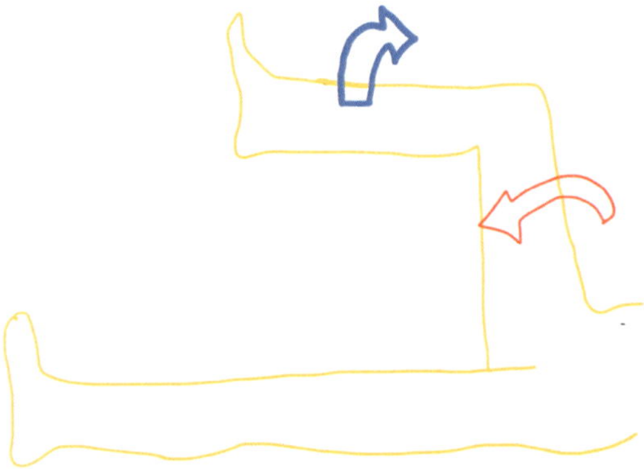

FIGURE 21.12.28 - Obturator Sign

V. Acute Appendicitis: Diagnosis
   A. Clinical: Alvarado scoring system
   B. Women of reproductive age with abdominal pain receive a beta-hCG pregnancy test to rule out ectopic pregnancy
   C. Leukocytosis with left shift, band cells
   D. Increased C-reactive protein
   E. Urinalysis: mild pyuria
   F. Imaging studies if uncertain
      1. CT scan with PO and IV contrast
         a) Enlarged appendix > 6 mm, fecalith, periappendiceal fat stranding, free fluid
      2. Ultrasound for children and pregnant women
         a) Enlarged appendix may be seen
         b) Peritoneal fluid or abscess in advanced cases

Alvarado score	
Feature	**Score**
Migration of pain	1
Anorexia	1
Nausea	1
Tenderness in right lower quadrant	2
Rebound pain	1
Elevated temperature	1
Leucocytosis	2
Shift of white blood cell count to the left	1
Total	**10**

TABLE 21.12.2 - Alvarado Score

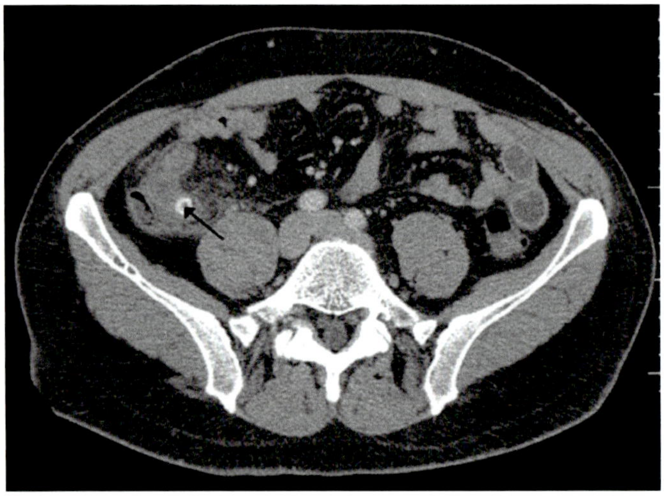

FIGURE 21.12.30 - CT Scan of Abdomen: Perforated Appendix

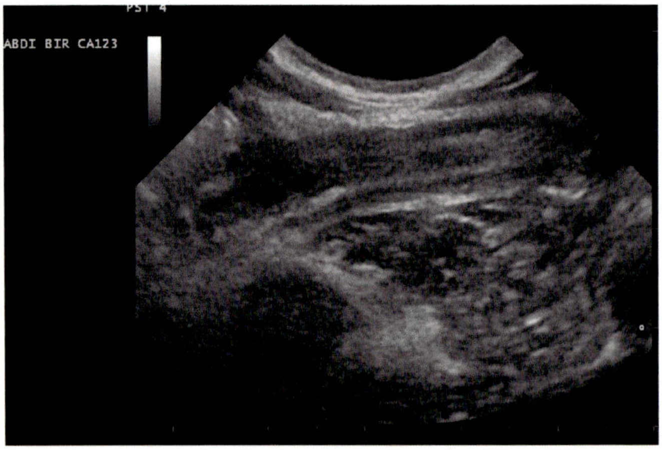

FIGURE 21.12.31 - Ultrasound of Abdomen: Acute Appendicitis

VI. Acute Appendicitis: Management
   A. Urgent open or laparoscopic appendectomy is definitive treatment
   B. NPO, IV fluids, analgesics, antiemetics
   C. Single dose of antibiotics covering anaerobic and gram negative bacteria
   D. Non-perforated appendicitis should not exceed antibiotic use over 24 hours

VII. Acute Appendicitis: Complications
   A. Perforated appendix
   B. Abscess formation
   C. Gangrenous appendicitis
   D. Inflammatory appendiceal mass
   E. Pylephlebitis

VIII. Perforated Appendix
   A. Free rupture of the appendix
   B. High fever, tachycardia, hypotension
   C. Rebound tenderness and guarding and decreased bowel sounds on physical examination
   D. Emergency appendectomy, intravenous antibiotics, give appropriate antibiotic once cultures are obtained

IX. Appendiceal Abscess
   A. Inflamed appendix surrounded by pus and necrotic tissue
   B. High grade fever, leukocytosis
   C. Localized RLQ pain and tenderness on physical examination
   D. Imaging: fluid collection surrounding appendix
   E. Abscess > 4 cm: drained → elective appendectomy 6 to 8 weeks later
   F. Abscess < 4 cm: antibiotics alone

X. Gangrenous Appendicitis
   A. Necrosis of the appendiceal wall
   B. Diagnosed intraoperatively
   C. High grade fever, tachycardia, tenderness
   D. Emergency appendectomy and intravenous antibiotics

XI. Inflammatory Appendiceal Mass
   A. Ill-defined mass of inflammatory periappendiceal tissue
   B. Tender mass localized in the right lower quadrant
   C. Intravenous antibiotics
   D. Surgery if no improvement after 48 hours of antibiotics

XII. Pylephlebitis
   A. Septic thrombosis of the portal vein or its branches that can lead to bowel infarction and death
   B. Sequelae of perforated appendicitis
   C. Fever, abdominal pain
   D. Broad spectrum antibiotics

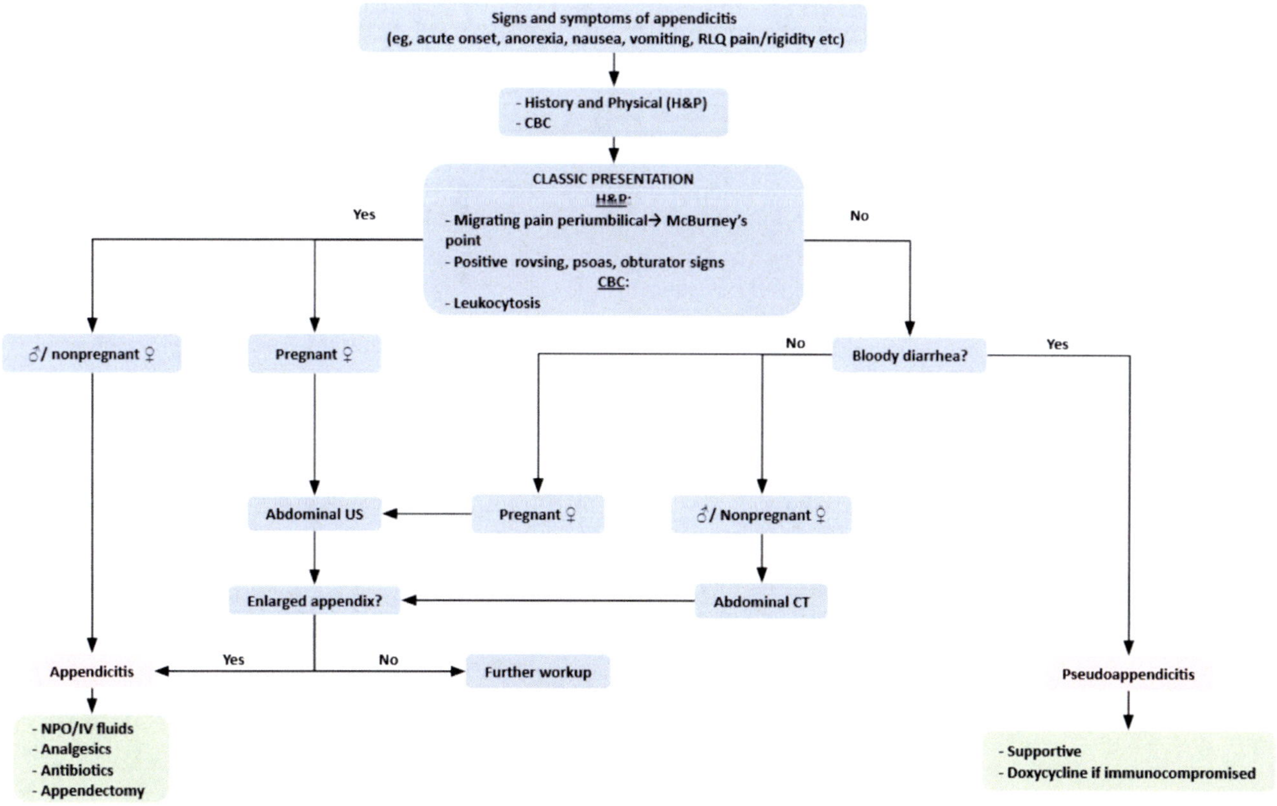

FIGURE 21.12.32 - Algorithm: Evaluation and Management of Acute Appendicitis

REVIEW QUESTIONS

1. How can a parasitic infection result in an abdominal abscess in the retrocecal area?
    - **A parasitic infection can result in an abdominal abscess in the following way: large parasite → obstruction → compromised vasculature → ischemia → perforation → abscess.**
    - A parasite(s) can become so large that they themselves cause obstruction, leading to vascular compromise.
    - The pathophysiology is similar to the process of a fecalith causing an obstruction.
    - The obstruction leads to distention and increased intraluminal pressure, thereby resulting in decreased venous system pressure, leading to vascular congestion and a compromised vascular supply leading to ischemia.
    - If left untreated, there is a weakening of the tissue wall which can result in perforation and potentially leading to abscess formation.

2. A 17-year-old obese woman is brought to the emergency department by her mother because of lower abdominal pain for the past 2-days. On physical examination there is significant right lower quadrant tenderness on palpation. She states the abdominal pain initially started at her belly button and has since moved to its current location. What diagnoses must you consider with this presentation and is any imaging warranted in this patient?
    - **Diagnoses considered with this presentation include appendicitis and ectopic pregnancy. In this patient, an ultrasound is warranted.**
    - This patient is presenting with concerns of appendicitis, especially due to the location of the pain and the age of the patient. However, before starting treatment of appendicitis, other life threatening conditions must be ruled out.
    - Ectopic pregnancy cannot be ruled out just by the history, so a urine pregnancy test must be done prior to imaging.
    - If a question describes a female patient with lower quadrant pain, a pregnancy test is always performed before ultrasound or CT scan to rule out ectopic pregnancy.
    - Then, if imaging is required, ultrasound is preferred for pregnant patients and children due to the contrast toxicity and radiation exposure that CT scans have.
    - Here ultrasound would be the preferred imaging.

3. A 27-year-old man comes to the emergency department because of abdominal pain for six days. Over the past 3 days he has also experienced nausea, and vomiting. Past medical history and family history is unremarkable. Vital signs show blood pressure of 90/60 mmHg, and pulse of 90 beats/min. Physical examination shows localized tenderness to palpation in the right lower quadrant. A CT scan of the abdomen is performed and shows a 3cm retrocecal well-defined fluid collection. Which of the following is the next best step in management after an IV fluid resusitation?

    A. Urgent laparotomy
    B. Proton pump inhibitors
    C. Intravenous antibiotics
    D. Analgesics

    - **The correct answer is option C.**
    - This patient presents with abdominal pain for almost a week.
    - Vitals signs reveal the patient is hypotensive and tachycardic.
    - Physical examination shows RLQ tenderness, which hints at appendicitis as a potential diagnosis.
    - CT scan is suspicious for abscess formation due to the defined retrocecal fluid collection.
    - In cases of appendiceal abscesses, IV antibiotics are indicated over surgery, making C the correct answer.
    - However, he should be stabilized from the standpoint of his hypotension first, which is why antibiotics would be given after an IV fluid bolus.
    - An appendiceal abscess must first be managed with intravenous antibiotics if it is less than 4 cm in size and drained percutaneously if the abscess is larger than 4 cm.
    - Morbidity and mortality is lower with this approach than with immediate surgery.
    - Option A is incorrect because urgent laparotomy is needed to prevent perforation, but since perforation has already occurred and resulted in abscess formation, IV antibiotics are indicated.
    - Option B is incorrect because proton pump inhibitors are a mainstay treatment for acute gastritis and peptic ulcer disease.
    - Option D is incorrect because although analgesics are given for pain management, the underlying condition needs to be addressed. Analgesics will be given, but intravenous antibiotics ultimately lowers the morbidity rate in patients with abscess formation from appendiceal rupture and will be the next best step in this case.

Emergency Medicine | Section 6: Abdominal Pain & Acute Abdomen

I. Abdominal Pain: Pathophysiology

   A. Visceral nerves: colicky pain, dull, and diffuse pain

   B. Somatic sensory nerves: sharp, localized pain with guarding

   C. Mechanical distension → rupture → leak in peritoneum → acute abdomen

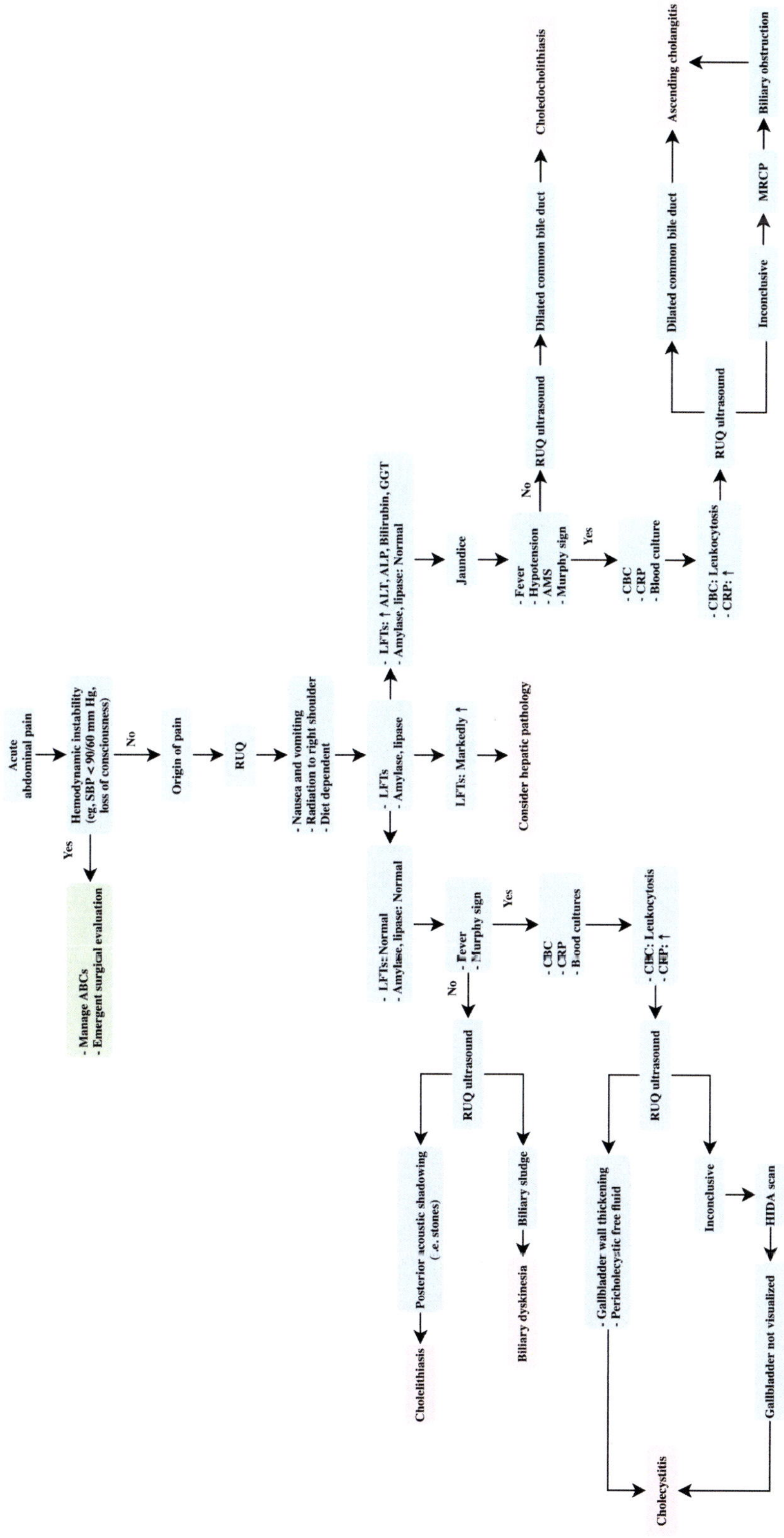

FIGURE 21.12.33 - Algorithm: Right Upper Quadrant Abdominal Pain

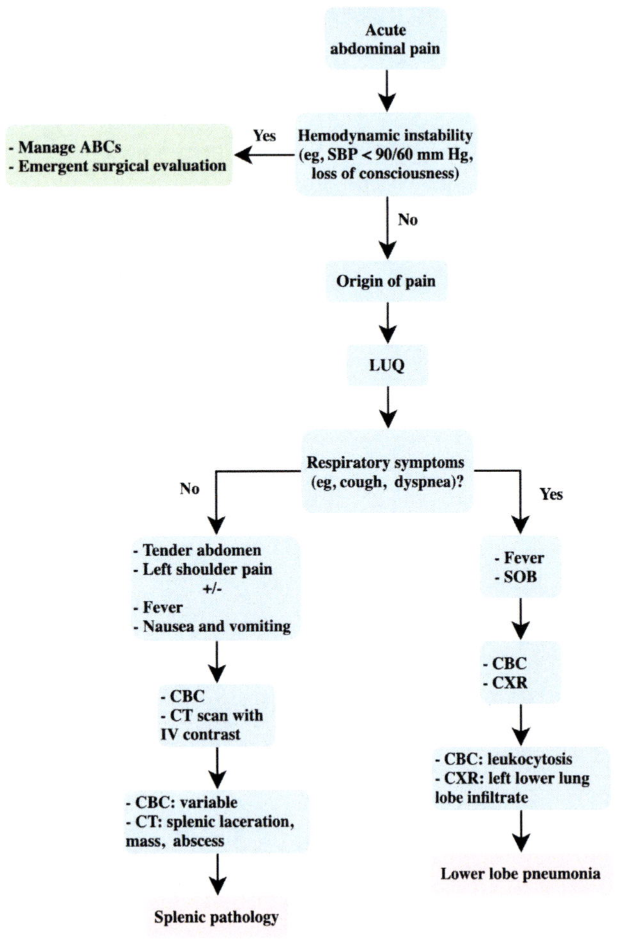

FIGURE 21.12.34 - Algorithm: Left Upper Quadrant Abdominal Pain

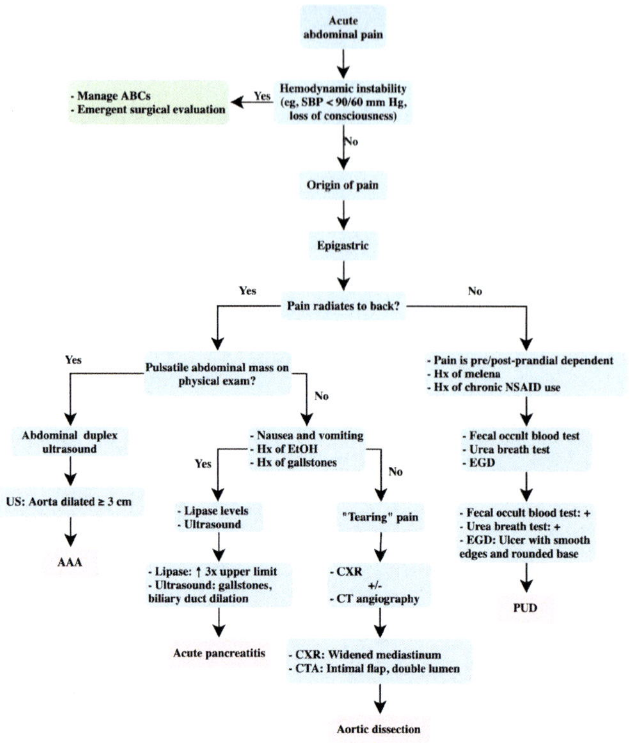

FIGURE 21.12.36 - Algorithm: Epigastric Abdominal Pain

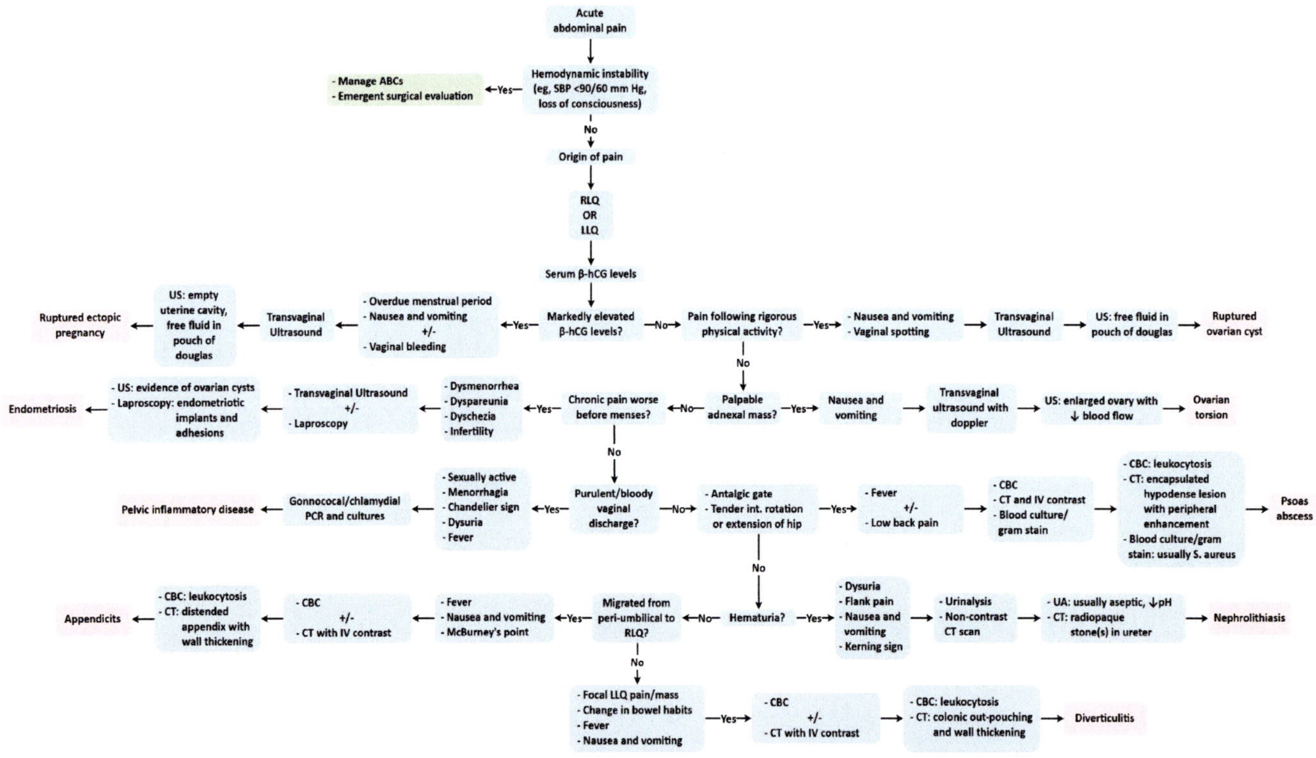

FIGURE 21.12.35 - Algorithm: Right Lower Quadrant and Left Lower Quadrant Abdominal Pain

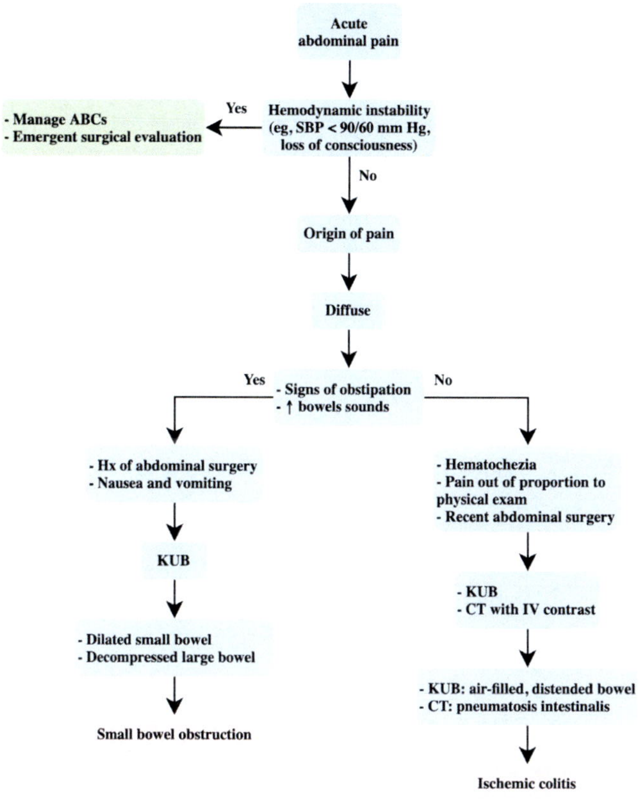

FIGURE 21.12.37 - Algorithm: Diffuse Abdominal Pain

II. Acute Abdomen
   A. Severe abdominal pain
   B. Acute onset < 5 days
   C. Thorough history and physical exam
   D. Peritoneal signs and shock call for immediate intervention
   E. Clinical diagnosis
   F. Tender abdomen with guarding and rigidity
   G. Absent bowel sounds
   H. Abdominal X-ray: free air under diaphragm
   I. If inconclusive, abdominal CT scan confirms diagnosis
   J. Pelvic ultrasound if positive β-hCG
   K. Hemodynamically unstable patient
      1. Emergent laparotomy
   L. Stable patient
      1. Treat underlying cause
      2. NPO, NGT, IV fluids, Foley catheter, abdominal exams, serial scans
      3. Parenteral analgesics and antiemetics, empiric antibiotic therapy

REVIEW QUESTIONS

1. A 45-year-old G5P5 woman was brought to the emergency department by her partner because of abdominal pain for the past 4 hours. She has had similar pain episodes in the past that previously resolved spontaneously. Vital signs are significant for a temperature of 102.2° F (39° C). Palpation of the right subcostal area causes pain on inspiration. Abdominal ultrasound is unremarkable. What is the next best step in the diagnosis of this patient?
   - **The next best step in the diagnosis is to obtain a HIDA scan.**
   - This multiparous woman over the age of 40 years complains of right upper abdominal pain for the past 4 hours.
   - She has had similar pain episodes in the past that used to resolve spontaneously.
   - These episodes are most likely consistent with the biliary colic.
   - Vital signs are significant for a fever of 102.2° F (39° C).
   - Palpation of the right subcostal area causes pain on inspiration.
   - This phenomenon is known as Murphy's sign and is present in patients with acute cholecystitis.
   - Fever further supports the diagnosis of acute cholecystitis rather than biliary colic in this patient.
   - However, abdominal ultrasound is unremarkable.
   - If the patient is suspected to have acute cholecystitis but the ultrasound is unremarkable, the best next step in the diagnosis is HIDA scan.
   - Failure of gallbladder visualization on HIDA scan suggests the cystic duct obstruction and confirms the diagnosis of acute cholecystitis.

REVIEW QUESTIONS

2. An 18-year-old male college student is brought to the emergency department by his friend because of severe left upper quadrant pain for the past hour. The pain started when someone hit him in the abdomen while playing rugby. The patient has a past medical history notable for a sore throat and severe fatigue for the past month. Vital signs show blood pressure of 80/65 mmHg and heart rate of 135 beats/min. What is the most likely cause of this patient's current symptoms?

- **The most likely cause of the patient's current symptoms is splenic rupture.**
- This 18-year-old college student reports severe left upper quadrant pain for the past hour.
- The pain started when someone hit him in the abdomen while playing rugby.
- The left upper quadrant pain and the history of trauma raises suspicion for splenic injury.
- Additionally, he has a past medical history of sore throat and severe fatigue for the past month, suggestive of infectious mononucleosis.
- Infectious mononucleosis can cause splenomegaly and predispose the patient to traumatic splenic rupture.
- Vital signs are significant for hypotension with the blood pressure of 80/65 mmHg and the tachycardia with the heart rate of 135 beats/min.
- Hemodynamic instability with left upper quadrant pain is most consistent with splenic rupture.

3. A 65-year-old man is brought to the emergency department by his daughter because of severe upper abdominal pain radiating to the back for the past 30 minutes. He has been smoking 3 packs of cigarettes per day for the past 40 years. Vital signs are significant for a blood pressure of 85/70 mmHg and a heart rate of 136 beats/min. Physical examination shows epigastric tenderness with a pulsatile abdominal mass. What is the next best step in the diagnosis of this patient?

- **The next best step in the diagnosis of this patient is to obtain an abdominal ultrasound asap to confirm AAA rupture.**
- This 65-year-old man reports severe upper abdominal pain radiating to the back for the past 30 minutes.
- He has an extensive smoking history predisposing him to vascular disease.
- Vital signs are significant for hypotension with blood pressure of 85/70 mmHg and tachycardia with heart rate of 136 beats/min.
- Physical examination shows epigastric tenderness with pulsatile abdominal mass suggestive of an abdominal aortic aneurysm with vitals concerning for rupture.
- Abdominal ultrasound will confirm the AAA rupture and vascular surgery should be consulted immediately.

REVIEW QUESTIONS

4. A 7-year-old boy is brought to the emergency department by his parents because of vomiting and right lower abdominal pain for the past hour. Vital signs are significant for a temperature of 100.4° F (38° C). Extension and internal rotation of the right hip as well as palpation of the left lower quadrant all exacerbate the right lower quadrant pain. What is the best treatment option for this patient?

   - **The best treatment option for this patient is urgent appendectomy.**
   - This 7-year-old boy presents with vomiting and right lower abdominal pain for the past hour.
   - His vital signs are significant for a fever of 100.4° F (38° C).
   - Extension and internal rotation of the right hip as well as palpation of the left lower quadrant all exacerbate the right lower quadrant pain.
   - Pain exacerbation on extension of the right hip is known as psoas sign.
   - On the other hand, worsening of the pain on internal rotation of the right hip is called obturator sign.
   - If palpation in the left lower quadrant exacerbates the right lower quadrant pain, this phenomenon is known as Rovsing's sign.
   - Positive psoas sign, obturator sign, and Rovsing's sign all suggest the diagnosis of acute appendicitis.

5. A 25-year-old woman is brought to the emergency department by her mother because of vomiting and abdominal pain for the past 4 hours. Her past medical history includes laparoscopy for ruptured ectopic pregnancy 2 years ago. Vital signs include temperature of 104° F (40° C), blood pressure of 80/60 mmHg, heart rate of 155 beats/min, and respiratory rate of 16 breaths/min. Physical examination shows diffuse abdominal pain with rebound tenderness, rigidity and guarding. Serum β-hCG is undetectable. The abdominal X-ray shows dilated bowel loops and air-fluid levels along with air under the diaphragm. Intravenous fluids and antibiotics are promptly initiated. Which of the following is the next best step in the management of this patient?

   A. Pelvic ultrasound
   B. Abdominal CT scan
   C. IV metoclopramide
   D. Emergent laparotomy

   - **The correct answer is option D.**
   - This 25-year-old woman is brought to the emergency department because of vomiting and abdominal pain for the past 4 hours.
   - Her past medical history includes laparoscopy for ruptured ectopic pregnancy 2 years ago which predisposes her to abdominal adhesions and bowel obstruction.
   - Vital signs indicate she is febrile and hemodynamically unstable.
   - Physical examination shows diffuse abdominal pain with rebound tenderness, rigidity and guarding. These findings are consistent with an acute abdomen and peritonitis.
   - The abdominal X-ray shows dilated bowel loops and air-fluid levels along with air under the diaphragm, indicating small bowel obstruction complicated by bowel rupture and pneumoperitoneum.
   - The next best step in the management of a hemodynamically unstable patient with an acute abdomen is emergent laparotomy.
   - Option A is incorrect. Although this patient is at risk of ectopic pregnancy based on her past history, serum beta-hCG is undetectable making this diagnosis unlikely. Plus, the patient is hemodynamically unstable and requires emergent intervention without wasting time.
   - Option B is incorrect because abdominal CT scan will not change the management of this patient. She will still require laparotomy so performing CT scan in this particular case would be a waste of time.
   - Option C is incorrect. Although this patient needs antiemetic for vomiting, metoclopramide is contraindicated in patients with bowel obstruction. This is because metoclopramide increases GI motility and exacerbates the symptoms of bowel obstruction.

Burn Degree	Tissue Involvement	Clinical Features
First degree (superficial)	- Epidermis	- Resembles a sunburn: localized, tender, blanching erythema - No blisters - Intact capillary refill
Second degree (partial thickness)	- Epidermis and parts of dermis	- Tender, edematous, mottled, skin - Blisters present
Third degree (full thickness)	- Epidermis and all of dermis	- Painless, white, charred, leathery areas of skin - No blanching
Fourth degree	- Epidermis, dermis, and all underlying tissue (e.g. adipose, muscle, bone)	- Painless, white, charred, leathery areas of skin - No blanching - Disfiguring

TABLE 21.12.3 - Thermal Burns

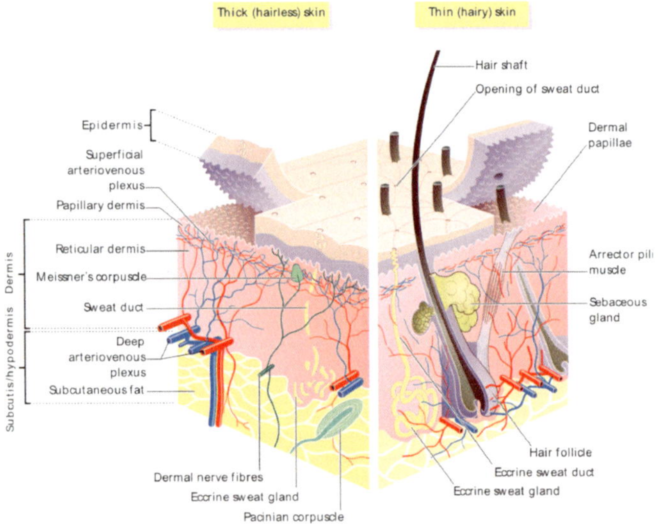

FIGURE 21.12.38 - Layers of Skin

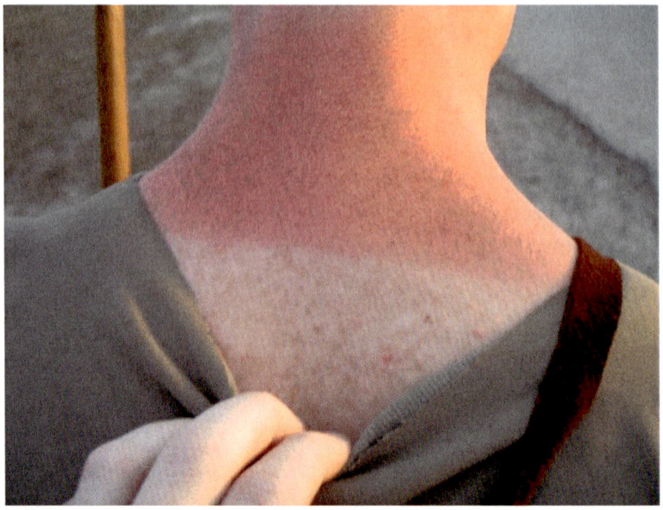

FIGURE 21.12.39 - First Degree Burn

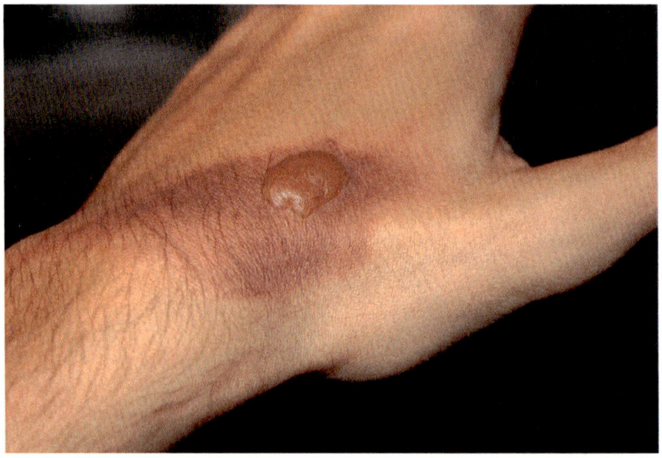

FIGURE 21.12.40 - Second Degree Burn

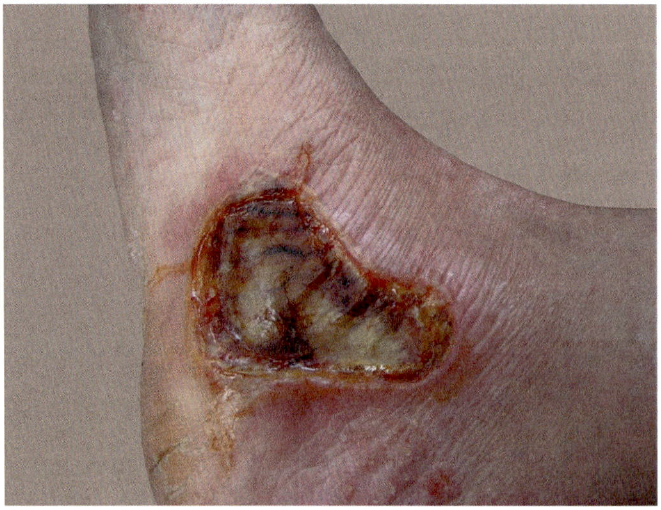

FIGURE 21.12.41 - Third Degree Burn

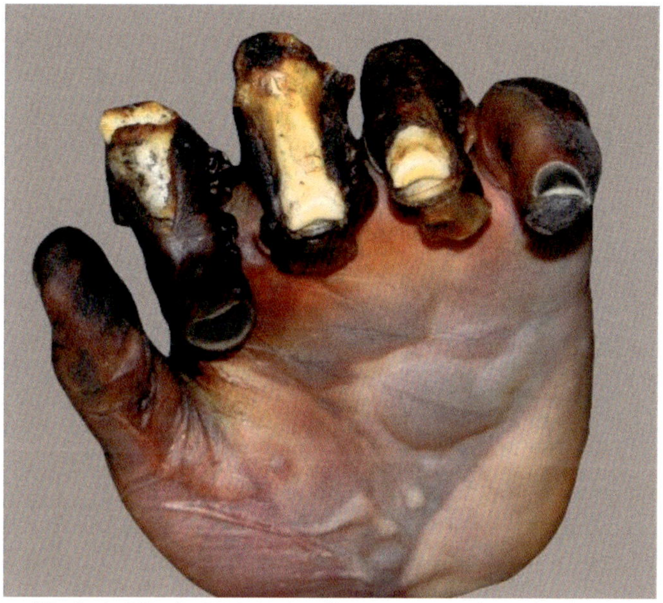

goga312 at Russian Wikipedia, CC BY-SA 3.0 <https://creativecommons.org/licenses/by-sa/3.0>, via Wikimedia Commons

FIGURE 21.12.42 - Fourth Degree Burn

I. Chemical Burns
    A. Alkali burns
        1. More damaging and lead to coagulation necrosis
    B. Acid burns
        1. Lead to liquefactive necrosis
    C. Treatment
        1. Decontamination and irrigation
        2. Transferral to burn center

II. Electrical Burns
    A. Examples: lightning strikes, electrical outlets
    B. Acute complications
        1. Cardiac arrhythmias (e.g. asystole, ventricular fibrillation)
        2. Muscle necrosis and myoglobinuria
        3. Renal failure
    C. Chronic complication: cataracts
    D. Treatment: monitor for arrhythmias, transfer to a burn center

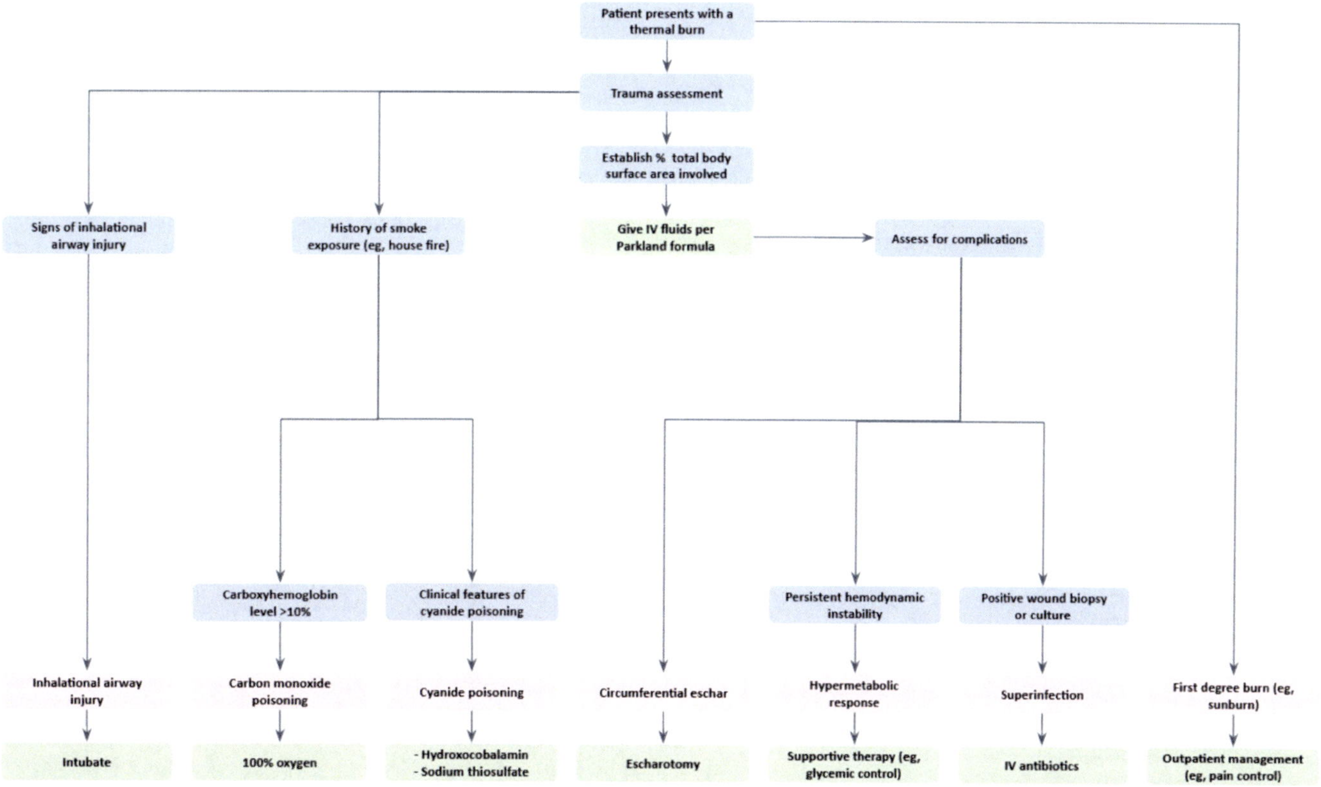

FIGURE 21.12.43 - Approach to Burn Injuries in the Emergency Department

Findings Suggestive of Inhalational Airway Injury
- Carbonaceous sputum
- Signs of oropharyngeal inflammation (e.g. pharyngeal erythema)
- Facial burns
- Singed eyebrows or nasal hairs
- Change in voice quality (e.g. stridor)

TABLE 21.12.4 - Features of Inhalational Airway Injury

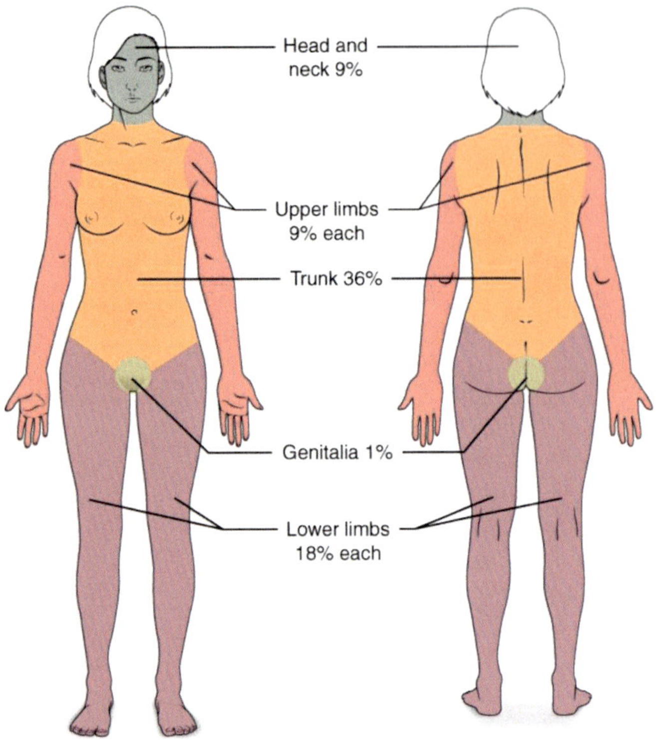

OpenStax College, CC BY 3.0 <https://creativecommons.org/licenses/by/3.0>, via Wikimedia Commons

FIGURE 21.12.44 - Rule of 9s

III. Parkland Formula
   A. Used to manage patients with second or third degree burns covering > 20% of their total body surface area (TBSA)
   B. Estimates total fluid needs within the first 24 hours per the equation:
      1. Total fluid requirement = TBSA (%) x weight (kg) x 4 cc/kg
      2. Give half of fluid requirements within first 8 hours
      3. Give second half within the next 16 hours
   C. Titrate intravenous fluids to achieve adequate urine output

IV. Circumferential Eschar
   A. A full-thickness (third degree) circumferential burn that disrupts venous and lymphatic drainage
   B. Increases risk for acute compartment syndrome distal to the burn
      1. Treat with escharotomy

V. Hypermetabolic Response to Burn Injury
   A. Moderate-to-severe burn injuries lead to release of inflammatory mediators and stress hormones (e.g. catecholamines, cortisol)
   B. Clinical features
      1. Tachycardia, hypertension, hyperthermia
      2. Hyperglycemia (due to insulin resistance)
      3. Increased tissue catabolism (e.g. muscle wasting)
   C. Diagnosis is clinical
   D. Address the underlying burn injury (e.g. early burn excision)
   E. Offer supportive therapy
      1. Beta blockers to control blood pressure and heart rate
      2. Insulin to control hyperglycemia
      3. Nutritional support to offset increased catabolism

VI. Superinfection
   A. Superinfection of a burn injury should be suspected when
      1. A second degree burn progresses to a third degree burn during inpatient stay
      2. There is green pigment around the burn wound
      3. There is black necrotic skin around the burn wound
   B. Most common pathogens: *Pseudomonas aeruginosa* and gram-positive cocci (e.g. *Staphylococcus aureus*)
   C. Diagnosis
      1. Positive wound culture
      2. Punch biopsy with > 100,000 bacteria/gram of burned tissue
   D. Treatment: IV antibiotics (e.g. aminoglycosides, vancomycin)
   E. Complication: burn wound sepsis

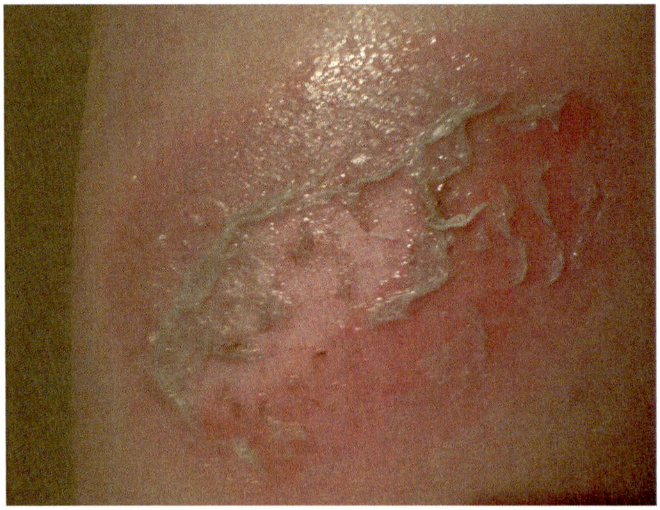

Pumpmeup, CC BY-SA 3.0 <https://creativecommons.org/licenses/by-sa/3.0>, via Wikimedia Commons

FIGURE 21.12.45 - Burn Wound Infection

VII. Burn Wound Sepsis

A. Burn wound sepsis diagnostic criteria

1. Temperature < 36.5° C (97.7° F) or > 39° C (102.2° F)
2. Systolic blood pressure < 90 mmHg, despite resuscitation
3. Heart rate > 90 beats per minute
4. Respiratory rate > 30 breaths per minute

B. Treatment: broad-spectrum IV antibiotics (e.g. piperacillin/tazobactam)

1. Consider coverage against MRSA (e.g. vancomycin)

VIII. Burn Injury Management Pearls

A. Lactated ringers is the IV fluid of choice for burn patients

1. Normal saline increases risk for hyperchloremic metabolic acidosis

B. Prophylactic topical antimicrobials (e.g. silver sulfadiazine) can be useful

1. No benefit of using oral or intravenous antibiotics prophylactically

C. Consider stress (Curling) ulcer prophylaxis (e.g. PPIs, H2-blockers)

D. Consider tetanus vaccination

REVIEW QUESTIONS

1. What is the degree of burn injury to this patient's palm?

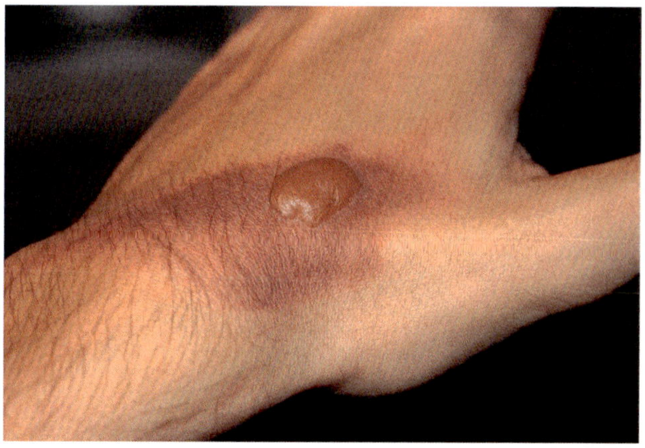

- **This patient's palm injury is a second degree burn.**
- It is a second degree burn because of the notable blisters.
- First degree burns do not exhibit blisters, and third or fourth degree burns tend to appear either extensively charred or white and leathery, which isn't the case on this patient's palm.
- The clinician could ask the patient if the palmar lesion is painful or not. Presence of pain would be consistent with a second degree burn, whereas absence of pain would be more consistent with a third degree burn.

Indications to Transfer Patients to the Burn Center
- Inhalational injury
- Electrical or chemical burns
- Burns affecting face, hands, feet, or perineum
- Second degree burns affecting > 10% of total body surface area
- Third degree burns
- Suspected child abuse

TABLE 21.12.5 - Indications to Transfer Patients to the Burn Center

REVIEW QUESTIONS

2. A 25-year-old patient is brought to the emergency department by his friend with second and third degree burns covering the back of his head and neck, his entire back, and the posterior aspect of his left leg. His weight is 143 lbs. What is the minimum amount of fluid that this patient should be given in the first 24 hours?

- **The minimum amount of fluid that this patient should be given is 8 liters in the first 24 hours.**
- The first step is to calculate the percent of the total body surface area affected by the burns. The "back of his head and neck" equates to 4.5%, "his entire back" equates to 18%, and "the posterior aspect of his left leg" equates to 9%.
- In sum, 31.5% of this patient's total body surface area has been injured by burns.
- The next step is to use this number along with his weight in kilograms in the Parkland formula. Calculations show 8,190 cc or 8,190 mL of fluid, which means that this patient should receive roughly 8 liters of fluid in the first 24 hours.
- Per the Parkland formula, half of this fluid should be given in the first 8 hours and the other half should be given over the next 16 hours. Therefore, the patient should receive about 4 L or 4000 mL of fluid in the first 8 hours, which means that the patient will need to receive 500 mL of fluid per hour in the first 8 hours.
- The remaining 4 L of fluid should then be given over the next 16 hours, which means a rate of 250 mL of fluid per hour.

REVIEW QUESTIONS

3. What are the clinical features that should prompt suspicion of compartment syndrome of an extremity?

   - **Clinical features that should prompt suspicion of compartment syndrome of an extremity are pain, paresthesias, pallor, pulselessness, poikilothermia, and paralysis.**
   - The clinical features of compartment syndrome can be remembered with the mnemonic of "Six Ps": pain, especially on passive stretching of the extremity, paresthesias, pallor, pulselessness, poikilothermia, and paralysis.
   - Pain and paresthesias are the earliest findings of compartment syndrome, and these symptoms should be taken very seriously in patients with circumferential eschars.

4. What is the primary way of distinguishing burn wound sepsis from hypermetabolic response to burn injury?

   - **The key difference is that burn wound sepsis requires a confirmed burn wound superinfection for diagnosis. In other words, patients must either have a positive culture or a positive wound biopsy.**
   - **Hypermetabolic response to burn injury, on the other hand, will cause refractory hemodynamic instability in the setting of negative cultures or biopsy results.**
   - Both of these complications of burn injuries can present with refractory hemodynamic instability.

5. A 27-year-old man is rescued from a burning apartment complex and brought to the emergency department via ambulance with extensive burns. He is unresponsive and vitals show temperature of 97.2° F (36.2° C), blood pressure of 87/55 mmHg, pulse of 110 beats per minute, and respiratory rate of 21 breaths per minute. Physical examination shows burns on his face and oropharyngeal erythema. There are partial-thickness and full-thickness burns on his back, abdomen, and lower extremities. The resident pages the burn unit in anticipation of transferring the patient to their care following initial stabilization. Which of the following is the next best in management while the patient is in the emergency department?

   A. Normal saline infusion
   B. Beta blockers
   C. Intravenous antibiotics
   D. Endotracheal intubation

- **The correct answer is option D.**
- This patient has extensive thermal burns.
- He is hemodynamically unstable and physical examination reveals extensive burn injuries. Importantly, he has burns on his face along with oropharyngeal erythema.
- Signs of oropharyngeal inflammation and facial burns are findings that are strongly suggestive of inhalational airway injury.
- During the trauma assessment of a patient with thermal burn injuries, identification of signs of inhalational airway injury should prompt urgent intubation because these patients are at high risk of developing airway edema and subsequent obstruction.
- Option A is incorrect because normal saline infusion is critical to first secure this patient's airway because of the high risk of airway edema and compromise in inhalational airway injury.
- Additionally, the fluid of choice in burn patients is lactated ringers, not normal saline. This is because normal saline can cause hyperchloremic metabolic acidosis when given in high amounts because of its supraphysiologic chloride concentration. Lactated ringers is a more balanced fluid that does not increase patients' risk for developing a metabolic acidosis.
- Option B is incorrect because beta blockers will likely be detrimental in this patient because he is quite hypotensive and is likely volume depleted.
- Option C is incorrect because intravenous or oral antibiotics are not useful in prophylaxis against burn wound superinfections; only topical antimicrobial agents are.

Emergency Medicine | Section 8: Immediate & Early Postoperative Fever

I. Postoperative Fever: Definition
  A. Fever > 100.4° F (38° C) after surgical procedure
  B. Self resolves in most cases

II. Postoperative Fever: Pathophysiology
  A. Tissue trauma, inflammation, bacterial toxins
  B. Activation of reticuloendothelial system
  C. IL-1, IL-6, TNF-alpha, IFN-gamma
  D. Preoptic nucleus of the hypothalamus
    1. PGE-2

III. Immediate Postoperative Fever: Etiology
  A. Within a few hours of surgery
    1. Malignant hyperthermia (< 1 hour)
    2. Febrile nonhemolytic transfusion reaction (1-6 hours from a blood transfusion)
    3. Pre-existing infection
    4. Preoperative or intraoperative tissue trauma

IV. Immediate Postoperative Fever: Clinical Features
  A. Malignant hyperthermia
    1. Muscle rigidity, fever, hypercapnia, acidosis
    2. Hyperkalemia, myoglobinuria
    3. Arrhythmia and renal failure
  B. Febrile nonhemolytic transfusion reaction
    1. Fever, chills
    2. Myalgia, nausea

V. Immediate Postoperative Fever: Diagnosis
  A. Malignant hyperthermia (clinically)
    1. Caffeine halothane contracture test, genetic testing
  B. Febrile nonhemolytic transfusion reaction (within 1-6 hours)
    1 Diagnosis of exclusion
  C. Pre-existing infection
    1. CBC, urinalysis, blood cultures
    2. Suspected source of infection (e.g. CXR for pneumonia)

VI. Immediate Postoperative Fever: Treatment
  A. Malignant hyperthermia
    1. Discontinue offending agent, cooling
    2. Dantrolene, high flow 100% oxygen
  B. Febrile nonhemolytic transfusion reaction
    1. Acetaminophen, leukoreduction, termination of transfusion
  C. Pre-existing infection
    1. Antibiotics

VII. Early Postoperative Fever: Etiology
  A. Early postoperative fever: days 0 - 3
  B. Atelectasis (e.g. collapse of a lung, absent gas exchange)
  C. Postoperative pneumonia (e.g. hospital-acquired or ventilator-acquired)
    1. Organisms commonly associated with postoperative pneumonia (e.g. *Pseudomonas*, *Klebsiella*, *Enterobacter*)
  D. Urinary tract infection (e.g. *E. coli*, *Enterococcus*)
  E. Surgical site infection (e.g. group A streptococcus, *Clostridium perfringens*)

VIII. Early Postoperative Fever: Clinical Features
  A. Common in both atelectasis and pneumonia
    1. Tachypnea, dyspnea, cough, hypoxemia
  B. Atelectasis
    1. Decreased breath sounds
  C. Pneumonia
    1. Increased breath sounds
  D. UTI
    1. Urinary urgency
    2. Suprapubic pain, costovertebral angle tenderness
  E. Surgical site infection (SSI)
    1. Pus
    2. Erythema, swelling
    3. Tenderness

IX. Early Postoperative Fever: Diagnosis
  A. Atelectasis or pneumonia
    1. Chest X-ray
      a) Collapsed areas (atelectasis)
      b) Consolidation (pneumonia)
    2. CBC
    3. Sputum and blood cultures
    4. Arterial blood gasses
  B. UTI
    1. Urinalysis (nitrites, leukocyte esterase, pyuria)
    2. Urine culture, CBC, blood culture
    3. Ultrasound
  C. Surgical site infection
    1. Physical examination (wounds, catheters, drain outputs)
    2. CBC, cultures, imaging studies

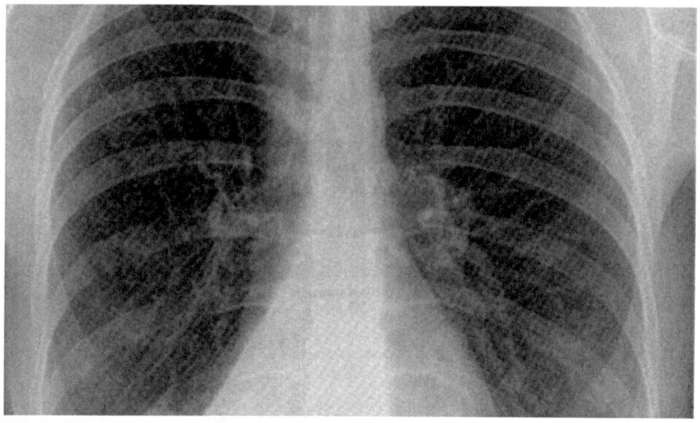

FIGURE 21.12.46 - Chest X-ray: Right Lower Lobe Atelectasis

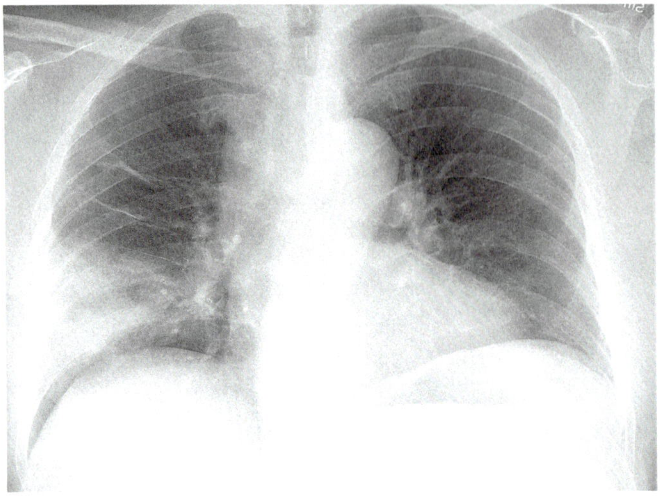

Mikael Häggström, M.D. - Author info - Reusing imagesWritten informed consent was obtained from the individual, including online publication., CC0, via Wikimedia Commons

FIGURE 21.12.47 - Chest X-ray: Right Middle Lobe Consolidation

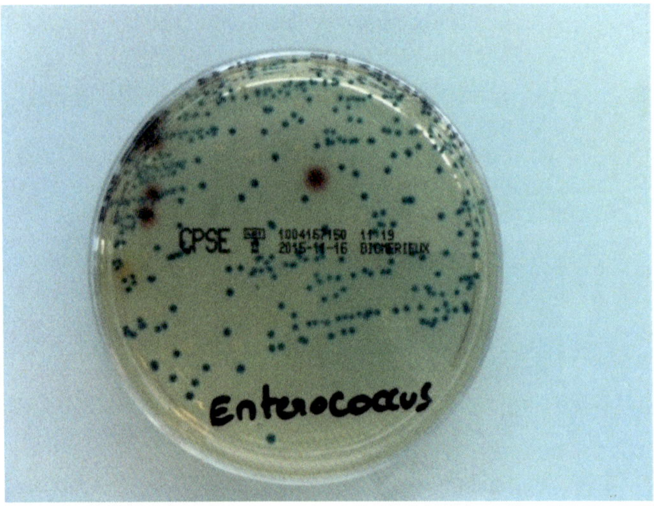

FIGURE 21.12.48 - Colonies of *Enterococcus* on Urine Culture

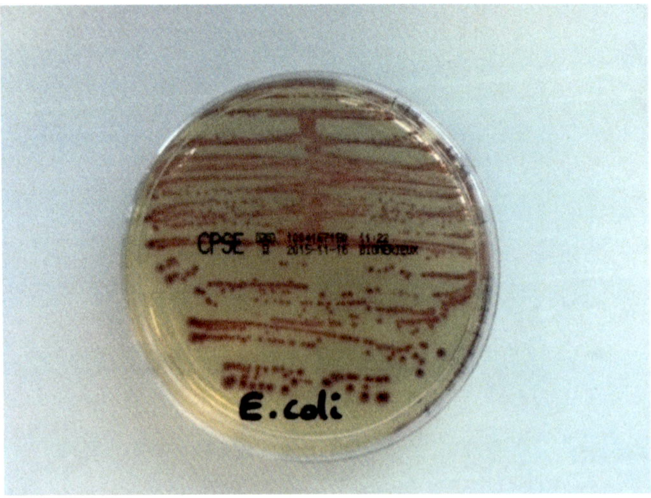

FIGURE 21.12.49 - Colonies of *E. Coli* on Specimen Culture

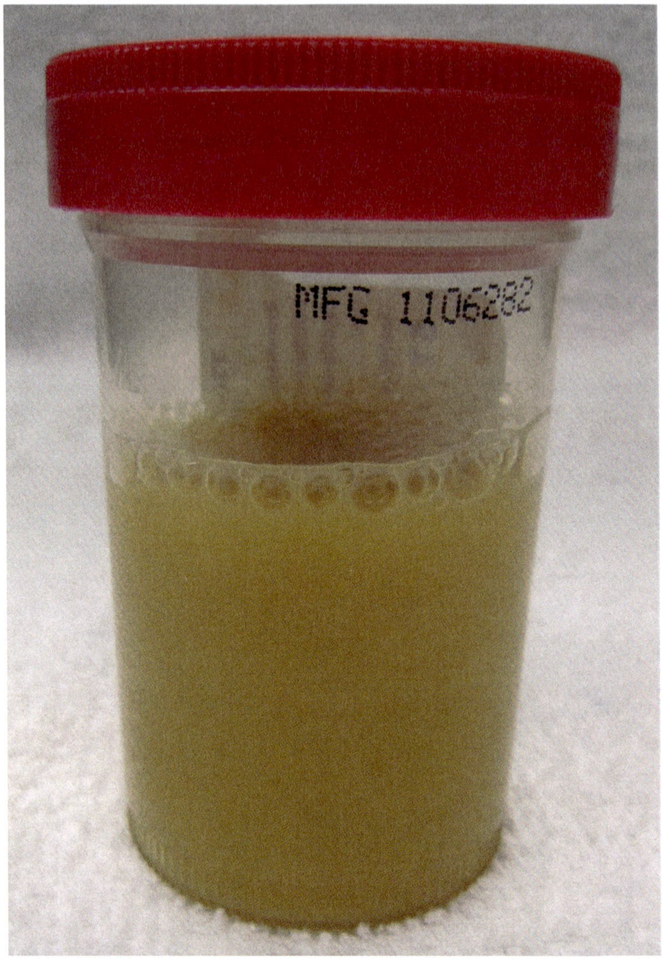

FIGURE 21.12.50 - Pyuria

X. Early Postoperative Fever: Treatment
   A. Atelectasis
      1. Deep inspirations, incentive spirometry
      2. Early mobilization, bronchodilators
      3. Chest physiotherapy
   B. Pneumonia
      1. Oxygen supplementation (SaO_2 < 94%)
      2. Empiric antibiotics (e.g. piperacillin-tazobactam)
   C. UTI
      1. Trimethoprim-sulfamethoxazole
      2. Cephalexin, ceftriaxone
      3. Fosfomycin
   D. Surgical site infections
      1. Superficial: delayed closure, incision & drainage, wound dressings
      2. Deep or severe: antibiotics and debridement

REVIEW QUESTIONS

?

1. A 45-year-old woman was admitted to the hospital and is now on postoperative day 2 following an uncomplicated cholecystectomy. She has now developed a low-grade fever as well as feelings of shortness of breath. Physical examination is notable for diminished breath sounds at both lung bases. The patient is asked to repeat the letter "E" while auscultating both lung bases and "E" is heard clearly. What is most likely the cause for these findings?

   - **The most likely cause for these findings is development of bibasilar atelectasis.**
   - The patient develops a low-grade fever and shortness of breath on postoperative day 2, which should prompt suspicion for atelectasis or pneumonia.
   - Physical examination reveals diminished breath sounds at both lung bases and negative egophony which is more suggestive of atelectasis than pneumonia.
   - Pneumonia typically will result in an abnormal egophony test, where the letter "E" is heard to sound like "A", indicating a consolidation.
   - A chest X-ray can be ordered to help distinguish between the two likely diagnoses.

2. A 24-year-old G1P1 woman develops a fever and chest pain three days after a complicated cesarean section in which she sustained significant blood loss. She describes her chest pain as sharp and worse when taking deep breaths. Vital signs show blood pressure of 130/75 mm Hg, temperature of 38.6° C (101.5° F), and pulse of 97 beats per minute. Lung examination shows crackles at the right lung base, while abdominal examination shows well-healing incisions without any abdominal tenderness. Pelvic examination is notable for a moderate amount of vaginal discharge that is not malodorous. There is no lower extremity edema or tenderness. Laboratory work-up shows hemoglobin of 9.7 g/dL and leukocyte count of 16,000/mm^3. Which of the following is the most likely diagnosis?

   A. Atelectasis
   B. Pneumonia
   C. Endometritis
   D. Urinary tract infection
   E. Wound infection

   - **The correct answer is option B.**
   - Three days after a cesarean section, this patient develops a fever and chest pain that appears to be pleuritic in nature.
   - Her high fever, pleuritic chest pain, crackles at the right lung base, and significant leukocytosis are strongly suggestive of pneumonia as the most likely diagnosis.
   - Option A is incorrect because atelectasis typically results in only a low-grade fever and does not cause such a stark leukocytosis.
   - Option C is incorrect because endometritis tends to present with lower abdominal pain and malodorous vaginal discharge. The moderate amount of vaginal discharge described is a normal finding in the immediate postpartum period and is known as lochia.
   - Option D is incorrect because the patient was not reporting symptoms suggestive of a urinary tract infection, such as dysuria, and she did not have any suprapubic tenderness on abdominal exam.
   - Option E is incorrect because the abdominal exam shows well-healing incisions without any drainage or oozing, making a wound infection less likely.

Emergency Medicine | Section 9: Late & Delayed Postoperative Fever

I. Late Postoperative Fever: Etiology
   A. Days 4 - 30
   B. Deep venous thrombosis
   C. Pulmonary embolism
   D. Drugs (e.g. vancomycin, beta lactams, phenytoin, heparin)
   E. Clostridium difficile
   F. Surgical site infections

II. Late Postoperative Fever: Clinical Features
   A. PE
      1. Sudden shortness of breath, pleuritic chest pain
      2. Tachycardia, hemoptysis
   B. DVT
      1. Sudden throbbing pain in calf
      2. Swelling
      3. Warm, red skin
   C. Drug fever
      1. Nonspecific symptoms (e.g. chills, fatigue)
      2. Diagnosis of exclusion
   D. Clostridium difficile
      1. Abdominal cramps, tenderness
      2. Watery diarrhea
      3. Recent antibiotic use

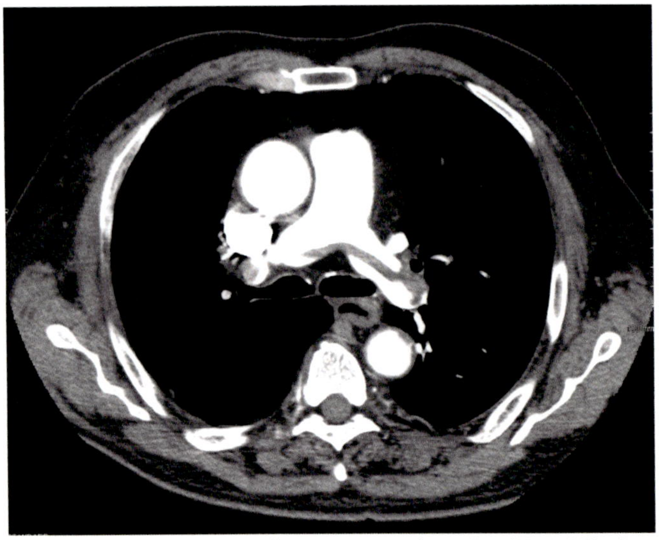

FIGURE 21.12.51 - CT Scan of Chest: Pulmonary Embolism

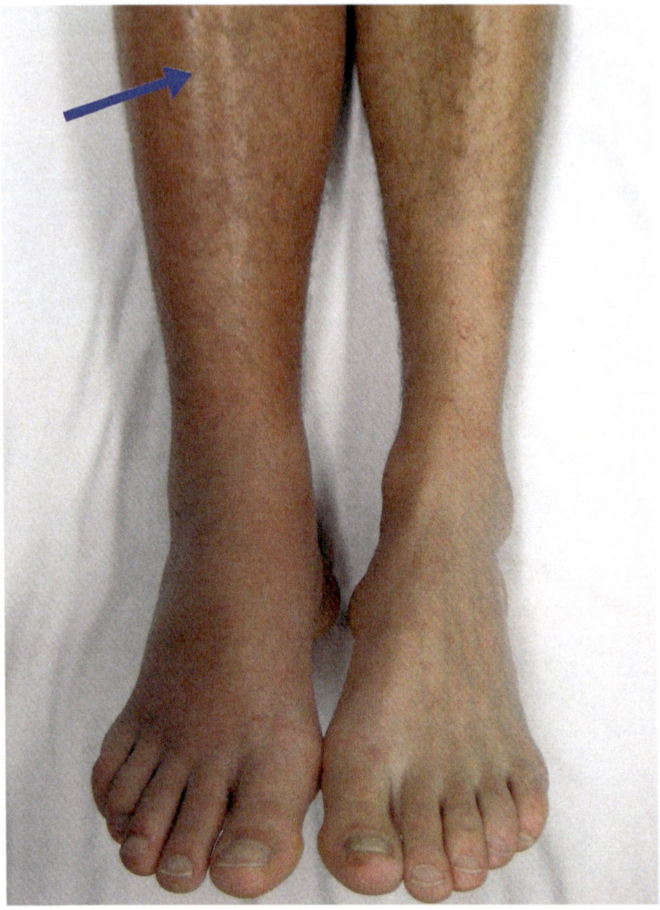

FIGURE 21.12.52 - Red and Swollen Leg in Deep Venous Thrombosis

III. Late Postoperative Fever: Diagnosis
   A. DVT and PE
      1. DVT: Doppler ultrasound
      2. PE: CT angiography (high likelihood), D-dimer (low likelihood)
   B. Clostridium difficile
      1. PCR (detects toxin B)
      2. X-ray or CT (wall thickening or perforation)

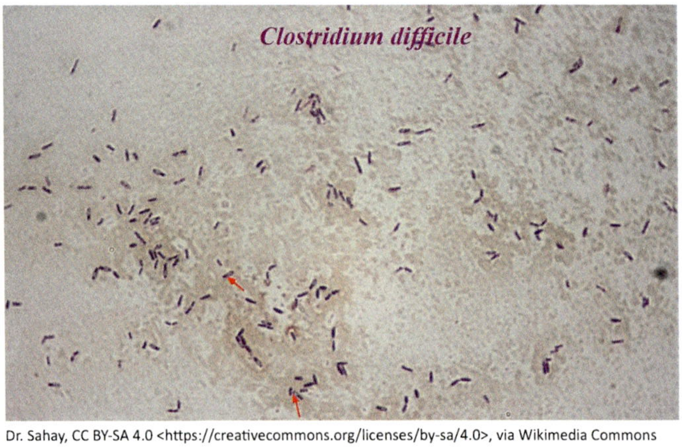

FIGURE 21.12.53 - Gram Stain of C. *Difficile*

IV. Late Postoperative Fever: Treatment
  A. DVT/PE
    1. Heparin
    2. Warfarin
    3. Thrombolysis/thrombectomy (severe)
    4. Inferior vena cava filters (contraindications to anticoagulation)
  B. C. difficile
    1. Discontinue offending medication
    2. Vancomycin
    3. Fidaxomicin
    4. Surgery (severe/refractory)

V. Delayed Postoperative Fever:
  A. > 30 days
    1. Unrelated to the surgery
    2. Infections of implanted devices
    3. Fistula

REVIEW QUESTIONS

1. A 55-year-old woman comes to her primary care physician because of severe watery diarrhea that started 3 days ago. 2-weeks ago she underwent an emergency cholecystectomy for gangrenous cholecystitis. She has been on broad-spectrum antibiotics since the surgery. She has a history of poorly treated type II diabetes mellitus. Vital signs show a temperature of 39° C (102.2° F), blood pressure of 130/80 mmHg, heart rate of 92 beats/min, and respiratory rate of 16 breaths/min. Physical examination shows nontender, nondistended abdomen without guarding and rigidity. Stool PCR for C. difficile toxin B is positive. Which of the following is the best treatment option for this patient?

    A. Erythromycin
    B. Vancomycin
    C. Metronidazole
    D. Exploratory laparotomy

- **The correct answer is option B.**
- This patient presents with watery diarrhea and high fever 2 weeks after cholecystectomy in the setting of recent antibiotic use.
- The timeframe of her fever is consistent with the late postoperative fever.
- She has been on broad-spectrum antibiotic regimen since the surgery.
- Additionally, stool PCR for toxin B is positive.
- All these findings are consistent with the diagnosis of pseudomembranous colitis caused by *C. difficile*.
- The best initial treatment option for uncomplicated pseudomembranous colitis is vancomycin.
- Option A, erythromycin, is incorrect because it is not used in the management of pseudomembranous colitis.
- Option C, metronidazole, is incorrect because it is mostly used in patients with fulminant C. Difficile colitis, characterized by hypotension, tachycardia, and signs of toxic megacolon.
- However, even in fulminant colitis, vancomycin and fidaxomicin are preferred over metronidazole.
- Option D, exploratory laparotomy, is indicated in patients with colonic perforation and peritonitis. This patient has normal abdominal exam findings, without signs of peritonitis or perforation and thus does not need surgical intervention.

TABLES & FIGURES

Made in United States
Orlando, FL
04 November 2026

90199925R00148